Contents

Foreword

Healthcare cannot be risk free. Nothing ever is. A complex system that involves one million general practitioner consultations per day, generating 1.5 million prescriptions and with an additional 100 000 visits by district nurses will inevitably result in errors. General practitioners know that the biggest risks occur when patients move across the different interfaces of care, at moments of handover – for example, primary and secondary care sectors. However, whilst healthcare cannot ever be risk free it is important that practitioners minimise the potential for risk at every point by introducing robust systems of clinical governance through effective leadership.

Many general practices already carry out risk management but they do not always recognise that they are doing this – it may be under the guise of medicines management or practice team appraisal. Risk management, however, can be made easier by having a structured approach to it and by applying that systemic attitude to many areas of clinical, managerial and organisational practice. Good systems for adverse incident reporting, alongside methods to deal appropriately with complaints, putting in place continuous staff development (ideally involving the whole team), analysing work load demand against practitioner capacity to deliver and having systems in place to review practice are all examples of risk management.

The benefits of a good risk management approach to care will impact on not just the practice but also more importantly on the patients, meaning that they are less likely to suffer from the adverse consequences of error.

This book is timely. We are currently at a crossroads in care; the high-profile events of Shipman and the subsequent six reports from the Shipman Inquiry will undoubtedly mean that practitioners, practices and primary care trusts will have to review all their systems where patients may be placed at risk. Patient safety must now be integral to all our thinking and should be firmly embedded throughout clinical care.

Sir Liam Donaldson
Chief Medical Officer
Department of Health
February 2005

About the editors

Keith Haynes is Director of MPS Risk Consulting Ltd and has worked for the Medical Protection Society since 1995. Prior to this he gained extensive experience in senior management positions within the NHS, latterly as Chief Executive of a major acute teaching hospital. As head of MPS Risk Consulting, Keith has been responsible for developing and managing a highly successful portfolio of risk management services, as a result of which it has been possible to produce this book. He is also a visiting senior lecturer with the University of York and a Fellow of the Faculty of Medicine, University of Manchester.

Malcolm Thomas was a partner in a general practice at Guidepost in South East Northumberland for nearly 14 years. He has held a number of appointments in medical and GP education (relating to both under- and post-graduates), and is currently an Associate Director of Postgraduate GP Education in Newcastle upon Tyne. An early interest in improving quality of care was satisfied in the practice as clinical lead partner (when such people were rare). He worked with the King's Fund Organisational Audit programme before being recruited to MPS Risk Consulting four years ago, which brought him together with Keith Haynes. His main area of specialised interest lies in improving communication between clinicians and patients. This led him to found Effective Professional Interactions Ltd, which has given him his second major current role.

List of contributors

Sandy Anthony SRN, BA, PGC in Health Services Management (Claims Handling and Risk Management)
Managing Editor
Medical Protection Society

Maureen Baker CBE, DM, FRCGP
Director of Primary Care
National Patient Safety Agency;
Honorary Secretary
Royal College of General Practitioners

Paul Bowden BSc (Hons), MBBS, MRCGP
GP Principal and Appraiser, Tunbridge Wells;
EPA Health Service Ombudsman;
Associate Consultant, MPS Risk Consulting

Jane Cowan MBBS, DCP, DCH, MRCPI, FRCPCH
Medicolegal Adviser
MPS Risk Consulting, Leeds;
Visiting Lecturer
Department of Health Sciences
University of York

Mark Davies BSc, MRCP, MRCGP
Part-time GP
Hebden Bridge, West Yorkshire;
Medical Director, Yorkshire Pennine Doctors on Call (PENDOC) (1999–2004);
Clinical Lead
National Booking Team
National Programme for Information Technology (NPfIT)

Mike Deavin SRN, RMN
Complaints and Legal Services Manager
James Paget Healthcare NHS Trust
James Paget Hospital, Norfolk

Mark Dinwoodie MA, MBBS, DGM, DRCOG, DFFP, DCH, D Med Ed, MRCGP
General Practitioner and GP Trainer, Bath;
GP with a Special Interest in Cardiology;
Associate Consultant for MPS Risk Consulting

Richard Fieldhouse MBBS, MRCGP, DRCOG
Chief Executive Officer
National Association of Sessional GPs;
Freelance GP

Jamie Harrison MA, MBBS, FRCGP
General Practitioner;
Associate Director of Postgraduate GP Education
University of Newcastle

Judith Harvey D Phil, BM, BCh
Freelance GP;
Council Member, National Association of Sessional GPs;
Author of Royal Society of Medicine's *Handbook of Practice Management*;
Former GP principal and LMC Chair, Buckinghamshire

Keith Haynes LLB (Hons), MSc, DipHSM
Director
MPS Risk Consulting, Leeds;
Visiting Senior Lecturer
Department of Health Sciences
University of York;
Honorary Fellow
Faculty of Medicine, University of Manchester

John Hickey MBBS, FRCA
Chief Executive
Medical Protection Society
London and Leeds

Brian Hurwitz BA (Cambridge), MBBS, MA, MSc, MD (London), FRCP, FRCGP
General Practitioner;
D'Oyly Carte Chair of Medicine and the Arts
King's College, London

John Jeffries MSc, DMS
Consultant in Health and Safety;
Formerly Managing Director of R&D Associates (Training) Ltd

Peter Mackenzie MA, MBBS, MRCGP, DRCOG, PgDLaw
Medico-Legal Adviser
Medical Protection Society

Peter Nicklin MEd, MBA, FInstLM
Patient Safety and Clinical Risk Adviser
MPS Risk Consulting;
Director, Institute of Leadership and Management;
Honorary Senior Fellow
Faculty of Medicine, University of Manchester;
Former Director, Clinical Risk Management Programmes, University of York

Julie Price BA, RGN, Dip HE (Practice Nursing)
Clinical Risk Manager
MPS Risk Consulting, Leeds

John Sandars MSc, FRCGP, MRCP CertEd
Senior Lecturer in Community-based Education
Medical Education Unit
The Medical School
University of Leeds

Malcolm Thomas MB, BChir, MRCGP
Founder and Director
Effective Professional Interactions Ltd;
Associate Director of Postgraduate GP Education
Newcastle upon Tyne;
Former Associate Consultant in Clinical Risk Management, MPS Risk Consulting

Tim van Zwanenberg EdD, FRCGP
Professor of Postgraduate General Practice;
Director of Postgraduate General Practice Education
University of Newcastle upon Tyne

Nigel Watson MBBS, FRCGP
General Practitioner, New Forest;
Chief Executive
Wessex Local Medical Committees;
Representative of Hampshire and Isle of Wight
General Practitioners Committee of the British Medical Association

Paul Wilding MBChB, MRCP (UK)
Medical Director
NHS Direct (West Yorkshire);
Former Director, Pennine Doctors On-Call (PENDOC)
GP out-of-hours co-operative

List of abbreviations

ACPC	Area Child Protection Committee
AHRQ	Agency for Healthcare Research and Quality
AIMS-ICU	Australian Incident Monitoring Study in the Intensive Care Unit
AMA	American Medical Association
AvMA	Action against Medical Accidents
BANs	British Approved Names
BMA	British Medical Association
BMI	body mass index
BMJ	*British Medical Journal*
BNF	*British National Formulary*
CAB	Citizens Advice Bureau
CD	controlled drug
CHAI	Healthcare Commission (formerly known as Commission for Health Audit and Inspection)
CHI	Commission for Health Improvement
CME	continuing medical education
CMO	Chief Medical Officer
CNST	Clinical Negligence Scheme for Trusts
COSHH	Control of Substances Hazardous to Health
CPD	continuing professional development
CPP	Committee on Professional Performance
CPU	central processing unit
CRHP	Council for the Regulation of Healthcare Professionals
CRM	clinical risk management
CRSA	clinical risk self-assessment
CSCI	Commission for Social Care Inspection
CSM	Committee on the Safety of Medicines
DISQ	Doctors Interpersonal Skills Questionnaire
DMD	Drug Misuse Database
DNA	did not attend
DVDS	Domestic Violence Data Source
EDI	electronic data interchange
EHR	electronic health record
EPR	electronic patient record
ESCA	Effective Shared Care Agreements
FPP	Fitness to Practise Panel
GMC	General Medical Council
GMP	Good Medical Practice
GMS	General Medical Services
GPC	General Practitioners Committee
GPR	GP registrar
HFEA	Human Fertilisation and Embryology Authority
ICAS	Independent Complaints Advisory Service
IM & T	information management and technology

INR	international normalised ratio
IT	information technology
IVF	*in-vitro* fertilisation
JCAHO	Joint Commission on Accreditation of Healthcare Organisations
JCPTGP	Joint Committee for Postgraduate Training for General Practice
LAN	local area network
LHB	local health board
LMC	Local Medical Committee
MCA	Medicines Control Agency
MCQ	multiple choice question
MDA	Medical Devices Agency
MDR	Misuse of Drugs Regulations 2001
MDU	Medical Defence Union
MHRA	Medicines and Healthcare Products Regulatory Agency
MMAT	Medicines Management Action Team
MMS	Medicines Management Services
MPO	medical protection organisation
MPS	Medical Protection Society
MSO	midstream urine specimen
MTRAC	Midland Therapeutic Review and Advisory Committee
NAO	National Audit Office
NASGP	National Association of Sessional GPs
NCAA	National Clinical Assessment Authority
NHS	National Health Service
NHSIA	NHS Information Authority
NHSLA	NHS Litigation Authority
NICE	National Institute for Clinical Excellence
NMC	Nursing and Midwifery Council
NPC	National Prescribing Centre
NPSA	National Patient Safety Agency
NRLS	National Reporting and Learning System
NSF	National Service Framework
NSPCC	National Society for the Prevention of Cruelty to Children
OOH	out-of-hours
OOHS	out-of-hours services
OSCE	objective structured clinical exam
PACT	Prescribing Analysis and Cost
PALS	Patient Advice and Liaison Services
PAMS	professions allied to medicine
PAT	performance assessment team
PCO	primary care organisation
PCT	primary care trust
PDP	personal development plan
PGD	patient group directive
PGEA	Postgraduate Education Allowance
PMS	Personal Medical Services
PPA	Prescription Pricing Authority
PPDP	practice professional development plan
PSNC	Pharmaceutical Services Negotiating Committee

QPA	Quality Practice Awards
QTD	Quality Team Development
RAM	random-access memory
RCA	root cause analysis
RCGP	Royal College of General Practitioners
rINNs	recommended International Names
RPSGP	Royal Pharmaceutical Society of Great Britain
SHA	strategic health authority
SIGN	Scottish Intercollegiate Guidelines Network
TOS	Terms of Service
UKMI	UK Medicines Information Agency
UPS	uninterruptible power source

Introduction

Keith Haynes and Malcolm Thomas

Why did we write this?

Medical care is a risky business. Few are really told this at medical school. Ask other health professionals and their experience is no different. They are not told that healthcare is a risky business either.

Sometimes you might be reached in a small way by the medical protection organisations. You might have taken their information to be exclusively directed at your risk of being sued. But in any event it didn't apply to you because you were going to be a good doctor or nurse – right? You might be forgiven therefore for not having paid closer attention.

It might be that you have come to know what some people already knew then. The fundamental nature of clinical care consists of working with risk. Individuals and their organisations are managing risk in every clinical encounter, and are themselves exposed to risk.

It is our intention in this book to show you:

- where these risks arise
- how you can analyse them
- what you can do to reduce them.

We mean to do this for individuals and for organisations, so the plan is that this book will be useful to both.

How have we gone about this?

The book has three sections.

The first section (Chapters 1 to 5) sets the scene. It covers the background and theory behind clinical risk management. You should find out from these chapters the current context for managing clinical risk, and develop an overview of the underlying theory and evidence.

The second section (Chapters 6 to 20) examines the main risks. In Chapter 6, the experience of MPS Risk Consulting and its associate consultants is backed up by published studies and the experience of other organisations. The result is a comprehensive introduction to the main areas of risk in primary care in the UK.

We then go on to treat each major area of risk to a chapter of its own, written by an author experienced in the relevant field and providing a blend of the theoretical and the practical.

The final section (Chapters 21 to 25) examines some particular solutions in more detail. This is either because they are not limited to single areas of risk (e.g. significant event audit) or because they are so important (e.g. communication).

A note about style

We have aimed for a consistent style in briefing our authors and editing their work. However, we have not felt the need to impose total uniformity.

The introductory chapters are, to some extent, essays. Therefore we have deliberately allowed the authors' voices to come through.

Even the more practical chapters treat a diversity of subjects in a variety of ways. Once again we have not felt the need to go further than to ensure that each chapter is clear enough to achieve its purpose.

How should you use this book?

You could, of course, read the book from cover to cover. We hope that some people will do this, and it should provide you with a practical, well-referenced and comprehensive guide to the subject if you do so.

However, the book has been written so that individual chapters and sections are coherent and stand on their own.

For example, the opening section plus Chapter 6 would provide a good theoretical introduction to the management of clinical risk in general and clinical risk in UK primary care in particular.

The 'single-topic' chapters (Chapters 7 to 20) are written to stand on their own, and can usefully be consulted for theory and practical advice about the relevant topic. Most of these chapters follow the same basic pattern as the whole book – that is:

- background
- theory
- practical advice and tips.

The chapters in the final section contain possible 'solutions' for either individual practitioners or organisations. Clearly these can be read in conjunction with any amount of the preceding material. For example, if your health centre has had a significant event relating to laboratory results, then you might particularly be interested in Chapter 10 (Results Management) and Chapter 24 (Significant Event Audit).

What next?

We hope that you will find our book interesting, thought-provoking and practical. We anticipate that many readers will choose not to read it from cover to cover at their first sitting. We hope that readers will keep the book to hand for future reference – for example:

- to help in practice and personal development planning
- to respond to risks identified, either ad hoc or as a result of a systematic enquiry
- to help to prepare for a visit from the Commission for Health Audit and Inspection (CHAI), now known as the Healthcare Commission.

Acknowledgements

The editors of this book met when Keith Haynes employed Malcolm Thomas as an Associate Consultant in Clinical Risk Management for MPS Risk Consulting, which he heads. This relationship has led to the book. Malcolm would like to thank Keith for taking him on, listening to his suggestions and supporting his development.

The editors would like to thank the authors of the individual chapters for their efforts in responding to initial and subsequent editorial requests. They have done an excellent job in producing texts that have been a pleasure to edit, and they have brought the vision to life.

We would like to thank the staff of MPS Risk Consulting for providing so many of the authors, for supporting Keith in his editorial role and for collating the manuscript. Many people other than the chapter authors and those specifically acknowledged have helped us with advice and support. To all, thanks.

In particular, we would like to identify two colleagues who have made a special contribution. This project literally would not have happened without Annys Cole of MPS Risk Consulting, who has been guardian of the manuscript and nerve centre of the operation. We would also like to thank Dr John Hickey, of the Medical Protection Society (MPS), for his encouragement and support in this venture.

Malcolm has a long history as a GP educationalist. Many colleagues and teachers have helped his professional development. He thanks them all, from his first experiences as a GP registrar to his current incarnation as Managing Director of Effective Professional Interactions.

He would also like to thank colleagues at the Postgraduate Institute for Medicine and Dentistry in Newcastle, in particular Professor Tim van Zwanenberg and Dr Jamie Harrison, for their enthusiastic encouragement and practical help.

Both editors would like to thank and acknowledge the help and support of Radcliffe Publishing. It is a pleasure to work on a manuscript knowing that the publishers seem so keen.

On a personal note, Malcolm would like to thank his wife (Ann) and children (Matthew and Christopher) for allowing him to spend evenings and weekends at the computer, writing and editing. Seeing their names in print will be significant recompense for the boys.

On a similarly personal note, Keith would like to thank his wife Mary for her support in the months that it has taken to edit the book, and many of his colleagues at MPS Risk Consulting who have offered their support and help.

Finally

We hope and expect that you will enjoy this book. We have been fortunate to have so many expert authors contribute to it. The credit for its usefulness is due largely to them.

We have checked all matters of fact for accuracy and taken second opinions. However, in a work of this scope it is unlikely that we have rooted out all errors. The responsibility for these lies with the editors, and we would be very pleased to hear from you if you find any mistakes. If we are fortunate enough to produce a revised edition, we shall benefit from this feedback.

As many of our readers know the provision of healthcare takes place in a rapidly changing environment and although we have tried to be as current as possible at the time of going to press, this has been one of our greatest challenges.

Finally, the views expressed herein are those of the authors and editors, and not necessarily of the organisations with which they are associated.

Section 1

Chapter 1

Risk management in primary care: why bother?

Maureen Baker

Key learning points

- Primary care is moving from delivery by un-coordinated, small-scale institutions to delivery by larger, more diverse organisations with increasingly close relationships to the new primary care trusts (PCTs).
- Risk is now seen both by practices and by PCTs as something that can be analysed and managed.
- The concept of clinical governance has developed in line with this evolution.
- Risk management is the fundamental component of clinical governance.
- The National Patient Safety Agency (NPSA) has recently been set up to support the development of patient safety. It too has risk management as one of its core principles.

Introduction

'Risk management', 'patient safety' and 'significant events' – are these just the latest in a succession of buzz words and phrases to be perpetrated in the primary care sector? Just what do these terms mean to hard-pressed clinicians and teams? And why on earth should we bother? Moreover, if we take on this agenda, are we not just setting ourselves up for complaints, criticism and litigation? These are the kind of questions we might expect to be raised by any number of clinicians and professionals in the primary care sector. Colleagues who are under pressure to deliver essential services might well wonder what on earth any of this has to do with them, and why they should expend time and energy in this field when there are so many other calls upon their time.

But such cynicism would, in this instance, be misplaced. An understanding and application of the principles of risk management and patient safety will not only protect patients from unintended harm, but will also support health professionals. Dedicated doctors, nurses and healthcare professionals are always appalled to learn that patients have been harmed when undergoing treatment at their hands. These can be very traumatic experiences for anyone to go through. By introducing systems that allow us to understand, analyse and manage the risks inherent in our brand of healthcare, we can develop safer systems for delivering primary care. So we should bother, not only for the sake of patients, but also on behalf of ourselves, our colleagues and our teams.

Background

Primary care services for a community have often been provided in the past from a number of small businesses based in that community. However, as we know, this situation is now changing. These small businesses were GPs, dentists, community pharmacists and optometrists who were independently contracted to a health authority and who were supported by their own employed clinical and administrative staff and by attached staff employed by health authorities or community or acute NHS trusts. There was little management control, provided that contractors worked within their terms and conditions of service. Most primary care professionals had no risk management systems as such, and had very little training in these concepts. Their main links to risk management had traditionally been with the medical protection organisations that indemnified them against legal action. Within this context, GPs and primary care professionals understood and managed clinical risk – GPs have been referred to as the 'risk-sink for the NHS'.[1] However, the idea of looking at systems in primary care, with the aim of identifying and managing the risks inherent to those systems, had not been articulated. In this chapter the various factors that have been exerted to move us away from this position and examine the origins of the patient safety movement in the UK will be described. The implications of the safety agenda for patient care and for supporting professionals will then be explored.

Litigation and complaints

In years gone by, complaints and claims against general practitioners were rare, but over the last 15 years, the number of complaints and claims has escalated steeply. For instance, in 1989 there were 38 claims against GP members of the Medical Protection Society (MPS), compared with 500 in 1998, representing a 13-fold increase.[2] More recently, we know that in the year 2000 to 2001 there were 140 000 formal complaints about NHS services, of which 95 000 related to hospital services.[3] It is difficult to estimate the cost of claims against GPs and primary care practitioners. However, data from the NHS Litigation Authority show that annual NHS clinical negligence expenditure rose from £1 million in 1974–75 (that is, £6.33 million at 2002 prices) to £446 million in 2001–02. We can therefore see that primary care professionals operate within a system whereby complaints and litigation are increasing across the NHS.

For most professionals, complaints and claims against them are profoundly negative experiences which often cause personal upset and anguish. It has been estimated that 38% of doctors who are the subject of a claim suffer clinical depression as a result.[4] Safer working practices resulting in a lower risk of adverse events not only protect patients, but also help professionals to minimise the personal trauma that arises from complaints and litigation.

Clinical governance

The concept of clinical governance was introduced in the document *A First Class Service* in 1998.[5] In this document, clinical governance was described as 'a framework through which NHS organisations are accountable for continuously improving the quality of their services and safeguarding high standards of care by creating an environment in which excellence in clinical care will flourish.' Clinical governance was to be the central focus for assuring the quality of care provided by NHS services. In the years since the introduction of this concept, clinical governance has become embedded within the ethos and working practices of primary care. Primary care organisations (PCOs) all have clinical governance structures, and the Chief Executive of the PCO has personal accountability for clinical governance, as do the Chief Executives of all NHS trusts. In addition, every practice is expected to have a clinical governance lead, and to participate in clinical governance activity across the PCO.

Clinical governance sets out to improve the quality of service to patients, to improve patient safety and to involve patients in healthcare. The National Clinical Governance Support Team in England uses the concept of the seven pillars of clinical governance. These are:

- risk management
- education, training and continuing professional development
- use of information
- clinical audit
- clinical effectiveness and research
- patient involvement
- staffing and staff management.

Risk management is therefore regarded as a fundamental component of clinical governance, and practices need to understand and apply the principles of risk management in their everyday work.

Primary care organisations

With the advent of PCOs in the early 2000s, attitudes to risk in general practice have changed. In many respects, PCOs have a closer relationship with individual practices than did the old health authorities. There is also now an expectation that practices will work collaboratively across a PCO area, for the benefit of patients. Changes in attitudes have also been greatly influenced by the concept of clinical governance and the accountability that Chief Executives of NHS organisations, including PCOs, hold for clinical governance issues. The majority of GPs are still independent contractors, and GPs are still by and large indemnified by the medical protection organisations, but PCOs now have a role in the risk management process, and as a result have been introducing the concepts of risk assessment and risk management within the PCO. An increasing number of PCOs now have clinical risk management systems and have either made or are making arrangements for patient safety incident reporting. Likewise, a number of PCOs are supporting significant event audits within and across primary care teams, and are also developing systems for conducting root cause analysis for critical incidents. In this climate, a proactive approach to developing risk management within practices is inevitable.

Professional codes

Although not explicitly directing professionals to undertake risk management, the professional codes that relate to primary care practitioners do require that practitioners engage in those activities that help to promote performance. *Good Medical Practice for General Practitioners* is the document that interprets *Good Medical Practice* (the professional code for doctors issued by the General Medical Council (GMC)) for the discipline of general practice.[6] In the section entitled 'Keeping up to date and maintaining your performance', this states:

> The other ways in which you maintain high-quality clinical care need to reflect the breadth and nature of the discipline. In maintaining good care you should therefore be aware of a range of ways of monitoring and improving care (e.g. significant event audit, risk management) and involve all your team members in maintaining and improving the quality of care which your practice provides. Clinical governance provides a framework that may help you to do this.

Therefore risk management is defined as a professional activity in which GPs are expected to participate. Other professional codes also refer to risk management. For instance, the publication *Medicine, Ethics and Practice* produced by the Royal Pharmaceutical Society of Great Britain (RPSGP)[7] also has a section on risk management that states:

> Pharmacists should ensure that they have robust risk management procedures in place.

Risk management is therefore clearly defined as a professional activity for a variety of primary care professionals.

The patient safety movement

In 2000, the Chief Medical Officer (CMO) for England, Professor Sir Liam Donaldson, published a document entitled *An Organisation With a Memory*.[8] This was the report of an expert group on learning from adverse events in the NHS. The report presented the evidence from the UK and other countries (especially Australia and the USA) regarding the consequences of adverse events and in particular the lack of systems in the NHS that allowed there to be learning from adverse events. This report also looked at the subjects of human error and risk management as applied in other industries, such as the aviation and nuclear power industries. The working party concluded that the NHS could gain great benefit by applying these principles to healthcare.

Following the publication of this influential report, and its follow-up *Building a Safer NHS for Patients*,[9] the NPSA was established as a Special Health Authority in June 2001 to co-ordinate efforts to report, and learn from, mistakes and problems that affect patient safety.

Seven steps to patient safety

As part of the remit described above, the NPSA has published guidance for NHS organisations on the steps that they should take to improve patient safety.[10] The seven steps are set out below.

1 *Build a safety culture.* Create a culture that is open and fair.
2 *Lead and support your staff.* Establish a clear and strong focus on patient safety throughout your organisation.
3 *Integrate your risk management activity.* Develop systems and processes to manage your risks and identify and assess things that could go wrong.
4 *Promote reporting.* Ensure that your staff can easily report incidents locally and nationally.
5 *Involve and communicate with patients and the public.* Develop ways to communicate openly with and listen to patients.
6 *Learn and share safety lessons.* Encourage staff to use root cause analysis to learn how and why incidents happen.
7 *Implement solutions to prevent harm.* Embed lessons through practices, processes or systems.

So . . . there are seven pillars of clinical governance, and now seven steps to patient safety. Seven must be the magic number! However, note that risk management is firmly incorporated in both of these guides to quality and safety.

Applying risk management in primary care

Primary care teams and practices have always generated a great deal of innovation in healthcare. Dedicated professionals are continuously reviewing their practice and considering ways in which to change systems and procedures to enhance patient care. Risk management techniques should be viewed as tools in the change management process that help practices and teams to identify, assess and manage the risks inherent in change. Indeed, risk management can also be applied to existing practice to establish what risks might be associated with current systems and whether practices need to make changes or to stick to what they are doing. Risk management can be applied to both clinical and non-clinical activity, and can be utilised in every primary care role. It has often been the case that primary care teams have felt pressurised into adopting all of the bright new ideas that come their way, sometimes due to fear that by not doing so they will be viewed as conservative and non-progressive. By using risk management techniques, teams can weigh up the risks inherent in changing practice, or in not changing, and determine a way forward whereby identified risks can be avoided or managed.

Conclusion

In this chapter the context in which risk management should now be viewed as a core activity for professionals and practices has been identified. We have seen that risk management is a key component of clinical governance and of the patient safety culture. Risk management in primary care does not equate to being risk averse – by its very nature primary care is a risky business. Rather, it should be seen as a method that allows practices and primary care teams to understand the risks inherent in their systems and processes, and the risks associated with introducing change or deciding not to implement change. By undertaking risk management in the primary care setting, we should expect there to be safer and therefore better-quality care for patients. Primary care professionals go to work in the morning to look after their patients and to provide a good service. Risk management is an important and useful tool to help them in this endeavour.

References

1 Haslam D (2003) 'Schools and hospitals' for 'education and health'. *BMJ.* **326**: 234–5.
2 Dyer C (1999) GPs face escalating litigation. *BMJ.* **318**: 830b.
3 Department of Health (2003) *NHS Complaints Reform: making things right.* Department of Health, London.
4 Department of Health (2003) *Making Amends: a consultation paper setting out proposals for reforming the approach to clinical negligence in the NHS.* Department of Health, London.
5 Secretary of State for Health (1998) *A First Class Service.* Department of Health, London.
6 Royal College of General Practitioners (2002) *Good Medical Practice for General Practitioners.* Royal College of General Practitioners, London.
7 Royal Pharmaceutical Society of Great Britain (2003) *Medicine, Ethics and Practice: a guide for pharmacists.* Royal Pharmaceutical Society of Great Britain, London.
8 Chief Medical Officer (2000) *An Organisation With a Memory.* Department of Health, London.
9 Department of Health (2001) *Building a Safer NHS for Patients.* Department of Health, London.
10 National Patient Safety Agency (2003) *Seven Steps to Patient Safety.* National Patient Safety Agency, London.

Chapter 2

Risk management, patient safety and a medical protection organisation

John Hickey

Key learning points

- Medical protection organisations (MPOs) are key stakeholders in the evolving patient safety agenda.
- Whilst an MPO's role is about protecting and safeguarding an individual clinician's interests and character, it is equally about ensuring the maintenance of high standards of professional practice, the prevention of negligence and malpractice, and the provision of risk management advice.
- The aetiology of complaints and litigation lies just as much in individual performance (communication, behaviour, attitude) as it does on competence (clinical skills).
- Patient-centred communication may be the best risk-management tool.
- In the event of an adverse outcome, an expression of regret or sorrow by the clinicial is *not* an admission of liability.
- Once an adverse outcome has occurred, clinicians need to learn to say 'sorry' to re-establish the doctor-patient relationship.

> I've made a career of studying the reasons doctors get sued for malpractice. While all doctors make mistakes, some who injure their patients never see a summons, and many who've done no harm are hauled into court.
>
> (LS Mangels, 1991[1])

Introduction

There are many stakeholders with an interest in the evolving patient safety agenda. Not least among them are the MPOs, which between them indemnify most of the UK's 33 500 general practitioners. Unlike an insurance company, the Medical Protection Society (MPS) holds discretionary funds owned by members, who comprise a broad body of healthcare professionals. A governing council comprises medical, dental and 'lay' representatives.[2] We bear the financial costs of negligence claims, as well as advising and counselling members who face a range of other actions taken against them in relation to their professional practice. We have been doing this for well over 100 years, which gives us a perspective on patient safety and the issue of clinical risk.

Patient safety has always been intrinsic to our work. Back in the nineteenth century, we were concerned to protect members and an innocent public from 'quackery'. Today, 'preventing avoidable harm to patients' is a value embedded in our mission statement. For decades we have offered a rich and varied educational programme which includes medical school lectures, a quarterly membership journal devoted to risk management, publications focusing on common pitfalls of practice and a dedicated risk management consultancy, advisory and training service. In recent years we have also opened and made available our database of claims for research purposes.

Our memorandum and articles of association[3] also clearly state that our objectives are to 'protect, support and safeguard the character and interests of medical practitioners'. The same document also includes the objective to 'take or assist in taking all proper proceedings (legal or otherwise) to maintain high standards of professional practice and to prevent negligence and malpractice'. While our role is about protecting and safeguarding an individual doctor's interests and character, it is equally about ensuring the maintenance of high standards of professional practice, the prevention of negligence and malpractice, and the provision of risk management and educational services. We believe that patient safety therefore remains intrinsic to what we do. As an organisation we support and defend our members who, in the view of expert opinion, have not been negligent. Nevertheless, however careful they are doctors can – and do – make mistakes. In these circumstances, patients who have suffered avoidable harm through the negligent acts or omissions of our members should be fairly and justly compensated. This is also why we believe that all clinicians should be appropriately indemnified to ensure that any patient who has been negligently harmed does not go uncompensated.

Of course, sometimes it is difficult to achieve a balance between 'protecting' a member's interests and those of the patient. Although we endeavour to protect our members' interests and the needs of the patient, these aims may sometimes seem to be in conflict, particularly if we take as our starting point the right of an individual (in our case the member) to representation and a fair hearing.

In addition, the business of litigation is adversarial in nature, and some have claimed that clinical negligence litigation has done very little to improve patient safety. Despite the so-called 'litigation explosion' in the developed world, there is absolutely no evidence that this has made healthcare safer. In fact, it can be argued that willingness to discuss adverse outcomes and look for the root causes has been hampered by the climate of fear induced by litigation and has actually made the system less safe. As Professor Sir Ian Kennedy has noted, clinical negligence works against the interests of patient safety:

> It provides a clear incentive not to report, or to cover up an error or an accident. Once this happens no one can learn from it and the next patient is exposed to the same or similar risk.[4]

Patient safety: a new perspective

To date much of risk management (and this book) has focused on systems, and this seems only right when much of the evidence following adverse incidents points to systemic failures. Although individual human factors will be involved in the error, we are being encouraged to look at the wider system and to move away from individual blame. However, even this can be problematic, and James Reason cautions against an over-reliance on viewing everything in terms of systems error. He suggests that ultimately this could lead to a 'learned helplessness' on the part of the individual: 'it was the system at fault and not me'.[5]

In the past, risk management was concerned mostly with clinical skills and competence, was clinician centred and existed largely within a voluntary framework. The focus today is on patient safety, with a shift in emphasis to the part that performance issues play, such as teamworking, systems design and effective doctor–patient communication delivered in an environment of increased accountability and regulation (*see* Table 2.1).

Table 2.1 Risk management and patient safety

Past	Present
Clinical risk management	*Patient safety*
Competence	Performance
Individual oriented	Team and systems oriented
Voluntary code	Regulatory framework
Clinician centred	Patient centred

All this represents something of a shift in emphasis for MPOs, too. The MPS has repeatedly advocated good communication in its practice advice to members. However, it might be argued that to date MPOs have paid insufficient attention to the aetiology of complaints and litigation. In particular, there is increasing international evidence that effective communication between doctor and patient and the ability to apologise when things have gone wrong can lead to a reduction in complaints and litigation in the first place. Of course, when we receive a complaint we only see the tip of the iceberg. The particulars of the claim will rarely give us an insight into the 'performance issues' that may have led to it, and once the adversarial process begins it is fought out in the area of competence – applying the Bolam test to the competence of the individual medical practice. As Professor Sir Ian Kennedy suggests it is therefore far too late at this stage for any contribution to be made to patient safety. When we scrutinise complaints and claims against members, we identify with Robert Bunting's description of precipitating and predisposing factors:[6]

- *precipitating factors* – adverse outcomes, iatrogenic injuries, failure to provide adequate care, providing incorrect care, system errors, mistakes
- *predisposing factors* – rudeness, delays, inattentiveness, miscommunication, apathy, no communication.

In our experience it is the predisposing factors that motivate patients to complain or claim, but of course when the details reach the media it is the precipitating factors that are most frequently cited.

I would therefore like to explore the role that more effective communication can play and the impact of saying sorry when an adverse outcome has occurred in reducing litigation and complaints. This may be the most effective risk management individual practitioners can be involved in.

Patient-centred communication

Despite our educational activities exhorting, explaining and illustrating best clinical practice, we have continued to experience a heavy caseload of claims and complaints. What has started to become apparent from research is that patients may sue or complain even when they have not been treated negligently. The handling of such cases can be very expensive both for the protection organisation (even when it does not lead to a final compensation award) and for the clinician involved. It is estimated that 38% of doctors who are litigated against suffer clinical depression.[7] Doctors have always known from experience that patients may take legal action if they have an outcome they were not expecting or a poor outcome. What has probably been less well understood is that complaints are frequently made in cases where there is simply a lack of rapport and understanding between doctor and patient. In other words, it is not just about clinical competence – it is also about patients' perceptions of the way in which they were treated, both clinically and as a person. Put simply, the evidence shows that patients tend not to sue people they like. Let us take a brief tour of the research.

Studies have repeatedly shown that the quality of medical care is poorly correlated with the occurrence of negligence lawsuits.[8–10] In the seminal Harvard Practice Study,[8,9] 3.7% of the hospital admissions reviewed resulted in an adverse outcome, of which one in four was, in the judgement of the authors, due to negligence. However, only 12% of those patients who suffered negligence filed a lawsuit, whereas 88% did not. Interestingly, two out of three claims were made by patients who had not even experienced an adverse outcome, or who had an adverse outcome that could not be considered to be due to negligence.

In another study,[10] no difference could be found in the clinical outcomes of those doctors who had never been sued and those who had been sued frequently (whether for small or large amounts).

A number of studies have shown an association between poor communication and negligence claims.[11–15] The communication problems most frequently identified were inadequate explanation of the diagnosis or treatment,[11–14] and patients feeling ignored.[12–14] Other communication problems included doctors not understanding patient and family perspectives, doctors devaluing patient and family views, patients feeling deserted[11] and patients feeling rushed.[12]

Using an experimental study of members of the public viewing videotaped consultations, Lester and Smith[15] demonstrated that poor doctor communication could be a risk factor in negligence claims and their findings suggested that good communication might decrease the likelihood of such claims. Taking this approach a stage further, Levinson *et al.*[16] analysed the relationship between poor communication and negligence claims through direct observation, and they identified specific communication behaviours that potentially reduce the risk of litigation. The behaviours of doctors who had not been sued are compared with those who had been sued[12] in Box 2.1.

Box 2.1 Differences in communication behaviours between doctors who have been sued and those who have not

Doctors who had not been sued	*Doctors who were sued . . .*
• Asked the patient questions	• Patient felt rushed
• Laughed	• Patient received no explanation
• Explained the process of the consultation	• Patient felt ignored
• Patient perceived sufficient time had been spent	• Patient felt less time was spent
Levinson *et al.*[16]	Hickson *et al.*[12]

The lesson for an MPO is that effective communication is at the heart of the doctor–patient relationship, and that attention to acquiring and maintaining communication skills is an effective part of risk management. It also offers the prospect of a more satisfactory outcome for the patient. Malcolm Thomas's excellent chapters on communication skills in this book begin to highlight some of the key techniques and behaviours that can be employed to build relationships with patients, develop rapport and change consultations into a more enjoyable and genuinely communicative experience for both parties.

Communication: the art of the apology

Apologising when something has gone wrong has been a mainstay of MPS advice to members for very many years. Our response to *Making Amends* explained that 'MPS has long advised doctors and dentists who have made a mistake to provide a full explanation, apologise to the patient and consider what they might do to prevent similar errors occurring in the future'. Box 2.2 summarises the position we adopt.

Box 2.2 The legal position and advice

- An expression of regret/sorrow is not the same as an admission of liability.
- Even an admission of liability is considered within the context of other evidence.
- An empathic explanation of the facts surrounding an adverse outcome is not an admission of liability.
- All medical protection organisations advocate better communication before and after an adverse event.
- Abandonment and poor communication after an adverse outcome are risk factors that medical protection organisations are keen to see reduced.
- Following a serious adverse outcome you can always seek advice from your medical protection organisation.

Other healthcare bodies also advocate open disclosure and an apology when there has been an adverse outcome. The NHS Litigation Authority (NHSLA) advocates that:

> ... it is both natural and desirable ... to express sorrow or regret at the outcome. [These] ... would not normally constitute an admission of liability ... not our policy to prohibit them, nor dispute any payment ... solely on the grounds of such an expression of regret.[17]

The GMC, in its response to *Making Amends*, stated:

> The GMC's *Good Medical Practice* places a duty on doctors to explain to patients who have suffered harm during medical treatment. We believe it would be simpler and clearer for clinicians to explain all adverse events to the patients they affect, as well as reporting them to the employing body and/or to an appropriate body such as the NPSA.[18]

Nevertheless, when I speak of this to audiences, I am frequently surprised how little understood or accepted it is. There is resistance, and a fear that they will inadvertently admit liability. There is growing international evidence to suggest that effective discussions after an adverse outcome might reduce the risk of litigation. There is certainly no evidence that such discussions increase it. The impact, therefore, of getting doctors to put this into practice is considerable.

The open, honest and timely disclosure of medical error to patients needs to become something which doctors take in their stride, in so far as:

- every healthcare professional at some stage in their career will need to conduct these conversations
- there is a clear ethical and professional imperative to disclose information when a patient has been harmed by medical treatment
- it helps the patient to recover psychologically and move on
- any hint of less than open disclosure undermines the trust on which the doctor–patient relationship is based.

What the MPS has become interested in is how to encourage doctors to put this particular communication skill into practice as a preventive measure – to contain patients' litigious intent by attending to their human needs for explanation and empathy.

For many years, patient representative groups (e.g. the Association against Medical Accidents, AvMA) have been making the same points. Most patients seek an explanation for what has occurred, together with an apology and reassurance that steps are being taken to prevent a recurrence if the end result was caused by clinician error. They only consult a lawyer when they meet a defensive attitude and are unable to obtain an explanation from the treating clinician. In the words of Charles Vincent, 'The lack of an explanation, and an apology if appropriate, may be experienced by the patient as extremely punitive and distressing, and may be a powerful stimulus to complaint or litigation'.[19]

The lesson for an MPO is that the ability of doctors to deal with an adverse outcome effectively and to say sorry is the most effective part of what has been called 'self-protective risk management'.[20] It also offers the prospect of a more satisfactory outcome for the patient. In this sense, open disclosure is in our view a 'mutually protective' act of risk management.

So if we are to be more open about adverse outcomes, how do we recognise them and how frequent are they? There are numerous definitions of an 'adverse outcome', but the following are probably as good as any:

> An unintended injury caused by medical management rather than the disease process.[8]

> An unintended or unexpected incident that led to harm.[21]

Thus adverse outcomes include outcomes due to negligent or inappropriate care, as well as unavoidable outcomes and complications of care. How common are they? Studies in developed countries suggest that the rate is about 10% (i.e. 900 000) in England each year. The NPSA estimates that these incidents contribute to 72 000 deaths each year,[21] and that 50% of these are preventable.

The concept of open disclosure has developed with three components.

- First, when unintended harm occurs, it involves informing patients and carers about what has gone wrong in an empathic way, which includes an expression of regret.
- Secondly, it involves in-depth analysis of the problem, including root cause analysis of severe problems.
- Thirdly, it involves a commitment by individuals and organisations to fix the system problem identified.[22]

At least 90% of patients want to be told all of the circumstances following an adverse incident.[23,24] Interestingly, 32% of doctors said that they would disclose complete details of the error, although 70% believe that they should give full details[25] and 33% reported that they would provide misleading or incomplete information if the error led to mortality.[26] In another study, house staff discussed only 24% of serious errors with patients.[27]

So why do clinicians find it so difficult to be open about mistakes and errors? The barriers to more open disclosure remain very real, and include fear of litigation, loss of professional reputation, difficulty in determining why a poor result has occurred, fear of patient reaction, difficulty in acknowledging that one may have made an error and, in the case of the death of a patient, criminal prosecution. Newman looked at the deeper, more personal feelings, which included shame, fear, self-doubt, isolation and sadness.[28] Mizrali looked at the observed behaviour of doctors when faced with a serious adverse outcome.[29] Initially there may be denial, when the doctor may pretend that the outcome did not happen or perhaps redefines the error in terms that make it appear not to be a mistake at all. Another response is discounting the error by shifting the blame from oneself on to external factors (e.g. the NHS and lack of resources, other healthcare workers or even the patient). Finally, distancing can occur, when reminders and possibly even any discussion with the patient might be avoided.

If an elderly patient slips in the street and fractures their neck of femur, the average GP would instinctively demonstrate an empathic response and an expression of sorrow, so why is this not the case when there has been an adverse outcome of care? For most people, *I'm sorry* is spoken almost reflexively throughout the day to express respect, regret and compassion. Yet for us physicians, the words *I'm sorry* can be among the hardest to say. Although all the evidence suggests that patients clearly want to talk about an adverse outcome and that an empathic discussion frequently improves patient satisfaction and care outcomes and reduces the likelihood of litigation, doctors find this difficult – even (or particularly) when there has been no error.

So how can we help? Policies, directives and exhortation from the NHS, the GMC or an MPO are not self-executive and do not necessarily change doctors' behaviour. However, education and coaching might do so. O'Brien and colleagues at the Cognitive Institute in Brisbane[30] have developed a model known as ASSIST© which appears to be a valid and reliable method of coaching doctors in discussing adverse outcomes with their patients. The approach is underpinned by the communication skills discussed in this book. Its key component is a sequential and structured dialogue with the patient (*see* Box 2.3). This coaching technique is being used extensively by medical insurers in Australia and New Zealand to assist their doctors in managing adverse outcomes more effectively.

Box 2.3 The ASSIST© model

- Acknowledge – that there has been a problem and you are aware of the patient's distress. Express empathy and concern.
- Sorry – express your regret and sorrow.
- Story – ask the patient to tell their story, what they know about the adverse outcome and what they have experienced.
- Inquire – allow the patient to ask questions. *Then* you can add any information that you feel is important for them to know in an honest and transparent way.
- Solution – allow the patient to generate suggestions as to how the situation should be managed. Offer additional suggestions to assist the patient.
- Travel – express your willingness to continue to care and increase contact. Do not resist any patient request to change to another doctor.

Source: *Mastering Adverse Outcomes*, Cognitive Institute, Brisbane, Australia[30]

Conclusion

The MPS takes seriously the point made by the CMO[31] that, in the past, learning opportunities may have been wasted. We are exploring positive interventions to share further our learning with the membership at large, with the developers of undergraduate curricula and with those few members who face serial complaints and claims. We, too, recognise that in the aftermath of the Bristol Inquiry 'all has changed, changed utterly'. A new order is emerging for patient safety which requires new and innovative approaches from MPOs.

Given the overwhelming evidence that many complaints and much litigation are rooted in poor communication skills, what should an MPO do? Well, it could take the view that this is the responsibility of the universities, postgraduate deaneries or other professional organisations. Conversely, it might conclude that the massive financial and personal costs associated with 'fighting' these debilitating and frequently unnecessary cases, which are borne by the MPOs, their members and the NHS, could be better spent on patient care. In short, we have the strongest incentive to remedy this problem.

References

1 Mangels LS (1991) Tips from doctors who've never been sued. *Med Econ.* **68**: 56–8, 60–4.
2 Palmer RN and Selvadurai N (2000) The UK medical protection and defence organisations. In: M Powers and N Harris (eds) *Clinical Negligence* (3e). Butterworths, London.
3 Medical Protection Society (2001) *Memorandum and Articles of Association.* Medical Protection Society, London.
4 *The Report of the Public Inquiry into Children's Heart Surgery at the Bristol Royal Infirmary 1984–1995: learning from Bristol*; http://www.bristol-inquiry.org.uk/final_report/report/index.htm
5 Reason J (2004) *Engineering a Safety Culture.* Patient Safety 2004. National Patient Safety Agency Conference, Birmingham, February 2004.
6 Bunting RF *et al.* (1998) Practical risk management for physicians. *J Health Risk Management.* **18**: 29–53.
7 Department of Health (2003) *Making Amends.* Department of Health, London.
8 Brennan TA, Leape LL, Laird NM *et al.* (1991) Incidence of adverse events and negligence in hospitalized patients: results of the Harvard Medical Practice study. I. *NEJM.* **324**: 370–6.
9 Localio AR, Lawthers AG, Brennan TA *et al.* (1991) Relation between real practice claims and adverse events due to negligence: results of the Harvard Medical Practice study. III. *NEJM.* **325**: 245–51.
10 Entman SS *et al.* (1994) The relationship between malpractice claims history and subsequent obstetric care. *JAMA.* **272**: 1588–91.
11 Beckman HB, Markakis KM *et al.* (1994) The doctor–patient relationship and malpractice: lessons from plaintiff depositions. *Arch Intern Med.* **154**: 1365–70.
12 Hickson GB, Clayton EN *et al.* (1994) Obstetricians' prior malpractice experience and patients' satisfaction with care. *JAMA.* **272**: 1583–7.
13 Vincent C, Young M *et al.* (1994) Why do people sue doctors? A study of patients and relatives taking legal action. *Lancet.* **343**: 1609–13.
14 Hickson GB, Clayton EW *et al.* (1992) Factors that prompted families to file medical malpractice claims following perinatal injuries. *JAMA.* **267**: 1359–63.
15 Lester GW and Smith SG (1993) Listening and talking to patients: a remedy for malpractice suits? *West J Med.* **158**: 268–72.
16 Levinson W *et al.* (1997) Physician–patient communication. The relationship with malpractice claims among primary care physicians and surgeons. *JAMA.* **277**: 553–9.
17 NHS Litigation Authority (2002) *Apologies and Explanations.* Circular 02/02. NHS Litigation Authority, London.
18 General Medical Council (2003) GMC response to *Making Amends.* Press release, 31 October 2003. General Medical Council, London.
19 Vincent C (2003) Understanding and responding to adverse events. *NEJM.* **348**: 11.
20 Kraman S and Hamm G (1999) Risk management: extreme honesty may be the best policy. *Ann Intern Med.* **131**: 963–7.

21 National Patient Safety Agency (2004) *Seven Steps to Patient Safety*. National Patient Safety Agency, London.

22 Fallowfield L (2003) *Communications with Patients in the Context of Medical Errors*. National Patient Safety Agency, London.

23 Witman AB *et al.* (1996) How do patients want physicians to handle mistakes? A survey of internal medicine patients in an academic setting. *Archives Int Med.* **156**: 2265–9.

24 Hingorani M *et al.* (1999) Patients' and doctors' attitudes to the amount of information given after unintended injury during treatment. *BMJ.* **318**: 640–1.

25 Vincent J (1998) Information in the ICU: are we being honest with our patients? The result of a European questionnaire. *Intensive Care Med.* **24**: 1251–6.

26 Novack DH *et al.* (1989) Physicians' attitudes towards using deception to resolve ethical problems. *JAMA.* **261**: 2980–6.

27 Wu AW, Folkman S *et al.* (1991) Do house officers learn from their mistakes? *JAMA.* **265**: 2089.

28 Newman M (1996) The emotional impact of mistakes on family physicians. *Arch Fam Med.* **5**: 71–5.

29 Mizrali T (1984) Managing medical mistakes: ideology, insularity and accountability among internists in training. *Soc Sci Med.* **19**: 135–46.

30 O'Brien M (2003) *Mastering Adverse Outcomes*. Cognitive Institute, Brisbane, Australia.

31 Department of Health (2000) *An Organisation With a Memory*. Department of Health, London.

Chapter 3

Policy framework and background

Peter Nicklin

Key learning points

- The extent of preventable harm caused to patients by their medical management has only recently been openly acknowledged.
- Healthcare policy, regulation and legislation aimed at improving patient safety have been significantly shaped by the findings and recommendations of the 'Bristol Inquiry'.
- Since 2000 an increasing number of patient safety organisations and agencies have been established, that have direct relevance to the provision of primary care.
- The effectiveness of these radical reforms to the regulation of patient safety has yet to be fully evaluated.

Introduction

The NHS employs approximately 1.3 million people, and of these over 10% are engaged in general practice. It would be reasonable to assume that the overwhelming majority of NHS staff are motivated by a benevolent desire to contribute to the care and cure of those using the service. Paradoxically, it is estimated that 10% of the 8.5 million patients admitted to hospitals in England and Wales each year experience a preventable adverse event,[1] and as many as 30 000 patients may die as a result of these incidents. The frequency of 'medical error' in primary care, where the majority of contacts with patients take place, has not been the subject of such rigorous scrutiny and is less well understood. However, the available evidence suggests that as many as 11% of prescriptions may be flawed,[2] and a MORI survey of the general public[3] reveals that 5% of individuals report being harmed by their medical care.

Beyond the individual patient's suffering and the anguish of the staff involved, it is variously estimated that the cost of medical error (additional treatment, prolonged stay in hospital and negligence claims) is £2–3 billion per annum. In 1975, about 500 clinical negligence claims were made against the NHS. By 1999, this had risen to around 10 000.[4] In accounting for this logarithmic increase, Walshe[5] offers a series of dynamically related explanations, including a wider trend towards litigiousness, easier access to the law for redress, a loss of public affection for the NHS (a preparedness to criticise), and the increased complexity and volume of care being delivered. The latter is pithily captured by Cyril

Chantler's assertion that 'Medicine used to be simple, ineffective and relatively safe. Now it's complex, effective and potentially dangerous'. However, there is no simple correlation between these factors and the perceived scale of failure in the NHS. Even when medicine was 'safe, simple and ineffective', errors and violations were common. In 1967, Barbara Robb published her savage indictment of the care of the elderly in hospital,[6] and this was followed in rapid succession by a series of harrowing reports of neglect, incompetence and cruelty in the country's mental hospitals (e.g. Ely, Farleigh, Whittingham, South Ockenden, Napsbury). Speaking of these, Clare[7] suggests that 'It is not at all certain that these highly publicised scandals actually contributed to the development of an informed public opinion . . .'. Indeed, the public seem to have been placated, reverted to their position of innocence and accepted quality 'as given' by the NHS. And then there was the Bristol Inquiry, Alder Hey, Harold Shipman . . . and 'all changed, changed utterly'.

Quality in the 'new' NHS

In this chapter we shall briefly review and analyse the Government's 'patient safety' policy imperatives and consider the role and function of some (of the many) agencies and regulators that have been spawned in the aftermath of 'Bristol' to improve quality in the 'new' NHS.

In December 1997, just 6 months after displacing a long-serving Conservative administration, the Labour government published its White Paper entitled *The New NHS: Modern, Dependable*.[8] This placed particular emphasis on 'quality', introduced the notion of 'clinical governance' and gave notice of the government's intentions to address 'patient safety' by ensuring that:

- clinical risk reduction programmes of high standard are in place . . .
- adverse events are detected and openly investigated, and the lessons learned promptly applied . . .
- lessons for clinical practice are systematically learned from complaints made by patients . . .
- problems of poor clinical performance are recognised at an early stage and dealt with to prevent harm to patients . . . .[8]

Although strong on aspiration, the White Paper lacked substance. However, its critics were silenced (or stunned) when in the summer of 1998 the Government filled in the detail.

In July 1998, the Government consulted on its health service quality strategy in *A First Class Service: Quality in the New NHS*,[9] prompted in part by the general and chronic decline in public confidence in the service, and according to the Government because 'a series of well-publicised lapses in quality have prompted doubts in the minds of patients about the overall standard of care they may receive'.

In the years since its implementation, *A First Class Service* has inevitably deviated in the detail (to which we shall return), but the principles still hold good.

Setting, delivering and monitoring standards

The overall thrust of the NHS quality framework is a dynamic system for *setting, delivering and monitoring standards* (*see* Figure 3.1), as summarised opposite.

- *Clear national standards* through the establishment of the *National Institute of Clinical Excellence (NICE)* to provide clear guidance on clinical (and cost-) effectiveness of health interventions, and the development of *National Service Frameworks (NSFs)* to raise standards of care and reduce inequalities.
- *Effective local delivery* of these standards through a system of *clinical governance* (a system through which healthcare organisations are accountable for continuously improving the quality of services), robust systems of *continuing professional development (CPD)* for health professionals, and the 'modernisation' of *professional self-regulation.*
- *National monitoring systems* – the establishment of the *Commission for Health Improvement (CHI)* (to undertake a rolling programme of clinical governance reviews of all NHS organisations in England and Wales and to investigate serious service failures), an *NHS Performance Framework* and a *National Patient Survey.*

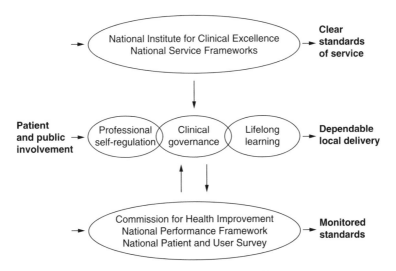

Figure 3.1 Setting, delivering and monitoring standards.[9]

Since 1998, a plethora of patient safety policies, regulations and reforms has been spawned – far too many to consider in detail in a single chapter (later chapters will amplify the detail). So in this chapter we shall focus on some of the organisations that most directly impact on the patient safety agenda, namely:

- the National Institute for Clinical Excellence (NICE)
- the Healthcare Commission
- the National Patient Safety Agency (NPSA)
- the National Clinical Assessment Authority (NCAA)
- the Council for the Regulation of Healthcare Professionals (CRHP).

However, before proceeding it would be useful to consider (in summary) some reports that have influenced and complemented the policy initiatives which the Government has introduced.

An Organisation With a Memory[10]

In 2000, the CMO (for England) reported on the findings of an expert group tasked to 'examine the extent to which the NHS currently has the capacity to learn from incidents and service failures, and to recommend steps which might be taken to help ensure similar events can be avoided in the future'. In providing the context of its findings, the expert group candidly revealed the scale of clinical error in the NHS, concluded that the health service consistently failed to learn from its errors, and criticised its passive and closed culture. The report identified four key areas that the NHS must address:

- a unified mechanism for reporting and analysis when things go wrong
- a more open culture in which errors or service failures can be reported and discussed
- mechanisms for ensuring that, where lessons are identified, the necessary changes are put into practice
- a much wider appreciation of the value of the system approach in preventing, analysing and learning from errors.

Building a safer NHS

Government reports of this type are normally shrouded in jargon and diluted or distorted by political editing. This report is possibly an exception, and the reader who has a serious interest in patient safety is urged to read *An Organisation With a Memory*.[10] Inevitably a report of this type is strategic in focus, and the operational detail followed in rapid succession. In *Building a Safer NHS for Patients*,[11] the Department of Health announced the formation of NPSA to collect and analyse information on adverse events, identify lessons to be learned, produce solutions and disseminate these to healthcare organisations.

Almost simultaneously, the Department of Health published *Assuring the Quality of Medical Practice*.[12] If the formation of the NPSA was viewed as a rational but potentially over-bureaucratic initiative, the directives contained in this publication were radical and represented a challenge to the medical profession. They heralded the introduction of mandatory CPD, appraisal and revalidation, and the establishment of the NCAA, which was charged with assessing doctors whose clinical performance was causing concern and providing an objective report on the problem and advice on what action (if any) should be taken. In the aftermath of the Bristol Inquiry the Government strongly criticised medical self-regulation as being slow, lacking transparency and lacking accountability to the public. *Assuring the Quality of Medical Practice* affirmed the reform of the GMC and the formation of CRHP which would ensure that the individual professional regulatory bodies acted in a consistent manner, which presumably included being consistent with the Government's wishes. The formation of the CRHP had been 'trailed' in *The NHS Plan*[13] the previous year, in which it described its role in benign terms such as 'coordinating' and 'acting as a forum for common approaches' and then the wake-up call, concluding that 'were concerns to remain about the individual self-regulatory bodies, its role could evolve'!

The concepts of *clinical risk* and *patient safety* are relative newcomers to the UK healthcare policy and regulatory arena. The Clinical Negligence Scheme for Trusts

(CNST) managed by the NHSLA was introduced in 1995 and developed from a concern to limit the financial liability for clinical negligence of member trusts. In 1997, the CNST introduced assessed risk management standards intended to provide NHS trusts with financial incentives (a discount on subscription) to improve patient safety. There are three levels to the CNST standards, level 1 being the most basic and attracting a 10% discount, and level 3 being the most rigorous and attracting a 25% reduction. In 2003, the National Audit Office (NAO) report *Achieving Improvements Through Clinical Governance*[14] revealed that 'one in five trusts have not achieved any level, and most have yet to move beyond level 1'. This begs the question of what price (or what discount) should be paid for patient safety. The medical protection organisations have over a century of experience of (quite properly) defending their members from complainants and litigants, and may have occasionally defended what might now be seen as indefensible. However, more recently they have assumed a more proactive and prophylactic role in terms of protecting patients and contributing to the emerging patient safety agenda. And prior to the Bristol Inquiry the academic community paid relatively little attention to the question of medical error, its causation and patient safety. Subsequently, scientific scrutiny of these issues has intensified. In 2003, a systematic review of over 4500 papers conducted by the NHS Centre for Reviews and Disseminations at the University of York concluded that 'the quality of original research appeared to be variable . . . often the studies lacked focus . . . were conducted on a small scale' . . . . [and] 'the current research evaluating the effectiveness of reporting systems is limited and in the main of poor quality'.[15]

The Bristol Inquiry

With regard to patient safety, most if not all roads lead back to Bristol, and when Sir Ian Kennedy presented the *Report of the Public Inquiry into Children's Heart Surgery at the Bristol Royal Infirmary, 1984–1995* in July 2001, the recommendations contained few surprises, as the Government had already established the essential principles in *A First Class Service*[9] and had constructed the regulatory mechanisms and legislative framework over the previous three years. However, the report did criticise the NHS clinical negligence system, describing it as part of the 'culture of blame' and recommending that 'It should be abolished . . . should be replaced by an effective system for identifying, analysing, learning from and preventing errors and other sentinel events'. In June 2003, the CMO published *Making Amends*,[3] a consultation paper setting out proposals for reforming the approach to clinical negligence in the NHS. At the centre of a complex series of recommendations is a proposal to establish a less confrontational and fairer 'NHS Redress Scheme' which would investigate the alleged harm, provide an explanation, develop and deliver a package of remedial care and provide payments for pain and suffering. It also proposed a statutory 'duty of candour' requiring clinicians and health service managers to inform patients about actions that have caused harm. In return they would be exempt from disciplinary action (unless there is a criminal offence). *Making Amends* comes from the same stable as *An Organisation With a Memory*, and is recommended reading for the patient safety enthusiast!

On 18 July 2001, the Secretary of State for Health commended the Kennedy Report (*Learning From Bristol*) and the majority of its recommendations to the House of Commons. Kennedy had recommended the establishment of an 'overarching' Council for the Quality of Healthcare to coordinate the many agencies and regulators that were now competing to monitor, audit and inspect the NHS. In the event, on 31 March 2004 the Commission for Health Improvement 'ceased operating', and the following day its responsibilities were assumed by a new Healthcare Commission (formerly known as the Commission for Health Audit and Inspection, CHAI) which simultaneously acquired functions that had previously been exercised by the National Care Standards Commission, the Audit Commission and the Mental Health Act Commission, and which assumed a key role in the NHS Complaints procedure. In October 2003, John Reid had advised a Commons Health Select Committee that he intended to rationalise the many 'arm's-length' NHS agencies that had proliferated in recent years. It is anticipated that more of these functions will migrate to the CHAI. Thus at a stroke the NHS has its 'overarching Council for Quality', with Sir Ian Kennedy at the helm as its chairman.

Kennedy also recommended the establishment of a regulatory body for NHS managers. The Government agreed to consider this, but responded by producing a *Code of Conduct for NHS Managers*,[16] the first principle of the code being to 'make the care and safety of patients my first concern and act to protect them from risk'. How this code is being assimilated into primary care and particularly by independent contractors is far from clear, but there is strong anecdotal evidence that few practice managers are aware of the existence of the code of practice, and that even fewer of their employing general practitioners are aware of it.

All of this amounts to a complex, dynamic and potentially bewildering set of arrangements which have posed significant challenges not only to healthcare organisations and the professions, but also to the 'new regulators' – this has proved to be a very crowded arena, and the potential for replication (if not competition) is an issue that still has to be resolved. We shall consider just how effective these policies have been later, but just what do all of these regulators do and what are the implications for primary care?

Regulation, regulation, regulation . . .

National Institute for Clinical Excellence (NICE)

This organisation was established in April 1999 with the aim of advising the NHS (and its users) on technologies that are both clinically and cost-effective. Its guidance is intended to improve the quality of care by promoting 'evidence-based practice', to reduce the wide variations in treatment ('postcode rationing') and to limit the use of costly technologies (particularly pharmaceuticals) when cheaper and equally effective alternatives are available. The NICE guidance is intended to be objective and to provide the best available evidence irrespective of the cost to the NHS, and since October 2001 it has been mandatory for purchasers. Some NICE decisions have been controversial and have attracted the attention of the media, the guidance on Viagra, Relenza, beta-interferon and Taxane being notable examples. And although many believe that NICE seeks to ration GPs' choice of treatment, under the NICE regime prescribing costs for general practice prescribing have risen by 10% year on year. However, when GPs refer their patients to local NHS trusts, will they be NICE compliant? Research conducted at the University of York[17] suggests that the answer is a resounding maybe! Issues that influenced adoption of the guidance included affordability (direct and infrastructure costs), national and local priorities and the acceptability of the guidance to local clinicians and managers.

Commission for Health Improvement (CHI) and the Healthcare Commission (CHAI)

CHI was formed in April 2000 to undertake a rolling programme of clinical governance reviews of all NHS organisations and to investigate serious service failures. By 2004, CHI had completed well over 300 reviews, including 62 primary care trusts. The reviews currently focus on seven key components of clinical governance:

- patient and public involvement
- clinical audit
- risk management
- clinical effectiveness programmes
- staffing and staff management
- education, training and CPD
- use of information.

These are scrutinised against explicit criteria and rated by an analysis of data/ policies provided by the trust, invited comments from the local community and the report of a team of trained reviewers (lay people and healthcare professionals) who observe the trust 'in action' and interview staff and patients. This includes visits to selected GP surgeries and other independent contractors. A report and recommendations are then published and made available on the CHAI website.

In March 2004, immediately prior to its demise, CHI published *What CHI Has Found in Primary Care Trusts*.[18] Embedded in many positive findings were some clinical risk management issues for general practice. Concerns included the following:

- *confidentiality* – 'one in five reviews found that private conversations can be overheard in general practice waiting areas'
- *complaints* – 'found that patients (and staff) are not always clear on how to complain or comment about their care'
- *medicines* – 'prescribed medicines are often not taken as advised by the prescriber . . . only half of patients felt they were involved enough in decisions about medication . . . only 61% felt they were given enough information about side-effects'
- *repeat prescriptions* – 'pose a risk to patients if left unmonitored'
- *communication* – 'PCTs still struggle to ensure that people from minority black and ethnic communities are well informed about health services . . . staff were not always aware of translation/interpretation facilities'.

These are not novel findings. They mirror MPS Risk Consulting's experience of conducting clinical risk self-assessments in over 200 general practices, and are discussed in detail in subsequent chapters.

As with all regulators, CHI had its critics, and although a survey conducted by the NHS Confederation[19] revealed that only 20% of respondents considered their CHI review to be negative, concerns were expressed about a range of issues.

Criticism included the major demands that the review process placed on organisations, insufficient clarity of purpose, the use of inappropriate criteria and, on occasions, a lack of seniority and relevant experience of review teams. However, the killer blow was delivered by the Kennedy report, which criticised CHI's lack of independence from Government and its limited scope and responsibilities. The NHS Reform and Healthcare Professions Act (2002) established the legislative platform for the setting up of CHAI with a wider role, greater independence and more 'teeth'. In 2005, CHAI will use revised criteria for its inspections.

National Patient Safety Agency (NPSA)

This was established in July 2001, and in February 2004 the NPSA launched its National Reporting and Learning System (NRLS) to enable NHS staff to report anonymously patient safety incidents (adverse events) and near misses either via the NRLS electronic platform or via the Internet. The NPSA will analyse this information, identify lessons to be learned, produce solutions and disseminate these to healthcare organisations. The benefit of reporting and learning from adverse events is self-evident, but in an NHS that is perceived by many as perpetuating a 'blame culture' it is an issue of ambivalence. Research in primary care consistently reveals significant under-reporting of incidents. According to a survey conducted by www.Doctors.net.uk in 2004, '82% of UK doctors have seen a colleague make a mistake or give sub-optimal care, but only 15% of serious incidents resulting in death or disability are reported'. However, 97% believe that a reporting system would improve patient safety, but '81% do not trust their NHS trust or the Department of Health to run such a system'. Incident reporting and *significant event audit*, which is incentivised in the 'new' GP contract, is the subject of a subsequent chapter.

The NPSA also has an active research and development programme which has included an investigation to improve the safety of GP computerised prescribing systems. The R&D programme and NRLS will provide information for the NPSA's series of Safety Alerts and Safer Practice Notices. The NPSA is also developing a range of online resources to help NHS staff to improve patient safety. These include an e-learning *root cause analysis* 'toolkit' and an *incident decision tree* to help managers to apply a fair and consistent approach to staff who have been involved in a patient safety incident.

National Clinical Assessment Authority (NCAA)

This was formed in April 2001 and describes its role as follows: 'To help doctors and dentists in difficulty, the NCAA provides advice, takes referrals and carries out targeted assessments where necessary'. The NCAA's assessment involves trained medical and lay assessors. Once an objective assessment has been carried out, the NCAA will advise on the appropriate course of action. The NCAA does not take over the role of an employer, nor does it function as a regulator. It is established as an advisory body, and the NHS employer organisation remains responsible for resolving the problem once the NCAA has produced its assessment'.

In announcing the rationale for a NCAA, the *NHS Plan* proclaimed that 'It will mean the end to the current arrangement where doctors can be suspended for years while concerns or allegations about their performance are investigated'.[13] In this author's view there is another compelling reason. The overwhelming majority of doctors enter medicine with benevolent intent, but for some their performance deteriorates as a sequela of occupational or domestic stress, more serious mental health problems or professional isolation. This does not go unnoticed by their colleagues, managers and subordinates. If reporting an adverse incident is difficult, 'blowing the whistle' on a colleague or your boss is a really tough call. Consequently, many doctors whose performance is causing 'some' concern drift into chronicity and the issue is only addressed when there is a dramatic failure and remediation is not possible. This represents not only a hazard to patients and the loss of a costly and scarce clinical resource, but also a tragic waste of an individual's career.

In its first year of operation the majority of referrals to the NCAA simply required advice, and it conducted approximately 20 full assessments. In addition to conducting its assessments and providing advice on subsequent action, the NPSA provides a range of resources to assist in the prevention and management of 'poor performance'. These include a comprehensive Web-based 'toolkit' to help NHS managers to deal with performance problems locally, and a leaflet for PCT staff entitled *Concerned About the Performance of a Colleague?*, which provides practical guidance on how to act if they have concerns about the performance of a colleague.

Another regulator (another acronym)!

The NAO identified 18 NHS bodies and 'arm's-length agencies' (plus all of the medical Royal Colleges) as having a legitimate voice on patient safety,[14] and although I can think of a few more, a brief word about just one will suffice here.

The Council for the Regulation of Healthcare Professionals (CRHP)

This is a statutory overarching body, covering all of the UK and separate from Government, which was established in April 2003. It promotes best practice and consistency in the regulation of healthcare professionals by the nine regulatory bodies. And you may recall that (in the words of the NHS Plan) 'were concerns to remain about the individual self-regulatory bodies, its role could evolve'! At the time of writing (July 2004) there is very little information on the CRHP website other than the report of a 'scoping exercise' to inform the Council of the size, regulations, constitution and other similarities and differences of the healthcare regulatory bodies, to enable it to establish its work programme and priorities. In addition, it presented itself at the High Court on two occasions in March 2004 to test its 'new' statutory powers of appeal against disciplinary decisions made by the GMC and the Nursing and Midwifery Council (NMC). It was found that 'not guilty findings' and 'lenient sanctions' could be referred to the court by the CRHP. This is definitely an organisation to keep an eye on, as it will certainly be keeping an eye on your profession.

And is this improving patient safety?

The implications of much of what has been discussed above will be amplified in subsequent chapters. However, for the casual observer the post-Bristol patient safety policy framework manifests itself as a confusing and shifting maze of acronyms (and of course before this book is published it will have changed again).* But the crucial question must be 'Is all of this improving patient safety?' Although we have established that the evidence base is pretty weak, the results of the regulators' reports might suggest that elements of patient safety are improving.[14] However, there will be no quick fix (so beloved by politicians) – patient safety is a component of quality and, as Gorman has observed, 'A lot of people have fancy things to say about quality, including me, but it's just a day in, day out, ongoing, never-ending, unremitting, persevering, compassionate type of activity'. As they say, the jury is out.

* Following a radical review of the 'arms length bodies' in the autumn of 2004 the NCAA was assimilated into the NPSA and during the same period the Council for the Regulation of Health Professions (CRHP) re-titled itself as the Council for Healthcare Regulatory Excellence (CHRE).

References

1 Vincent C et al. (2001) Adverse events in British hospitals: preliminary retrospective record review. BMJ. **322**: 517–19.
2 Sandars J and Esmail A (2003) The frequency and nature of medical error in primary care: understanding the diversity across studies. Fam Pract. **20**: 231–6.
3 Department of Health (2003) Making Amends. A consultation paper setting out proposals for reforming the approach to clinical negligence in the NHS. Department of Health, London.
4 National Audit Office (2001) Handling Clinical Negligence Claims in England. The Stationery Office, London.
5 Walshe K (2001) The development of clinical risk management. In: C Vincent (ed.) Clinical Risk Management (2e). BMJ Books, London.
6 Robb B (1967) Sans Everything. Nelson, London.
7 Clare A (1976) Psychiatry in Dissent: controversial issues in thought and practice. Tavistock Publications Ltd, London.
8 HM Government (1997) The New NHS: modern, dependable. The Stationery Office, London.
9 Department of Health (1998) A First Class Service: quality in the new NHS. Department of Health, London.
10 Department of Health (2000) An Organisation With A memory. Report of an expert group on learning from adverse events in the NHS. The Stationery Office, London.
11 Department of Health (2001) Building a Safer NHS for Patients. Department of Health, London.
12 Department of Health (2001) Assuring the Quality of Medical Practice. Implementing Supporting Doctors, Protecting Patients. Department of Health, London.
13 Department of Health (2000) The NHS Plan: a plan for investment, a plan for reform. Department of Health, London.
14 National Audit Office (2003) Achieving Improvement Through Clinical Governance. The Stationery Office, London.
15 Westwood M et al. (2003) Patient Safety: mapping of the research literature. NHS Centre for Reviews and Disseminations, York.
16 NHS (2002) Code of Conduct for NHS Managers. Department of Health, London.
17 Cullum N et al. (2004) The Evaluation of the Dissemination, Implementation and Impact of NICE Guidance. University of York, York.
18 Commission for Health Improvement (2004) What CHI has Found in Primary Care trusts. Commission for Health Improvement, London.
19 NHS Confederation (2002) Reviewing the Reviewers: NHS experience of CHI clinical governance review. NHS Confederation, London.

Chapter 4

Education, appraisal and revalidation

Tim van Zwanenberg

> If the licence to practise meant the completion of his education, how sad it would be for the practitioner, how distressing to his patients.
>
> (Sir William Osler)

Key learning points

- Technological advances and greater complexity in clinical practice have increased risk. Keeping up to date is part of the job.
- Continuing education and accountability have become linked in a way that they never were before.
- The scope of CPD is wider than medical knowledge alone, involves lifelong learning, and must meet the needs of patients, practitioners and the NHS.
- Appraisal is a developmental process that results in the formulation of a personal development plan.
- Participation in a managed appraisal system provides a 'powerful indicator' of fitness to practise, and leads to revalidation.
- Clinical governance is a coherent range of interlinked processes which together assure the quality of clinical care. These processes include risk management and CPD. Each contributes to the other.

Introduction

General practice and primary care have changed enormously in recent times, in the wake of rapid medical and technological advances. General practitioners now have access to a far wider and more sophisticated range of investigations and treatments, and have increasingly taken on responsibility for the care of patients who would previously have been managed by consultants. Inevitably this direction of travel with its concomitant complexity has increased risk. Thus keeping up to date and abreast of developments is part of the job, and the active management of risk is a component of this.

However, it was not always so. At the inception of the NHS in 1948 there was still serious debate as to whether general practitioners required any continuing education at all. And one of the curiosities of the 1990 GP contract, with its imposition of compulsory retirement at the age of 70 years, was the revelation that there were still 19 GPs over the age of 90 years in practice. They would have qualified in the 1920s, before the advent of antibiotics, and yet would not have been obliged to undergo any further examination of their competence!

Over the lifetime of the NHS, ideas about education, learning and development have also evolved. These have enhanced our understanding of individuals, teams and organisations to the point where theory and empirical evidence from educational research have started to inform policy and practice (*see* Box 4.1).[1] The theory of adult learning, the idea of the learning cycle, the notion of organisational culture, increasing attention to the assessment of learners' needs, and the evaluation of learning have all had an impact in primary care. General practitioners are now much more overtly conscious and reflective learners than they were 50 years ago. Arguably much of this has stemmed from their experience of GP vocational training, where formative assessment of educational needs through the use of confidence rating scales and analysis of video recordings of consultations have become the norm.

Box 4.1 Ideas drawn from educational research and theory of adult learning

- Adults learn throughout their lives.
- The need to know is a powerful motivator for learning.
- Adults are competent to choose what and how to learn.
- Learning is more effective when it is undertaken for a stated reason.
- Learning is more effective when a method is identified and completed.
- Adults prefer learning activities that are problem centred and relevant to their situation.
- Experience is a rich learning resource, but exposure alone does not guarantee learning.
- Adults wish to apply new learning to their immediate circumstances.
- Learning is more effective when there is some follow-up after the learning activity.

'All changed, changed utterly'

Quoting from WB Yeats, 'all changed, changed utterly' was the title of Richard Smith's editorial in the *British Medical Journal* immediately following the GMC's verdict in the Bristol case.[2] In that article he forecast radical change in the way doctors are held to account. In truth there had been incremental development in both the contractual and professional regulation of general practitioners before then, but the incoming Labour Government of 1997 had a very large parliamentary majority and a mandate to 'modernise' the public services. Furthermore, quality in the NHS in general and the regulation of doctors in particular were to become major political priorities, as the Bristol Inquiry and other cases of doctors' misdemeanours unfolded, giving rise to lurid headlines in the popular press.

This has fundamentally influenced the way in which education has come to be viewed in the NHS. Increasingly, continuing education and accountability have become linked in a way that they never were before. On the plus side this means that education has become a serious business, and is no longer the private occupational therapy of the enthusiast. On the minus side there is confusion about the links between individual developmental processes (e.g. CPD and appraisal), individual professional regulatory processes (e.g. revalidation) and organisational processes (e.g. clinical governance). In particular, there are anxieties about intent in each case. Is the process intended to help to develop the many who are doing their best, or to detect the few whose performance is a cause for concern? In truth the answer is not simple because effective participation in all of these has come to be seen as an indicator of fitness to practise.

In an endeavour to shed some light on this confusion, the following and their interrelationships will be described:

- CPD
- appraisal
- revalidation
- clinical governance.

Most importantly, from the point of view of risk management, participation of clinicians in these activities is likely to lead to safer care for patients. And the processes of risk analysis and management fit well with the features of adult learning (*see* Box 4.1):

- learning based on problems of immediate relevance to practice (e.g. when things have gone wrong)
- learning from experience
- application of learning to immediate circumstances (i.e. clinical practice)
- follow-up of learning (e.g. through clinical audit).

Continuing professional development

Until quite recently, the learning that doctors undertook once they had completed their training was called continuing medical education (CME). However, three main factors have militated against the use of that term.[3]

- The content areas that doctors now study are broader than just clinical medicine.
- The learning that doctors share with other members of the primary care team means that much of the education is clinical rather than medical.
- There is a need to make continuing education effective in developing and assuring standards of practice.

Clearly doctors will always continue to learn more about clinical medicine throughout their working lives, and to refine and develop their clinical skills, but they increasingly need to address areas which are not primarily clinical at all, such as leadership, management (including risk management), audit, information technology and educational skills. These are professional rather than purely medical matters.

Equally, it is now commonplace for primary care team members to participate in various forms of inter-professional (learning from one another) and multi-professional (learning with one another) education, ranging from practice-based lunchtime sessions to protected learning time initiatives developed by primary care organisations. Patient care, particularly for patients with chronic conditions, is more team based, and this is reflected in guidelines and NSFs. Thus questions of management and aspects of practice policy are shared by the team or by certain members of the team. 'Working together and learning together' has become less of a slogan and more of a reality.

Finally, CPD, the now preferred term, encompasses a more systematic approach (see below) which lends itself to contributing to a more open and accountable service.

For general practitioners, the term first came to prominence with the publication of the previous CMO's report, *A Review of Continuing Professional Development in General Practice*, in 1998.[4] The report was important because it identified a range of shortcomings in the arrangements for general practitioners' CPD (e.g. poor assessment of educational need, often inappropriate learning methods, scant evidence on outcomes and fragmentation of resources), and it included a definition of CPD which was subsequently adopted across the NHS, with but minor amendment:

> a process of lifelong learning for all individuals and teams which enables professionals to expand and fulfil their potential and which also meets patients' needs and delivers the health and healthcare priorities of the NHS.

Its principal recommendation was that general practices should compile *practice professional development plans (PPDPs)* based on the service development plans of the practice, local and national NHS objectives, and on identified educational needs. Individual development plans for all members of the practice team would be incorporated, and would reflect both practice priorities and individual career aspirations. The plan would use practice-based and other novel forms of learning. Although often promised guidance on the implementation of the report's recommendations was never issued, many general practitioners, often with the assistance of GP tutors, have compiled their own *personal development plans* (PDPs) as a way of triggering their Postgraduate Education Allowance (PGEA).

The report signalled an important shift away from attendance at accredited events towards personal development planning and team-based, workplace-based learning as the main vehicles for CPD. It also highlighted the tripartite balance that needed to be struck in CPD between the needs of professionals, patients and the NHS. In embracing this philosophy, primary care has witnessed the further development of inter-professional education using techniques such as significant event audit as a means of learning from errors and near misses and reducing risk, and as a vehicle for developing teamworking (*see* Chapter 21).

According to Sylvester, 'the core of CPD is APPLE'.[1] He describes a modern and systematic approach to CPD in terms of stages in a process, emphasising that it is a single process (*see* Box 4.2).

Box 4.2 The stages of CPD

- Assessing and identifying educational needs
- Prioritising needs
- Planning learning activity
- Learning activity participation
- Evaluation or follow-up of learning activity

With CPD, clinicians should first assess their needs and prioritise them (*see* Box 4.3), and then plan their learning on the basis of those needs. The plan should be written down as a PDP, and appraisal facilitates this process. An evaluation of the learning can then be reviewed at a subsequent appraisal.

Box 4.3 Examples of methods for assessing educational needs

- Review of PDP
- Clinical audit
- Significant event analysis
- Prescribing, investigation and referral data
- Video analysis of consultations
- Clinical guidelines and protocols
- PUNs and DENs – a system devised by Richard Eve to log patients' unmet needs and doctors' educational needs[5]
- Complaints
- Patient surveys
- 360° peer feedback[6]

It is not surprising that some of the above examples of methods for assessing educational needs are identical to the tools used in risk analysis.

Appraisal

Appraisal is a well-established process in industry, commerce, the civil service and education, and has been introduced into different parts of the health service over the past decade or more. It is primarily an educational process that is based on dialogue and interaction with the appraiser, and which focuses on the development needs of the individual. It should be a structured process of facilitated self-reflection, and should allow the individual to review their professional activities comprehensively and to identify areas of real strength and areas of need for development.[7] Importantly for healthcare, there is some evidence, albeit in a hospital setting, of a positive association between effective appraisal and better outcomes for patients.[8]

Unfortunately, appraisal for doctors has been introduced into a perceived climate of anxiety, not least because the case for appraisal for doctors was first put by the CMO, Sir Liam Donaldson, in the context of 'preventing, recognising and dealing with poor clinical performance of doctors'.[9] Despite this, his definition of the process places it in an educational frame:

> Appraisal is a positive process to give someone feedback on their performance, to chart their continuing progress and to identify development needs. It is a forward-looking process essential for the developmental and educational planning needs of the individual.[9]

Annual appraisal is now a required activity for all doctors in the NHS. Furthermore, the GMC has determined that evidence of participation in a quality-assured appraisal system would be a 'powerful indicator' of continuing fitness to practise, and would thereby enable the doctor to have their license to practise extended for a further period by revalidation (see below).[10] This link with revalidation means that NHS appraisal is structured against the components of good medical practice as set out by the GMC (*see* Box 4.4),[11] with other sections added for research and management as appropriate.

Box 4.4 Components of good medical practice

- Good clinical care
- Maintaining good medical practice
- Relationships with patients
- Working with colleagues
- Teaching and training
- Probity
- Health

For many general practitioners, appraisal will be their first opportunity since graduating from vocational training to reflect with a sympathetic colleague on their performance and their development needs. There are three essential features of a successful appraisal, namely the reflection beforehand, the confidential discussion with the appraiser, and the formulation of an agreed PDP. The following steps need to be followed:

1 gathering information (*see* Box 4.3) and reflection (appraisee)
2 reviewing the information and planning the interview (appraiser)
3 appraisal interview with feedback on strengths and areas for development (appraiser and appraisee)
4 compilation of a PDP (appraiser and appraisee)
5 undertaking personal development (appraiser)
6 aggregating anonymised intelligence from PDPs to inform organisational development (appraisers).

There is standard NHS appraisal documentation for general practitioners, consisting of five forms which need to be completed as part of the process (*see* Box 4.5).

> **Box 4.5** Documentation for NHS appraisal
>
> * Form 1 – basic (personal) details
> * Form 2 – current medical activities
> * Form 3 – material for appraisal
> * Form 4 – summary of appraisal discussion with agreed action and PDP
> * Form 5 – detailed confidential account of appraisal interview (optional)

Appraisal is thus the process by which general practitioners and other primary care personnel can reflect on their daily work and needs, and formulate a plan of action. The skill of the appraiser is critical in enabling the process to be a positive and enriching experience. There is as yet little evidence of the benefits or otherwise of appraisal in general practice, but what evidence there is suggests that the process may make an important contribution to risk management. The following benefits were reported in one study of peer appraisal in general practice.

* It improves team cohesion, mutual support and honesty between team members.
* Positive feedback promotes well-being and enthusiasm in the team.
* It facilitates personal and professional development.
* It stimulates thought, reflection and further reading.
* It allows discussion of difficult topics in a safe environment.

The same report also noted that some doctors might find the process very threatening.[12] This has been reiterated by others, not least because of the link between appraisal and revalidation.[7] How then is the issue of poor performance to be tackled in the context of appraisal? The advice to the appraiser is quite simple. They are bound by the GMC guidelines, which state that:

> You must protect patients when you believe that a doctor's or other colleague's health, conduct or performance is a threat to them.[11]

In the unusual event that an appraiser has significant cause for concern about the appraisee's health, conduct or performance, they should stop the interview as these concerns must be addressed outside the appraisal process (*see* Chapter 15).

In summary, appraisal – which encompasses a regular and structured review of educational need (risk) – is potentially a critical vehicle for risk management at the level of the individual practitioner in primary care.

Revalidation

The GMC is the medical profession's self-regulating body, and as such is responsible for licensing doctors to practise in the UK. In May 2001, the Council confirmed that in the future and for the first time all doctors would have to demonstrate on a regular and periodic basis that they remained fit to practise in their chosen field. This process was termed revalidation, and through revalidation doctors would be entitled to remain registered with the Council and thereby remain licensed to practise. The introduction of revalidation was said to represent a significant change in the traditional approach to medical regulation, which until the 1990s had remained largely unchanged since 1858, when the Council was first established.[13]

The GMC originally proposed a three-stage process.

1 A folder of information describing what the doctor does and how well he or she does it. This would be regularly reviewed – annual appraisal would fulfil this in many sectors.
2 Periodic revalidation – a recommendation by a group of medical and lay people that the doctor remains fit to practise, or that the doctor's registration should be reviewed by the GMC.
3 Action by the GMC – in the majority of cases there would be revalidation of the doctor's register entry. In a minority of cases, there would be detailed investigation under the Council's fitness to practise procedures, which could lead to restrictions upon practice, suspension or erasure.[14]

In 2003, the GMC further clarified its approach. The system for the registration of doctors was being changed. In the past, the Medical Register showed who was properly qualified to practise medicine in the UK. This principle would continue, but in future the Register would be strengthened by a new system based on a licence to practise, supported by periodic revalidation. By the end of 2004 all doctors on the Register (except those who opted out) would have received their license from the Council, and by 1 January 2005 a license to practise would be required by law. By April 2005 the Council would be inviting doctors to be revalidated. It is anticipated that it will take five years for all doctors to be revalidated for the first time.[10]

Doctors can follow one of two routes to revalidation (or a mixture of both if needed, e.g. for doctors with portfolio careers), namely the appraisal route and the independent route. Most general practitioners are expected to follow the appraisal route. To do this they must show that during the revalidation period they have worked in a managed environment and participated in an annual appraisal system. As noted above, the appraisal system must be based on the principles of *good medical practice* (*see* Box 4.4) and be quality assured. Doctors should have been through at least one appraisal cycle before revalidation, and therefore should have started collecting material for their first appraisal by April 2004 at the latest.

The GMC will not normally want to see all of the information collected to support doctors' annual appraisals, but doctors should keep the information in a folder, as these will be randomly sampled by the Council.

A number of tools are being developed to help doctors to assemble supporting information for appraisal and revalidation, including self-report forms for probity and health, and a patient satisfaction questionnaire and professional colleague survey instrument (for 360° feedback).

Clinical governance

The original definition of clinical governance is well known.

> Clinical governance is a system through which NHS organisations are accountable for continuously improving the quality of their services and safeguarding high standards of care by creating an environment in which excellence in clinical care will flourish.[15]

However, in many ways the Royal College of General Practitioners' (RCGP) version is more accessible and captures the idea of a framework which covers a range of linked processes.

> Clinical governance is a framework for the improvement of patient care through commitment to high standards, reflective practice, risk management, and personal and team development.[16]

The concept of clinical governance was first proposed for the NHS in the 1997 White Paper, *The New NHS: Modern, Dependable*,[17] and was further elaborated a year later in *A First Class Service: Quality in the new NHS*.[18] Importantly, a statutory duty of quality was placed on NHS organisations, so that chief executives and their boards had to take clinical care as seriously as they did financial probity. The relationship between national standard setting and monitoring and local delivery was also spelled out (*see* Box 4.6).

Box 4.6 Setting, delivering and monitoring standards

	Quality mechanism
Clear standards of service	National Institute for Clinical Excellence National Service Frameworks
Dependable local delivery	Professional self-regulation Clinical governance Lifelong learning
Monitored standards	Healthcare Commission (formerly Commission for Health Audit and Inspection) National Performance Framework National Patient and User Survey

---

It is worth noting that dependable local delivery hinges on three linked processes. Lifelong learning is included in the definition of CPD, which in turn is a component of clinical governance and is facilitated by appraisal leading to revalidation – a process of professional self-regulation.

Clinical governance is an organisational system. It should provide a coherent range of processes which together assure the quality of clinical care. The processes cover four important domains, namely humane care, clinical effectiveness, risk management, and personal and professional development (*see* Box 4.7).[19] These domains are inevitably interdependent. Risk can undermine clinical effectiveness, whereas the proper implementation of evidence-based practice reduces the risk that patients will receive sub-optimal care.

Box 4.7 The component processes of clinical governance

Humane care
- What patients are looking for

Clinical effectiveness
- Evidence-based practice
- Disseminating and implementing evidence-based practice
- Quality improvement processes (e.g. clinical audit)
- Appropriate use of data (e.g. performance indicators)
- Managing information

Risk management
- Reducing risk
- Significant event analysis
- Lessons from complaints
- Tackling poor performance

Personal and professional development
- CPD
- Developing leaders
- Developing teamwork

Conclusion

For effective clinical risk management, clinicians need to be well-trained, lifelong learners who are prepared to acknowledge and tackle problems of performance, and who are able to learn from errors, complaints, significant events and near misses. They need to be forever vigilant and have a positive attitude to patient safety. Partly in response to a series of medical scandals, new processes have been introduced which together provide a matrix or framework that aims to improve the quality of patient care. Key elements of this are educational, and this is wholly appropriate. Medicine is a 'people business', and the people involved need to learn continually. Increasingly that learning needs to be systematised – not just serendipitous – to include a proactive approach to learning about risk analysis and management.

Postscript

In December 2004, after this chapter had been written, the Government announced that it was scrapping the April 2005 start date for revalidation and confirmed that it was to carry out a root-and-branch review of the scheme. The review to be carried out by the Chief Medical Officer, Sir Liam Donaldson, is expected to last at least six months and is likely to call for a toughening of the existing appraisal and proposed revalidation arrangements.

The review has been prompted by the publication in December 2004 of the Fifth Shipman Inquiry report in which the Inquiry chair, Dame Janet Smith, said that existing plans to grant revalidation if a GP had participated in 'educational' appraisals were not sufficient to prove fitness to practise.

References

1 Sylvester S (2001) Continuing professional development. In: J Harrison, R Innes and T van Zwanenberg (eds) *The New GP. Changing roles and the modern NHS.* Radcliffe Medical Press, Oxford.

2 Smith R (1998) All changed, changed utterly. *BMJ.* **316**: 1917–18.

3 Grant J (2000) Continuing professional development. In: T van Zwanenberg and J Harrison (eds) *Clinical Governance in Primary Care.* Radcliffe Medical Press, Oxford.

4 Department of Health (1998) *A Review of Continuing Professional Development in General Practice.* Department of Health, London.

5 Eve R (2003) *PUNs and DENs: discovering learning needs in general practice.* Radcliffe Publishing, Oxford.

6 Haman H, Irvine S and Jelley D (2001) *The Peer Appraisal Handbook for General Practitioners.* Radcliffe Medical Press, Oxford.

7 Conlon M (2003) Appraisal: the catalyst of personal development. *BMJ.* **327**: 389–91.

8 West MA, Borrill C, Csully J *et al.* (2002) The link between the management of employees and patient mortality in acute hospitals. *Int J Hum Res Manage.* **13**: 1299–310.

9 Department of Health (1999) *Supporting Doctors, Protecting Patients.* Department of Health, London.

10 General Medical Council (2003) *A License to Practise and Revalidation.* General Medical Council, London.

11 General Medical Council (1998) *Good Medical Practice.* General Medical Council, London.

12 Jelley D and van Zwanenberg T (2000) Peer appraisal in general practice: a descriptive study in the Northern Deanery. *Educ Gen Pract.* **11**: 281–7.

13 General Medical Council (2000) *Changing Times, Changing Culture.* General Medical Council, London.

14 General Medical Council (2000) *Revalidating Doctors: ensuring standards, securing the future.* General Medical Council, London.

15 Scally G and Donaldson LJ (1998) Clinical governance and the drive for quality improvement in the new NHS in England. *BMJ.* **317**: 61–5.

16 Royal College of General Practitioners (1999) *Clinical Governance: practical advice for primary care in England and Wales.* Royal College of General Practitioners, London.

17 Department of Health (1997) *The New NHS: modern, dependable.* The Stationery Office, London.

18 Department of Health (1998) *A First Class Service: quality in the new NHS.* The Stationery Office, London.

19 van Zwanenberg T and Edwards C (2004) Clinical governance in primary care. In: T van Zwanenberg and J Harrison (eds) *Clinical Governance in Primary Care.* Radcliffe Medical Press, Oxford.

Further reading

• Chambers R, Wakley G, Field S and Ellis S (2003) *Appraisal for the Apprehensive.* Radcliffe Medical Press, Oxford.

- General Medical Council, Department of Health (2004) *Appraisal and Revalidation*; www.revalidationuk.info
- Haman H, Irvine S and Jelley D (2001) *The Peer Appraisal Handbook for General Practitioners*. Radcliffe Medical Press, Oxford.
- Martin D, Harrison P, Joesbury H and Wilson R (2001) *Appraisal for GPs*. ScHARR, University of Sheffield, Sheffield.
- Martin D, Harrison P and Joesbury H (2003) *Extending Appraisal to All GPs*. ScHARR, University of Sheffield, Sheffield.
- Rughani A (2000) *The GP's Guide to Personal Development Plans*. Radcliffe Medical Press, Oxford.
- van Zwanenberg T and Harrison J (2004) *Clinical Governance in Primary Care*. Radcliffe Medical Press, Oxford.

Chapter 5

The theory and evidence base for clinical risk management

John Sandars

Key learning points

- Clinical risk management provides a structured process to improve patient safety.
- There is a wide variation in the reported frequency and nature of medical error in primary care.
- This wide variation is related to the specific contexts in which medical error is reported.
- Important lessons on how to identify medical error can be learned from experiences in secondary care and non-healthcare settings.

Introduction

The reduction of medical error and the improvement of patient safety has become a major priority for all healthcare providers. Clinical risk management provides a strategic approach to improving patient safety by identifying the frequency and nature of medical errors and then developing ways to reduce the likelihood of these errors occurring in the future. This process in an integral part of the NHS proposed approach to learning from errors and improving patient safety.[1]

Most of the work on clinical risk management has been undertaken in secondary care, especially in the USA, but recently the NHS has taken steps to improve patient safety in primary care. Primary care has not had a string of highly publicised medical errors, but it is the setting for the highest number of patient contacts within the NHS, and there is a large potential for medical errors to occur in the complex environment of primary care.

Clinical risk management

The theory of clinical risk management is quite simple. It acknowledges that all healthcare activity, by its very nature, carries a risk. Such risk can be due to a variety of causes, whether it is an accident, a mishap or a mistake. The systematic approach to clinical risk management consists of four steps:

- step 1 – the identification of risk
- step 2 – the analysis of risk
- step 3 – the treatment of risk
- step 4 – the evaluation of risk treatment strategies.

Identification of risk

Risk identification is fundamental, otherwise any strategy to reduce risk may be inappropriate! The most commonly used method is incident reporting, but more systematic methods can be used.

Analysis of risk

Risk analysis is the process of determining the impact of the risk and deciding whether something needs to be done to reduce the risk.

Treatment of risk

This step is concerned with doing something about reducing the risk. The possibility of risk may have to be accepted, but every effort should be made to establish whether it can be controlled or avoided by appropriate interventions.

Evaluation of risk treatment strategies

The final step, which involves determining whether all of the hard work has actually been effective, is crucial.

Clinical risk management and primary care: the present position

At the present time, clinical risk management in primary care by the NHS is mainly at the stage of identification of the risks. This should provide the foundation for the next steps of risk analysis and risk treatment to be developed. It is important that the NHS policy is guided by the available evidence, since this evidence, even though it has been derived from secondary care and non-healthcare settings, can still provide valuable lessons on how to identify risk successfully.

Some information is already available about the clinical risks in primary care, including such risks in the UK, and this should enable all involved in patient care to increase their awareness of the frequency and causes of medical error. We do not have a complete picture of medical error in primary care, but there is already sufficient to act upon to improve patient safety.

The frequency and nature of medical error in primary care: the evidence base

In 2001, the Department of Health commissioned the School of Primary Care at the University of Manchester to conduct a literature review in order to investigate the frequency and nature of error in primary care. A systematic approach was adopted to review the literature, and the following databases were accessed in July and August 2001: Medline (1966–2001), EMBASE (1988–2001) and the patient safety bibliography resource of the US National Patient Safety Foundation (1939–2001). In addition, a study of the claims database of the MPS was included.

Only 12 studies and one book chapter (which described a further four studies in the Netherlands) were identified. These studies are listed in Table 5.1.

Interpreting the evidence base

There was wide variation in the reported frequency and nature of medical errors in primary care. This appears to be related to several factors, and it is important that they are considered before the results of the studies are interpreted.

Purpose of data collection in the study

Studies were performed for a variety of purposes, ranging from a main aim of identifying the frequency and nature of error to studies designed to review administrative medico-legal databases.

Settings

There is little extensive research from the UK. Most studies were performed in a variety of countries, mainly the USA, Australia and the Netherlands, with differing primary healthcare systems.

Definitions of error

There were no consistent definitions of what constituted an 'error'. Some studies used a wider definition that encompassed actual and potential harm to patients, while others only considered errors that caused actual harm, including those which resulted in medico-legal action. The classification of harm was made by a variety of individuals, ranging from individual primary care doctors to community pharmacists.

Method of collecting data

Most studies were opportunistic, relying on the identification of incidents. The only studies that attempted to be systematic were those which used prescribing review, allowing an incident rate to be calculated.

Classification of errors

The depth of understanding of the causes of error varied across the studies. Most studies identified simple classifications, but more intensive interviews allowed a deeper insight into causation.

The results of the literature review

The studies demonstrated that error does occur in a primary care setting, ranging from 5 to 80 per 100 000 consultations. Most errors do not result in actual patient harm, and the errors mainly occur in the young and the elderly. These rates are likely to be an underestimate, as they were identified opportunistically.

Table 5.1 The identified studies of error in primary care

(a) Errors that occur during the process of care

Setting	Definition of error	Method
Australian general practice[2,3]	'an unintended event, no matter how seemingly trivial or commonplace, that could have harmed or did harm a patient'	Non-random sample of 325 general practitioners Voluntary contemporaneous incident self-reporting on purpose-designed incident-report form with free and fixed responses
US primary care clinics at an academic medical centre[4]	'incidents resulting in, or having a potential for, physical, emotional or financial liability to the patient'	Number of doctors not stated Anonymous mandatory reporting by all personnel. Events identified by a variety of methods, including patient complaints, medico-legal enquiries, observations by risk department and case conferences
US family physicians[5]	'an act or omission for which the physician felt responsible and which had serious or potentially serious consequences for the patient'	Random sample of 53 family physicians Qualitative semi-structured interviews
Netherlands general practice[6]	Not clearly defined (several studies described in book chapter, based on studies published by the authors in Dutch)	Study 1 – diagnosis compared with necropsy findings Study 2 – qualitative open-ended interviews Study 3 – analysis of coded morbidity data Study 4 – self-reporting of one error per month
US family practice[7]	'that was something that should not happen in my practice, and I don't want it to happen again'	Sample of 50 doctors Self-report of incidents using paper cards and computer
Sweden primary care[8]	'neglect that lies within his or her line of responsibility'	187 district physicians Database of complaints from either patient, relatives or Health Board
UK general practice[9]	'claims recently registered against general medical practitioners'	1000 consecutive registered claims on medical negligence insurance claims database
UK general practice[10]	'an event that is thought to be important in the life of the practice and which may offer some insight into the general care of the patient'	Case study of one primary healthcare team using significant event audit Qualitative interviews of core participants and observation of six significant event audit meetings

(b) Errors associated with medication use

Setting	Definition of error	Method
UK general practice and community pharmacists[11]	Opinion of community pharmacist and identification of 'items which did not conform to the criteria for prescription writing stated in the *British National Formulary*'	Review of 15 916 prescriptions written by eight general practitioners Identification by community pharmacist at dispensing
UK community pharmacists[12]	(a) 'all potential adverse drug reactions' (b) prescribing error 'a change in the dose, strength or type of medication which was probably not intended by the prescribing doctor'	(a) 64 406 dispensed items Community pharmacist review (b) 5906 prescribed items Community pharmacist review
UK community pharmacists[13]	'when a community pharmacist had to contact the prescriber during the dispensing process'	201 000 items dispensed 14 community pharmacists Frequency recording
Netherlands community pharmacists[14]	'prescription modifications by community pharmacists'	47 374 prescriptions 141 community pharmacists Frequency recording, with validation by original prescription

These errors were often caused by multiple interrelated factors, but the commonest factors appear to be related to diagnosis (range 26–78%) and treatment (range 11–42%). Contributory factors are often related to lack of coordination or communication between the various healthcare providers, and difficulties in making professional judgements. The important contribution of the patient and practice staff to error should also be noted. For example, the doctor may follow the request of the patient, but the consequence of doing so may actually harm the patient.

Individual doctors tend to recall more significant threats to patient safety, especially those that have a contributory cause which is related to significant human factors in the doctor, such as fatigue.

Systematic identification of prescription and prescribing errors has identified rates ranging from less than 1% to 11% of all prescriptions. Most errors do not cause actual harm, but are a potential threat to patient safety. The commonest error concerns the dose of medication. Thus the important role of the community pharmacist in the identification and rectification of error should be noted.

The Medical Protection Society (MPS) claims database

The medico-legal database of the MPS is a valuable source of information. This is the largest database of medical error, it relates to UK general practice, and analysis should give some indication of the priority areas for action, since most of the claims relate to serious or potentially serious harm to patients.

Using this database a study was carried out of 1000 consecutive formally registered claims against general practitioners in the UK.[9] The largest category was investigation and treatment (63%), followed by prescribing (19%).

Investigation and treatment

The findings can be summarised as follows:

- failure/delay in diagnosis (54%)
- wrong diagnosis (25%).

The largest category was malignant neoplasms, followed by diseases of the circulatory system and injuries.

Subgroup analysis identified consistent trends, such as over-reliance on normal investigation and lack of appropriate examination.

Prescribing

The largest category was failure to warn about or recognise drug side-effects, followed by medication and prescribing errors.

The main groups were related to the use of steroids in disease management, and allergy to antibiotic prescribing.

Alleged failures on the part of GPs

In a total of 449 claims the main categories were related to failure/delay in the following:

- hospital admission ($n = 118$)
- referral ($n = 116$)
- examination ($n = 69$).

Administration errors

These were noted in 4.8% of claims. The main categories were poor records, errors in communication and errors made by a receptionist or other employee.

Practice nurse error

This was noted in 3.2% of claims. The main categories were related to administering an injection or blood test, undertaking a procedure, and giving inappropriate advice.

Comment on the evidence base

The review of the literature identified two closely interrelated concepts that require further understanding if there is to be a thorough appreciation of medical error in primary care.

1 *The frequency of errors.* Identification of the true frequency requires a systematic process, similar to a mass screening programme for disease identification. Surveys have tried to capture the frequency in a hospital population, often by targeting specific groups, such as those receiving medication. However, such surveys are highly resource dependent, and opportunistic programmes have been widely introduced, which include primary care settings. Incident reporting, a type of opportunistic screening, does not give a true population frequency as it is limited to those incidents that are reported.
2 *The nature of error.* The definition of an 'error' will determine what is identified, and what constitutes an error varies considerably across various studies. To fully understand why errors occur, which is essential for preventing such errors in the future, requires some form of classification, but again this varies considerably.

Methods of identifying medical error: the evidence base

The literature review for the Department of Health also considered the various methods that have been used to identify medical error. Important lessons can be learned from the experience gained in secondary healthcare and non-healthcare settings.

Opportunistic incident reporting

Opportunistic incident reporting is the most widely used method for identifying medical error, and has been proposed by the NPSA as the main method for its clinical risk management strategy. It is useful to consider what the evidence shows.

Background

The concept of critical incident monitoring and reporting arose from studies in the Aviation Psychology Program of the United States Air Force during and after the Second World War.[15] Since that time the technique has been applied within a variety of industries, ranging from aviation to petrochemical processing. It is recognised that there is a continuum of incidents, ranging from apparently trivial incidents to near misses and full-blown adverse events. Major adverse events, or *sentinel events*, rarely occur, but *precursor events* or near misses occur more often. Studies of commercial aviation have shown that safety incidents associated with such near misses are very similar to those associated with full-blown disasters.[16]

Experience of incident monitoring in intensive-care units

A comprehensive system for the identification and analysis of adverse events in the intensive-care environment has been developed in Australia.[17] It is useful to consider this system as the development and evaluation have been extensively researched and there are useful lessons to be learned for primary care.

In 1993, the system was piloted in three intensive-care units and was designed to be non-threatening to all staff. An incident was defined as 'any event or outcome which could have reduced, or did reduce, the safety margin for the patient'. Information about an incident was gathered anonymously from staff involved in an incident using an incident report form. This form was designed to include a narrative section to elicit a description of the incident in the reporter's own words, and a multiple-choice section to elicit contextual details about the incident with regard to the type of incident, predisposing and limiting factors, staff and patient factors, patient outcome and suggestive corrective strategies. All staff (medical and nursing) were introduced to the concept of incident reporting, and there was continuous support from a local coordinator, in addition to a resource manual. The incident forms were freely available and were returned to a locked deposit box. Patient and staff confidentiality was ensured by excluding personal identification information from the report forms. A total of 129 incidents were reported, and 90% of participants showed a 'positive attitude' to the incident monitoring system.

The Australian Incident Monitoring Study in the Intensive-Care Unit (AIMS-ICU) was subsequently established nationally, and the first year of reporting was studied. Seven ICUs contributed 536 reports which identified 610 incidents, providing an insight into the nature of incidents. National reporting of data provides information related to wider practices and professional issues, but at the heart of the system is a local facilitated group review meeting to suggest preventive strategies and explore national study findings. Ongoing momentum of the project is assisted by regular local staff newsletters and poster displays.

Comment on incident-monitoring systems

The studies provide valuable insights into the features associated with successful systems, as well as some of the dilemmas. Many of these features are closely interrelated, and they will now be described briefly.

Reporting participation: mandatory vs. voluntary

After reviewing the incident-reporting systems present in healthcare in the USA, the Institute of Medicine recommended complementary mandatory incident-reporting systems and voluntary near-miss-reporting systems. Mandatory systems are usually related to accountability, and receive reports on errors that resulted in serious harm or death, tend to receive reports from organisations, and may release information to the public. In contrast, voluntary systems have a focus on safety improvement and may receive reports from organisations or frontline practitioners, are more likely to be confidential, and report near misses. Near misses provide an opportunity to identify 'cracks' in the system which may lead to major adverse events.

Mandatory systems have not been successful in gaining compliance with reporting requirements, and often little action is taken unless significant numbers of harmful events have been reported. There is an implication that an individual is at fault, yet analysis of most serious errors reveals multiple system failures and the involvement of many individuals.

Provision of anonymity vs. confidentiality

The main objective of any incident-reporting system is to gather information about the frequency and nature of adverse events, but often a major reason for not reporting adverse events is fear. This fear is multi-dimensional, including fear of embarrassment, fear of punishment and fear of litigation.

Voluntary reporting systems provide an opportunity for frontline practitioners to tell the complete story, especially the human factors associated with error, but this can only occur if there is an assurance that they will not be blamed or subject to litigation. Confidentiality, where information will not be disclosed outside the system, appears to be a prerequisite for any system. There is also a strong case for anonymous reporting in which individuals do not have to identify themselves or others. However, experience in Australia with many thousands of anonymous reports shows that many individuals who file anonymous reports are quite happy to own up to them at quality assurance meetings with peers. This concept of anonymity has been challenged as being undesirable. Analysts cannot contact reporters to obtain more information, and it may be difficult to guarantee anonymity. A system of anonymous incident reporting also does not confer a special privilege on doctors, since it does not replace existing legal or disciplinary procedures.

Definitions of adverse events

There is no uniform nomenclature, and this can be a major barrier to incident reporting, creating uncertainty about what types of incidents to report, but also affecting any data analysis. The detection of incidents that have either caused or have the potential to cause harm requires clear definitions. In *An Organisation With a Memory*, an adverse healthcare event and a healthcare near miss are clearly defined:[18]

> An adverse healthcare event is an event or omission arising during clinical care and causing physical or psychological injury to a patient.

> A healthcare near miss is a situation in which an event or omission, or a sequence of events or omissions, arising during clinical care fails to develop further, whether or not as the result of compensating action, thus preventing injury to a patient.

These definitions have been modified by the NPSA on incident reporting, yet still recognising the important distinctions:

An adverse patient incident is 'any event or circumstance that could have or did lead to unintended or unexpected harm, loss or damage'. If the incident resulted in harm, loss or damage then an 'adverse event' has occurred, but if no such consequence occurred it is called a 'near miss'.[19]

Reporting and documentation of incidents

The reporting of incidents is an obvious prerequisite for any incident-monitoring system. It is generally accepted that in all systems there is under-reporting. In a study of two obstetric units in the UK, less than 25% of designated incidents were reported.[20] A questionnaire designed to explore the reasons for low rates of reporting identified that although most staff knew about the incident-reporting system, almost 30% did not know how to find a list of reportable incidents, and there was considerable variation in their views about when they would report an incident. The main reasons for not reporting were fears that other staff members would be blamed, high workload, and the belief that the circumstances or outcome of a particular case did not warrant a report. Similar findings have been described in incident-reporting schemes in the USA, in which 30% of all adverse events in patients were not reported. In Taiwan, 82% of needlestick injuries were not reported, especially by medical staff, with the stated explanation that they were too busy or were unaware of the reporting requirement or mechanism.

Most incident-reporting systems maintain two methods for documenting incident reports, namely a paper incident-report system and a computerised database. A paper incident-report system can have problems associated with legibility of forms, confidentiality/security, misplacement of forms and delays in resolving the reported incident after it has been reported. A study comparing a point-of-service computerised system with a paper incident-reporting system identified several advantages of the point-of-service system. The benefits included real-time information and trending of occurrences, reduced liability by securing reports earlier, earlier problem resolution, and maintaining a higher level of confidentiality.

Classification and analysis of incidents

Incident analysis ought to uncover what happened during the occurrence of an incident, how it happened and, most importantly, why it happened. However, most incident analysis approaches only record the 'what' and 'how' of an incident occurrence.

Research into adverse incidents in other disciplines has shown that incidents are typically not caused by a single, unique factor, but by a complex combination of conditions and events. Any incident occurrence is precipitated by a number of factors that can be organised into a 'causal tree'. These causal factors are organised into a hierarchy that includes factors immediately preceding the incident (also called 'active failures') and those further removed from the incident (also called 'latent failures'). A complete understanding of 'how' an incident occurred can only be achieved by identifying both active and latent failures. This deeper understanding can be achieved by incident analysis, provided that there are methods to classify incidents, and this is the first step in developing a corrective strategy to prevent the occurrence of further incidents.

- Narrative description of incidents is a feature of most incident-reporting systems, but requires classification prior to analysis. This could be achieved by using existing classifications such as ICD-9 and the Read system, but they have been found to be unsuitable for this purpose.
- Categories for classification can be used as a multiple-choice section on reporting forms.

Feedback of findings to produce change

The ultimate aim of any incident-reporting system is to learn from the incidents to prevent them happening again, thereby improving the quality of patient care. An important factor is the time required for feedback.

Conclusion

Adverse event incident reporting has been used extensively in a variety of medical and non-medical settings, but little research has been undertaken in a primary care setting. Under-reporting of adverse events appears to be the main problem with incident-reporting systems, and this is associated with several interrelated factors. Reporting can be maximised by ensuring that the system becomes part of the organisational culture and that barriers to reporting are minimised. This can be achieved by encouraging the voluntary reporting of all near misses in an environment that is free from reprisal and that concentrates on identifying underlying system defects rather than individual error. All members of staff can be involved, but there is a need for regular prompting to report incidents and a mechanism that is both simple and takes place soon after the event. The importance of local review meetings to plan actions to remedy identified problems is emphasised, but there is also a role for national databases that can identify trends and allow policy to be developed.

Systematic identification of medical error

Incident reporting has been regarded as underestimating the extent of medical error, and since it is opportunistic there is no indication of the true extent. This dilemma has led researchers to develop other methods, including 'chart reviews', in which medical records are systematically studied in order to identify 'adverse events', and the direct observation of doctor–patient interaction.

No studies were identified from primary care, and the use of such methods appears to be unlikely except in research.

The use of medical audit and quality improvement data

Medical audit has now become established as part of the regulatory and quality improvement systems in healthcare (both primary and secondary). There is already a large amount of audit in primary care, but there has been little attention to its use in systematically identifying medical error. However, there is a huge potential for using existing systems of quality improvement and audit to identify, classify and reduce error in healthcare. A recent systematic review of the quality of clinical care in general practice emphasises that in almost all studies the processes of care did not reach the standards set out in national guidelines or set by the researchers themselves.

The potential for learning through existing channels for medical audit includes the following.

1 *Identification of critical incidents.* This can include significant event audit, but there are variants, such as practice mortality meetings. There are certain methodological issues related to such audits. First, background information may be difficult to obtain, especially since primary healthcare interfaces extensively with secondary care and other healthcare providers in the community. Secondly, medical records may be incomplete.

2 *Systematic identification by identifying shortfalls in the process of care.* This can be achieved by using care pathways, such as GP referral for suspected cancer. Identified shortfalls in care can be regarded as 'critical incidents' which can then be investigated and analysed by available techniques, depending on their severity, impact and potential to cause harm.

The use of medico-legal and complaints databases

Medical error is often highlighted through patient complaints and litigation. There are several problems associated with the use of such data. Most instances of adverse events do not result in complaints or malpractice claims, and many complaints and malpractice claims are unrelated to error. However, such data are accessible, contain clinically detailed information and may hold lessons that can be learned. Often the information is about major adverse events, such as those reported by the various defence organisations or the GMC.

Much of the data is held on databases by the various defence organisations. However, detailed analysis is not usually forthcoming, due to confidentiality issues and the fact that much of the data relates to identifiable individuals rather than to systems and their potential deficiencies.

A feature of current healthcare is the increased role of the consumer. Patient satisfaction with medical care is a measure of patient perception of the quality of that care, and may be used as a way of opportunistically identifying adverse events, both actual and potential. However, as with litigation claims, there is no clear relationship between adverse events and complaints. In a content analysis of 342 letters of complaint, it was impossible to determine in 29% of cases the nature of the complaint or what action the complainant wanted.[21] Patient complaints do provide important insights into the care provided, especially by giving an additional viewpoint.

The impact of litigation and patient complaints on doctors is often not appreciated. Studies of senior hospital clinicians and general practitioners in the UK highlighted the psychological effects experienced, including anger, distress and a feeling of being personally attacked. The doctors also described the impact on clinical practice, but this was not always detrimental. Most had subsequently attempted to improve communication with patients and staff and to keep better records. Adverse consequences included loss of confidence and a desire to withdraw from clinical practice.

The relationship between medical error and professional judgement

A clear understanding of the nature of error is essential for a full appreciation of why events that harm or have the potential to harm patients occur in the complexity that is characteristic of primary care. The word 'error' is a rather emotionally laden term, implying blame rather than simply representing any aspect of performance which, with hindsight, deviated from the ideal. The psychology of error highlights both the inevitability of error within any human performance and the fact that this is often highly 'context bound', where performance is influenced by the nature of the task and the circumstances and environment in which that task is being undertaken.[22]

Carrying out any action involves the setting of goals and intentions that drive performance. An 'error' is a flawed plan or action, and occurs when the planned sequence fails to result in an intended outcome. Such errors can be divided into two major categories, namely 'active' and 'latent'. Research into errors in numerous industrial settings has highlighted the importance of latent errors. Active errors are usually immediate precursors to an incident, and can be considered in three broad categories as follows.

1 *Knowledge-based errors.* These are the result of forming the wrong intention, or making the wrong plan, and are due to inadequate knowledge or experience.
2 *Rule-based errors.* These involve failure to apply a rule designed to avoid error, or the application of a badly designed rule.
3 *Skill–based errors (slips and lapses).* These are the result of 'absent-mindedness', and they occur in highly skilled people who have a large repertoire of subconscious responses but who fail to monitor their actions. The result is an action that was not intended.

Latent errors contribute to or 'shape' the intended plans and actions. Examples include the individual's physiological state, working environmental conditions, training, working policies and procedures, and socio-cultural factors.

The reality of professional practice is characterised by its complexity and by the inability to apply neutral knowledge to such situations. There are important implications, especially in primary care where undifferentiated problems often present, disease often presents at an early stage, patients often want to make major choices with regard to suggested management plans, and it is often necessary to juggle the available resources. Professional judgement, which lies at the heart of professional practice, is highly dependent on craft knowledge that has been acquired through professional practice. This is in contrast to technical knowledge, which is often not regarded by practitioners as being relevant to the demands that they face.

Research into accident causation, especially in aviation and other high-profile industries, has revealed the important contribution of 'human factors' as a cause of active error. It has been estimated that 90% of aviation accidents can be attributed to such factors. This does not mean that blame can be attached to individuals, but rather that error is inevitable and systems need to be in place to prevent such errors. In medicine, and especially in primary care, decisions are often made with an incomplete knowledge of all the available facts, without all of the investigations, respecting patient preferences and with little idea of the ultimate outcome. This is the reality of practising general practice.

To begin to understand the nature of error in primary care, it is important that these 'human factors' are identified. The exemplar studies of identifying adverse incidents show that the deeper aspects, such as practitioner fatigue or running late, can best be identified by employing a qualitative technique in which practitioners describe the reality of their world.

Conclusions

The existing evidence base on medical error in primary care is small, but the data that are available can provide valuable insights into the frequency and nature of such errors. There is a much wider evidence base that considers the experiences in secondary care and non-healthcare settings, providing important lessons to inform policy decisions in the development of systems for incident reporting, which is the foundation for clinical risk management in primary care.

References

1 Department of Health (2001) *Building a Safer NHS for Patients. Implementing* An Organisation With a Memory. Department of Health, London.
2 Bhasale AL, Miller GC, Reid SE and Britt HC (1998) Analysing potential harm in Australian general practice: an incident-monitoring study. *Med J Aust.* **169**: 73–6.
3 Bhasale A (1998) The wrong diagnosis: identifying causes of potentially adverse events in general practice using incident monitoring. *Fam Pract.* **15**: 308–18.
4 Fischer G, Fetters MD, Munro AP and Goldman EB (1997) Adverse events in primary care identified from a risk-management database. *J Fam Pract.* **45**: 40–6.
5 Ely JW, Levinson W, Elder NC, Mainous AG and Vinson DC (1995) Perceived causes of family physicians' errors. *J Fam Pract.* **40**: 337–44.
6 Conradi MH and de Mol BAJM (1999) Research on errors and safety in Dutch general and hospital practice. In: AR Rosenthal, L Mulcahy and S Lloyd-Bostock (eds) *Medical Mishaps: pieces of the puzzle.* Open University Press, Buckingham.
7 Dovey S, Green L and Fryer GF (2000) *Identifying Threats to Patient Safety in Family Practice.* (www.aafppolicy.org/posters/errors/). The Robert Graham Center, Washington, DC.
8 Kriisa I (1990) Swedish malpractice reports and convictions. *Qual Assur in Health Care.* **2**: 329–34.
9 Silk N (2000) *An analysis of 1000 consecutive UK general practice negligence claims* (an abridged version was published in the November 2000 issue of *Health Care Risk Report*). Unpublished report from the Medical Protection Society, Leeds.
10 Sweeney G, Westcott R and Stead J (2000) The benefits of significant event audit in primary care: a case study. *J Clin Govern.* **8**: 128–34.
11 Neville RG, Robertson F, Livingstone S and Crombie IK (1989) A classification of prescription errors. *J R Coll Gen Pract.* **39**: 110–12.
12 Shulman JI, Shulman S and Haines AP (1981) The prevention of adverse drug reactions – a potential role for pharmacists in the primary care team? *J R Coll Gen Pract.* **31**: 429–34.
13 Hawksworth GM, Corlett AJ, Wright DJ and Christyn H (1999) Clinical pharmacy interventions by community pharmacists during the dispensing process. *Br J Clin Pharmacol.* **47**: 695–700.
14 Buurma H, de Smet PAGM, van den Hoff OP and Egberts ACG (2001) Nature, frequency and determinants of prescription modifications in Dutch community pharmacies. *Br J Clin Pharmacol.* **52**: 85–91.

15 Flanagan JC (1954) The critical incident technique. *Psychol Bull.* **51**: 327–8.
16 Barach P and Small SD (2000) How the NHS can improve safety and learning. By learning free lessons from near misses. *BMJ.* **320**: 1683–4.
17 Beckmann U, West LF, Groombridge GJ *et al.* (1996) The Australian Incident Monitoring Study in Intensive Care: AIMS-ICU. The development and evaluation of an incident reporting system in intensive care. *Anaesth Intensive Care.* **24**: 314–19.
18 Department of Health (2000) *An Organisation With a Memory.* Department of Health, London.
19 National Patient Safety Agency (2003) *Seven Steps to Patient Safety.* NPSA, London.
20 Vincent C, Taylor-Adams S, Chapman EJ *et al.* (2000) How to investigate and analyse clinical incidents: Clinical Risk Unit and Association of Litigation and Risk Management protocol. *BMJ.* **320**: 777–81.
21 Lloyd-Bostock S (1999) Calling doctors and hospitals to account: complaining and claiming as social processes. In: AR Rosenthal, L Mulcahy and S Lloyd-Bostock (eds) *Medical Mishaps: pieces of the puzzle.* Open University Press, Buckingham.
22 Reason J (1990) *Human Error.* Cambridge University Press, Cambridge.

Section 2

Chapter 6

Some of the main risks in general practice: an overview

Keith Haynes

Key learning points

- Clinical risk management (CRM) is a key component of the clinical governance agenda in primary care.
- PCOs and practices still have some way to go towards realising the full benefits of CRM.
- Evidence shows that 76% of incidents in general practice are to do with systems failures and are potentially preventable.
- Risk assessments in 200 practices have identified a number of key risks, including areas such as confidentiality, repeat prescribing, managing test results, computerisation, staff safety, communication, Health and Safety, etc.
- Having identified these common areas of concern, it falls to risk management (and this book) to help to manage them better.

Introduction

The clinical governance requirements for PCOs are no different from those placed upon NHS trusts. The Health Act 1999 makes it quite clear that it is the 'duty of each primary care trust and each NHS trust to put and keep in place arrangements for the purpose of monitoring and improving the quality of health care which it provides to individuals'.

The challenge has been for PCOs to achieve this in what has been little more than a loose affiliation of representatives of primary care teams and practices. The key elements of clinical governance might be described as follows (*see* Figure 6.1):

- processes for recording and deriving lessons from untoward incidents, complaints and claims
- a risk management programme and system
- effective clinical audit
- evidence-based clinical practice
- a supportive, non-blaming culture that is committed to the concept of lifelong learning

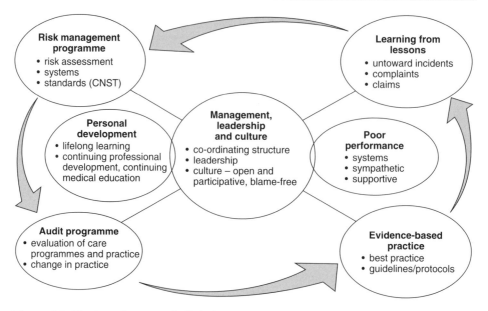

Figure 6.1 The key elements of clinical governance.

Of course, introduced in isolation none of these dimensions will provide effective clinical governance. The key is to ensure that each of these processes is connected and the loop is closed, providing a coherent and comprehensive clinical governance programme that is underpinned by sound leadership and management providing the right cultural climate.

CRM is a key component of the clinical governance agenda in primary care. As a tool for improving quality in healthcare generally, CRM has been around at least since 1994,[1] and was given a considerable boost when clinical governance was introduced in the late 1990s. However, the Commission for Health Improvement (CHI) (now the Commission for Health Audit and Inspection, known as the Healthcare Commission) has observed that PCTs and practices still have some way to go towards realising the full benefits of CRM. Observations so far have included the following:

> CHI found little evidence of formal learning mechanisms for PCT-employed staff in areas such as reported incidents. [The PCT should consider developing] a clinical risk management system that facilitates the management and monitoring of incidents and how to learn from them.[2]

CHI expects PCTs to 'increase awareness of risk management policies, extend the system of incident reporting across all staff groups and develop a system for near miss reporting.'[3]

Despite CHI's observations, some PCTs have embraced the potential of CRM as:

- a tool for reviewing systems and improving quality of services
- a mechanism for understanding current issues within practices (an important part of the learning necessary for fledgeling organisations)

- a means to enable them to support their practices to improve the quality of services.

In reality, the core unit for clinical governance is the individual general practice. The contents of this chapter (and the whole book) will be focused on the practice as the fundamental unit of CRM, and will be of considerable interest to PCTs as a result.

An approach to clinical risk management

To many, the very words 'risk management' suggest something rather sterile and uninteresting. This is unfortunate, as it is about improving the quality of patient care and ensuring patient safety. In essence, it is about good clinical practice. Thankfully, the language in this area is changing to embrace 'quality' and 'patient safety'.

Evidence shows that 76% of incidents in general practice are preventable, and that they are more to do with systems failures (e.g. abnormal test results that are missed or not acted upon, poor legibility of prescription, failure to review patient's history, etc.) than clinical judgement.[4] In another study, an overall error rate of 75.6 per 1000 appointments was reported, with the errors being classified into six categories, namely prescriptions, communication, appointments, equipment, clinical care and 'other' errors.[5] In total, 42% of the errors related to prescriptions, although only 6% of these were medication errors. Communication errors accounted for 30% and clinical errors accounted for 3%.

In response to this, MPS Risk Consulting has developed a Clinical Risk Self-Assessment (CRSA) process. It is based on an accepted risk management model that involves identification, measurement and control of risks, and it also draws on the Australian/New Zealand Risk Management Standards.[6]

The process involves a one-day practice visit by a trained MPS consultant. Ahead of the visit, the practice manager and a GP partner are asked to complete a fairly detailed questionnaire about the practice. This includes questions about the medical records system, repeat prescribing arrangements and how test results are handled, for example. Members of the MPS consultancy team (who are mainly practising GPs) then talk confidentially with individuals in the practice, including receptionists, practice nurses, the practice manager, GPs and other key staff. During these semi-structured interviews, issues raised by the pre-visit questionnaire are discussed and interviewees are invited to identify risks in their systems.

The heart of a CRSA is a half-day multi-disciplinary workshop which follows these exploratory discussions. Participants are asked to:

- identify risks that the practice team know have occurred or think could occur
- assess the likelihood and consequences of those risks occurring
- review the controls that are in place for managing those risks
- agree the actions that the practice team needs to take and what the key priorities are.

This is then followed up with a detailed report capturing the output.

The CRSA is a process that involves the whole practice team. It is not inspectorial, but rather it allows practices, within a facilitated, supportive environment, to identify for themselves the areas which they feel could cause problems.

Some of the common themes emerging: an overview

A wide range of risks has been identified by practices, and an analysis of the first 200 CRSAs has revealed a number of core areas of risk that were consistently identified by the practices (*see* Box 6.1).

Box 6.1 Most common risk areas

Confidentiality	85%
Test results	77%
Repeat prescribing	75%
Staff safety	72%
Communication within practice/message taking	51%
Health and Safety	50%
Record keeping	48%
Referrals	47%
Computers	45%
Communication with secondary care	41%

The main areas of concern identified by the practices will now be discussed.

Confidentiality (see Chapter 7)

Recurring themes include the following:

- problems imposed by the physical layout of the practice premises and the lack of confidential areas where patients could talk to receptionists
- visibility of computer screens, appointment and message books
- third parties requesting information such as test results, or collecting prescriptions for family members
- reliably identifying callers over the telephone before giving out confidential information.

Confidentiality is a risk identified by the majority of practices, and although there is an obvious concern about this important issue there is also a high level of awareness, and most non-clinical staff have contracts of employment containing standard confidentiality clauses. Many of the issues are environmental in nature (e.g. poor soundproofing in consulting rooms, reception desks with adjacent waiting areas), which are very difficult to change, although there are some things that practices could do, such as ensuring that computers are sited appropriately and that password-protected screensavers are used. Any practices that are fortunate enough to be designing or building new purpose-built accommodation are advised to ensure that they focus on the appropriate design components of any new build to ensure that the building is conducive to maintaining patient confidentiality.

However, although there is a high level of awareness of the need to maintain confidentiality, it is sometimes less certain whether practice staff fully understand some of the wider issues and implications, in particular the Data Protection Act and the implications for the physical security of records, Caldicott guardianship and the GMC guidance on confidentiality.

Repeat prescribing (see Chapters 11 and 25)

Recurring themes include the following:

- review dates being overridden, thus interfering with the effectiveness of the reauthorisation system
- difficulties in ensuring that patients are adequately monitored (a requirement of their condition, or the nature of the medication that they are taking)
- repeat prescribing data not being reviewed often enough to ensure that all medications on repeat are both necessary and appropriate
- prescribing from inadequate and illegible discharge summaries, following a change in the patient's medication by a member of the hospital staff
- identifying vulnerable patients who under- or over-use their medication.

The lack of an effective system for managing repeat prescribing remains a potential risk in many practices. The component elements of an effective repeat prescribing system, including adherence to a suitable protocol, are dealt with in Chapters 11 and 25. However, when reviewing the system, practices may wish to focus on the three stages of the process, namely requesting, reauthorising and issuing the repeat prescription.

Many practices allow repeat prescriptions to be requested by telephone. A balance needs to be struck between access to the practice, particularly in rural locations and for housebound patients, and the potential for mis-transcribing any requests for a repeat prescription. If requests are being received by telephone, then ideally the person receiving the request should be able to call up the patient's medication records on computer screen in order to avoid having to transcribe the details.

With regard to reauthorisation and review, it is very important that the limits which are being set for review are not overridden, and that the reauthorisation system is therefore effective. Many of the computer systems that are in place are integral to ensuring that patients on repeat prescriptions are monitored, particularly those on toxic therapies and those requiring regular blood tests. However, practices need to remember that the system will only be as good as those who use it (*see* Case study 6.1).

Case study 6.1: repeat prescribing

Between 1980 and 1992, Mr S received regular blood pressure checks for his hypertension and was on appropriate drug therapy. Up until 1991 all repeat medication had been recorded in the patient's records on a repeat prescribing card, but in 1991 the practice changed to using the computer for repeat prescribing.

Continued

Between 1992 and 1998 Mr S was on atenolol $56 \times 100mg$ 1 bd, and received a prescription every 2 months which he collected directly from his local pharmacy. The entry on the computer was 56 1 bd authorised for 12 repeats, so Mr S should have been seen biannually. In fact, over the 6-year period he was not reviewed at all.

Mr S died in 1998 from myocardial infarction.

The practice explained that repeat prescriptions are signed by all doctors in the practice, on the assumption that the patient is in the review system. In practice, the reception staff would inform the patient that they were due for review. However, in this case, in printing prescriptions from the repeat prescribing window on the computer they also reauthorised at the review point for another 12 prescriptions. Consequently, the patient passed three review points at 2-yearly intervals without being seen.

The systems which are put in place are only as good as the extent to which they are complied with.

Within our sample of 200 practices, hardly any practices ensure that a doctor reviews a repeat prescription that has been requested but not collected before it is destroyed, and records its non-collection.

A review by the doctor may reveal some clinically significant information which they would want to act upon. Failure to destroy the repeat prescriptions without the doctor reviewing them may have serious consequences.

Test results (see Chapter 10)

Recurring themes include the following:

- difficulties in ensuring that both patients and receptionists are aware when multiple tests have been done
- a lack of clarity about the extent of the patient's responsibility to contact the practice for their own test results, or for the practice to proactively contact patients themselves
- dealing with patients who have been asked to come in to discuss a test result, but who fail to attend
- dealing with third parties (such as family members) who request information about a patient's test results
- a lack of clarity about what the reception staff should say to a patient who phones for their test results.

Very few practices have a really effective, failsafe system for ensuring that test results are communicated to patients, although in most cases any patient with an abnormal test result would be contacted directly by their doctor. This is often a risk that has been managed by the usual approach to safety netting in general practice, namely asking the patient to contact the surgery within a specified time.

Case study 6.2: test results

Mr B went to see his GP, Dr D, after passing blood in his urine. Dr D found nothing else of note in the history, and he examined the abdomen, genitalia and prostate, all of which were unremarkable. Blood was visible in the sample that Mr B gave for a midstream urine specimen (MSU).

Mr B was about to move to a new area. Dr D noted this and recorded that he told Mr B to register with a new GP and to be investigated.

The MSU result showed only RBC+ and was filed in Mr B's notes (stamped by another practice member as normal). Two months later the notes were transferred to Mr B's new practice. A further 2 months passed and Mr B went to see his new GP, Dr J, after a minor car crash. The episode of haematuria had not recurred and was not mentioned.

Dr J kept her notes on a new record card. She did not see the previous entry about haematuria and there was no review of the notes.

It was another 4 years before Mr B came back to the surgery. He gave a history of recurrent long-standing gross haematuria. Urinalysis showed RBC++++, protein+ and WBC+. Dr J sent an MSU, checked the full blood count and urine and electrolytes, prescribed trimethoprim and referred Mr B to a urologist.

Mr B was found to have an invasive bladder carcinoma. He had a total cystectomy but died from metastatic disease less than a year later.

Ideally, a safe system for dealing with test results should aim to have the following components.

1   There should be a system for recording test results that are requested, which checks them off when they are returned. The premise is that if the practitioner requests a test, he or she ought to know that it has been done. A few practices have such a system in place, usually in a manual form. Other practices have a system, but only in relation to limited areas such as smear tests and histology samples. For the vast majority of practices it is often beyond the scope of their resources to run such a system in relation to all tests that they request. The ideal solution is to ensure, through the computer system, that any tests that have not had a posting back via lab-links are searchable. At present the computer systems that are in place in general practice do not provide this facility.

2   Clear information should be given to the patient about how he or she will be advised about the test and ideally information about the number of tests carried out, so that the patient can prompt practice staff when enquiring about results. This is to avoid the situation where a number of tests have been carried out and the patient is told that the result is normal, when other test results that have yet to be returned may be abnormal.

3   Most importantly, a system is needed for ensuring that action is taken on all test results before they are filed, particularly abnormal test results.

4   Clear instructions should be available to non-clinical practice staff so that they are not drawn into giving or interpreting clinical information.

Computers and record keeping (see Chapter 9)

Recurring themes include the following:

- problems associated with some members of the practice team using predominantly paper records and others predominantly the computer for recording clinical information
- confidentiality of computer screens
- integrity of the audit trail, which may be affected if users either share a password or do not log off when they have finished using a computer
- failure to make records of telephone consultations with patients
- lack of training in keyboard skills.

Some practices continue to use the Lloyd George or A4 record, while using the computer to record essential clinical information. Others have become 'paperless' and no longer use the Lloyd George or A4 record at all during the consultation. There are still other practices where some of the doctors will be using paper records during consultation and others will be using the computer to record their clinical findings. There are potential risks associated with this practice, as self-evidently this will result in clinical information sitting astride the two media. Practices that operate in this way are encouraged to move further in the direction of becoming paperless, and to support their staff in gaining the necessary computer skills.

Health and safety (see Chapter 20)

Recurring themes include the following:

- the need for formal health and safety assessments in many practices
- a requirement for improved understanding of overall responsibilities in relation to health and safety matters generally
- the absence of formal Control of Substances Hazardous to Health (COSHH) assessments
- the need for further training in health and safety matters
- other hazardous substances being stored in unlocked, low-lying cupboards
- specimens being handed to reception staff who are not immunised against hepatitis B.

There are varying degrees of understanding and activity in relation to health and safety issues in general practice. Often there is a lack of understanding of the responsibility placed on individuals within the practice for ensuring compliance with health and safety matters. Much more guidance and assistance is required to help practices to achieve acceptable standards.

Case study 6.3: health and safety

Mrs H visited the health centre with her three children, accompanied by her sister.

The first consultation with Dr J involved S, then 19 months old. Following that consultation he was accompanied by his mother out of the consulting room and returned to the waiting room.

The mother then took the second of her children to see Dr J, leaving her sister, S, and the remaining child in the waiting room.

After a short while the consultation was interrupted when it became apparent that the youngest child, S, had wandered unnoticed into the neighbouring procedure room where he had picked up a bottle of phenol and had obviously taken an amount of this substance orally.

The bottle of phenol had been left on a storage trolley approximately 2½ feet high, and the procedure-room door had previously been closed by the receptionist but was not locked. It was not practice to lock the door, and a key was not available.

Dr J was the only person in the health centre to use phenol for minor surgery, and was the last person to replace the phenol on the trolley. The phenol was normally stored on a high shelf in the procedure room.

S suffered severe internal burns and ulceration of his oesophagus and stomach mucosa, together with damage to the airways and right lung following aspiration of the stomach contents.

Staff safety and security

Recurring themes include the following:

- the safety of lone workers
- the need for systems for summoning assistance with which staff are familiar
- the need for training in how to deal with aggressive and violent patients.

This is an area of increasing concern to staff, even if there have been no specific incidents of violence within the practice. Practice staff often need support and training in how to deal with such situations. As a starting point, practices should review the Department of Health guidance on promoting a policy of low/zero tolerance so far as violent patients are concerned (www.nhs.uk/zerotolerance).

Communication (see Chapters 8 and 13)

Recurring themes include the following:

- poor systems for recording and passing on messages
- infrequent opportunities for the whole practice team to meet
- inadvertently forgetting to make a referral
- delayed, illegible and sometimes confusing information from secondary care.

Case study 6.4: missed referral

Mrs A suffered from depression and was seeing her GP, Dr P. During a consultation to review the efficacy of her lofepramine, Mrs A mentioned that she had had a lump on the side of her face for a long time. Dr P examined Mrs A's face and noted the presence of a mobile lump, 1 cm in diameter, over the left mandible. Dr P intended to refer Mrs A to her local oral surgery service for advice. Unfortunately, she forgot to dictate the referral letter at the end of the surgery.

Dr P's normal practice was to tell patients to contact her if they had not heard about a referral once a month had passed. Mrs A had several further appointments at the surgery over the next few weeks, but failed to attend any of them. She eventually came to see Dr P to discuss other matters, 4 months after the first consultation about the lump. The lump, and its assessment by the oral surgeons, was not mentioned in the consultation.

A month later, Mrs A was at the surgery again and saw Dr C. She mentioned that she had heard nothing from the oral surgeons. Dr C left Mrs A's notes out for Dr P with a note explaining the lack of an oral surgical opinion. Dr P realised her error and dictated the referral shortly afterwards. Mrs A was seen by the oral surgeon, Mr Q, within 2 weeks.

The lump was duly excised and a tissue diagnosis of acinic carcinoma was made. This required further somewhat radical surgery, involving bone grafting from the hip. Unfortunately this graft became infected, causing significant pain and disfigurement to Mrs A, and necessitating further surgery.

There are a variety of issues concerning 'communication' in general practice. At a basic level it is about the way in which messages are recorded and passed on in the practice. Sometimes it involves failure to write a referral letter. Many practices also complain that there are too few opportunities to get the entire practice team together because very often everyone is too busy going about their daily tasks. The benefits of creating time for the whole team to meet cannot be overstated.

There is great potential for risk at the interface between primary and secondary care. For example, many practices complain of the poor quality of discharge information and the lack of timely information upon discharge, including confusion about who has responsibility for the patient and who is to prescribe in certain circumstances. The potential for things to go wrong in this area as a result of poor communication is endless.

Conclusion

Our work with practices has confirmed that many of these issues are of concern to them. Having identified the issues, the next step is to offer some useful and practical guidance for managing these 'risks'. What follows, therefore, in this section of the book is a more detailed exploration of these common risks, together with practical guidance on how to manage them better. The final section of the book focuses on solutions for some of the main areas of risk.

References

1   NHS Executive (1994) *Risk Management in the NHS.* HMSO, London.
2   Commission for Health Improvement (2002) *CHI Clinical Governance Review, Central Manchester PCT*; www.chi.gov.uk
3   Commission for Health Improvement (2002) *CHI Clinical Governance Review, Hillingdon PCT and NHS Direct, West London*; www.chi.gov.uk
4   Bhasale AL *et al.* (1998) Analysing potential harm in Australian general practice: an incident-monitoring study. *Med J Aust.* **169**: 73–6.
5   Rubin G *et al.* (2003) Errors in general practice: development of an error classification and pilot study of a method for detecting errors. *Qual Saf Health Care.* **12**: 443–7.
6   Australian/New Zealand Standards (1995) *Risk Management.* Australian/New Zealand Standards, Sydney.

Chapter 7

In confidence

Sandy Anthony

Key learning points

- Breaching patient confidentiality is easy to do.
- Doctors and nurses are often the worst offenders.
- Good systems can help.
- So, too, can a well-designed environment.
- Staff training is vital.
- This chapter offers tips on effective staff training.

A nurse needed to give a patient a phone number. She jotted it down on a piece of scrap paper and handed it over. When the patient arrived home she found, on the reverse of the paper, the names and diagnoses of two other patients.

A hospital in the USA discovered that it had been consistently faxing confidential patient information to a restaurant in Tampa because the speed-dial number they were using had been entered wrongly. In another case, a receptionist transposed two digits while dialling, and faxed confidential patient information to a local car mechanic's shop.

Someone in a hurry left the original documents, containing patient-identifiable information, on a photocopier. As the copier had been housed in a public-access corridor, it is not known how many people saw the papers before they were discovered by another member of staff.

A man attending a busy outpatient clinic for an HIV test was taken into a cubicle next to a busy waiting room. When he told the phlebotomist what the blood test was for, she leaned out of the cubicle and called out to another member of staff, in full hearing of the patients in the waiting room, 'I can't do HIV tests'.

A laboratory worker had been given permission to use 'dirty paper' (i.e. papers that contained data, test results, and so on) as scrap paper for practising maths homework. She inadvertently took several of the papers home with her at the end of the day. She lived in a hostel and left the papers in a common room, where they were discovered and sent to the Department of Health. On examination, the papers were found to be laboratory reports concerning TB, STD and HIV/AIDS patient information.

All of the above are actual incidents reported in the USA,[1] but similar acts of carelessness are almost certainly happening in the UK, too, on a daily basis. They are all inadvertent breaches of confidentiality, and were all avoidable.

Each of the above scenarios demonstrates a lack of vigilance on the part of the personnel concerned. There may or may not have been systems, protocols and policies in place to prevent these breaches of confidentiality, but they all come to nothing if the people who are entrusted with making the system work are not committed to it. Moreover, it would be naive to believe that you can anticipate every possible opportunity for such breaches to occur and design appropriate protocols to prevent them. Gaps in the system only become apparent once a breach has occurred and there have been repercussions.

The lesson that can be learned from the above examples is that you can put good systems in place to minimise the risk of confidentiality breaches, but it will be a complete waste of time if you do not also invest in staff training. It is not enough just to get staff to sign a confidentiality agreement along with their employment contract. They need to understand what patient privacy means in practice, and they need to appreciate how important it is.

If you can rely on your staff to take these issues seriously and to act intelligently and use their initiative, then you can be reasonably confident that the risk of confidentiality breaches in your practice is negligible. Good, comprehensive training, supported by a clearly expressed practice policy, is therefore the single most important thing you can do to protect your patients' privacy.

Do not assume that it is only non-clinicians who need training, either. Even though nurses and doctors are bound by professional codes of conduct, they are often the worst offenders when it comes to breaching patient confidentiality. After all, they are privy to far more sensitive personal information than are non-clinical workers.

> A friend of mine was waiting to see her consultant in an outpatient clinic recently. While she was there, two nurses sat down a few seats away in the waiting room and started loudly discussing the contents of a patient's case file. His name was written in big black letters on the cover and my friend could easily read it from where she was sitting.

> A GP accosted a colleague in the corridor to ask his advice about managing a patient whose diagnosis was proving elusive. She gave him a quick run-down of the signs and symptoms and the investigations she had ordered. The conversation took place outside the door to the toilet, where another patient sat listening to every word.

Culture

It is much easier to be vigilant if you are working within a culture that supports the principle of patient confidentiality. This means that everyone within the team is committed to the concept, is alert to potential pitfalls and is prepared to act when they see patient privacy being compromised. This includes being up-front with colleagues if they see or hear them being careless.

A good way of inculcating such a culture is to devote a couple of hours to a risk assessment involving all members of the team. Getting people to identify weaknesses in your systems for handling confidential information, and suggesting improvements, engenders a sense of common purpose and helps to reinforce everyone's commitment. Get the session going by holding an open discussion around one or two hypothetical scenarios (*see* the sample scenarios on page 81). This helps people to translate the concept of 'confidentiality' from an abstract ideal into the everyday world of often conflicting demands.

When looking at your practice's systems, you might like to focus on the main trouble-spots – the environment, your paper systems, and protocols for dealing with particular situations.

The environment

You could work through the following checklist regarding the environment.[2]

- Are the medical records stored in a lockable room that is accessible only to authorised personnel?
- Are computer monitors positioned in such a way that they cannot be over-looked?
- Are printers and fax machines located in secure areas?
- Do you have special waste bins for the secure disposal of personal information? How often are they emptied (and by whom)? Where are they located?
- Are consultation rooms soundproof?
- Are there areas in which staff discussing patient care may be overheard?
- Do rooms with computer terminals have locks on the doors?
- Is the appointment book kept where it cannot be easily seen by patients?
- Is seating in the waiting room placed at a distance from the reception desk?
- Does the layout of the reception area discourage patients from queuing up at the desk?
- Do receptionists have access to a telephone out of hearing of waiting patients?
- Can the reception office be closed off from the waiting room if necessary (e.g. when only one person is on duty and she has to leave the room)?[2]
- If you use an answering machine, is it located so that casual listeners cannot overhear a message being left?

If the answer to any of these questions is no, discuss possible solutions among yourselves. You could consider, for example:

- playing background music in the waiting room
- installing thicker doors on consultation rooms
- allocating an area where patients can speak in confidence to the receptionist if they need to
- installing a glass screen across the reception desk. This has the added benefit of increasing staff security
- adjusting the height or width of the reception desk – if it is too wide, patients may have to raise their voices to be heard, and if it is too low, papers can be too easily seen

- if it is not possible to move a computer out of the range of sight of visitors, consider investing in flat screens that can only be viewed from the front.[2]

Administrative systems

Questions to ask yourselves about your administrative systems should include the following.

- Are levels of access to records restricted on a 'need-to-know' basis?
- Do you have a system for tracking the whereabouts of paper records?
- Do you have a robust audit trail for electronic records?
- Are laboratory samples and their accompanying documentation sent in sealed packages?
- Do you anonymise patient information as far as possible when conducting audits?
- Do all staff have passwords for computer access and do they change them regularly?

Policy and protocols

If you do not already have a written policy regarding confidentiality, you should seriously consider drafting one. Once you have a policy, do not just leave it on a shelf – make it work. Incorporate it into your staff induction and training materials, include excerpts from it in your practice leaflets, and review it annually to make sure that it is in line with current legislation (e.g. the Data Protection Act) and still relevant to your circumstances (e.g. expansion of the primary healthcare team).

Your policy should include the following:

- an explicit statement about your commitment to maintaining patients' privacy
- the levels of breaches that can occur – that is, (i) inadvertent, (ii) intentional without malice or personal gain, and (iii) intentional with malicious intent or for personal gain
- the effects of breaches – that is, (i) minor, with no harm to the patient, (ii) minor, with some harm to the patient, (iii) moderate, with harm to the patient and (iv) major, with severe harm to the patient
- the disciplinary sanctions that apply to breaches, depending on the level of breach and its effect
- what staff must do if they become aware of a breach or potential breach of confidentiality.

Your protocols should include the following:

- secure storage of, and access to, medical records
- procedures for use of computers, especially passwords, access privileges and use of screensavers, etc.
- information that can and cannot be given over the telephone – this could also include specimen forms of words for politely refusing to divulge information if it is not appropriate to do so
- information that can and cannot be given over a mobile phone

- procedure for sending faxes
- procedure for sending patient information via email
- descriptions of materials that can be sent by ordinary mail, and those that should be sent by a more secure method
- procedure for sealing confidential packages and documents to be mailed
- receipt of test results and procedure for communicating them to the patient
- procedure for contacting patients at home or at work (e.g. do not leave a message or say who is calling if the patient is not available).

Access and information flows

The days when the doctor and a receptionist were the only people who would handle a patient's records are long gone. Not only have primary healthcare teams expanded, leading to many more caregivers contributing to patient care, but also there is a clamouring for access from outside the practice. These simple doctors' *aide-mémoires* have developed into a valuable resource in their own right, especially if they are computerised.

At the practice level, computerised patient records can be used for various audits to measure performance, to identify target groups of patients and to help to profile patient populations. This is likely to increase markedly over the next few years, not least because of the new GP contract.

Interested parties from outside the immediate care team include social services, local authorities, PCTs, researchers, epidemiologists and the Department of Health. Each has its own agenda and requirements. Social services, for example, are likely to be more interested in individual patients, and it may be that there are grounds for sharing certain information with them in the patient's interests. Researchers, too, may want direct access to the content of patients' records, along with their names and contact details. PCTs and the Department of Health, on the other hand, will probably be satisfied with anonymised information.

Patient information therefore takes two forms, namely identifiable and anonymised, and it is used for the following purposes:

- the delivery of healthcare – this includes clinical audit
- meeting wider medical objectives – this includes (along with medical research) financial audit, health-service management and social care
- to protect the interests of wider society.[3]

Anonymised information is not confidential, so any disclosures should be anonymised as far as is possible. However, in many circumstances only identifiable information can be used, and if so, the following general rules apply.

- As the information is collected with the express purpose of providing healthcare for the patient, you have the patient's implied consent to share the information with fellow professionals, within the context of patient care. Even so, controls are still necessary, and access should be granted on a strict need-to-know basis. This is easier to implement if the records are computerised, because most systems will allow you to set different levels of access, depending on the role of the team member.
- The demarcation between healthcare and social care is often blurred, so sharing information with other agencies beyond the healthcare team, even

though it may be very much in the patient's interests, is less clearly legitimate. You will therefore need to obtain the patient's express consent for such disclosures. However, there will often be cases where the patient lacks the capacity to give consent, and in these circumstances you may go ahead and share the information if it is in the patient's best interests, carefully documenting your reasons for doing so. You should have an information-sharing protocol that is agreed with the other agencies with whom you deal.

- Disclosure of identifiable patient information for medical (i.e. other than healthcare provision) purposes should be made only with the patient's express consent. The patient should be made aware of the use that would be made of their details, they should be given the opportunity to ask questions, and they should be told that they have the right to withhold consent. Various combinations of leaflets, notices, letters and one-to-one discussions can all be employed to notify patients.

- Disclosure for other (non-medical) purposes encompasses a collection of scenarios, including police enquiries, solicitors' requests for medical records, insurance reports, occupational health reports, complaints procedures, notifications to the DVLA, reports to coroners' courts and court orders. In almost all cases you will need the patient's explicit consent before you disclose information. The exceptions are those that place a statutory duty on you to impart confidential information, namely, complying with a court order, assisting the coroner and reports to the DVLA. You may also disclose confidential information about a patient without their consent if it is in the public interest. However, even in circumstances in which you do not need the patient's consent before disclosing information, as a matter of courtesy you should, if possible, tell the patient what you are doing and why.

Conclusion

There is no doubt that protecting patient privacy has become more complex in recent years because there are generally so many more people involved in a patient's care. Another trend that looks set to occupy more of the foreground is the use of patient information for non-clinical purposes or for reasons other than direct patient care. There seem to be ever more bodies clamouring for such information – health planners, auditors, epidemiologists, and so on. The rule here is to provide only anonymised data unless there is clear support for including identifiable information – for example, when reporting notifiable diseases.

Despite the above considerations, maintaining patient confidentiality is largely a straightforward application of common sense. Getting it right depends more on the awareness and commitment of all members of staff than on rigid controls.

References

1   *Serious Confidentiality Breach*, 4 June 2002, www.chbc.com; Florida Department of Health, Bureau of Laboratories, *Investigative Report #01-172: Alleged Breach of Confidential Patient Information*, 17 December 2001; South Dakota Academy of Family Physicians, *Breaching Patient Confidentiality – easier than you think*, www.sdafp.org; *Reporting, Correcting Privacy Breaches: Hospital's HIPPS training comes to life*, www.aishealth.com.

2   Anthony S (2002) Confidentiality: simple risk-management measures. In: J Tingle (ed.) *Patient Confidentiality*. Emis Professional Publishing, London.

3   Department of Health (2003) *Confidentiality: NHS code of practice*. Department of Health, London.

Appendix 7.1: Scenarios for discussion at a team workshop

A patient picks up his medical records from your desk and starts to read them. Should you let him proceed?
(Points to consider: mention of third parties in the notes, and potentially damaging information.)

You are a GP registrar. You notice two of the practice's principals in a local pub and realise that they are a little the worse for wear. They are discussing – more loudly than they probably realise – a particularly troublesome patient. What should you do?

A 15-year-old girl makes an urgent appointment. She wants the morning-after pill, which you prescribe. The following day her mother (who is a good friend of yours) phones and asks to speak to you. She has found the patient information leaflet in her daughter's room and wants to know what is going on. Should you tell her?
(Point to consider: Gillick competence.)

You are working in reception and your nextdoor neighbour comes in for an appointment. She looks upset when she comes out of the consultation room. Later that day, you inadvertently see a referral letter saying that her doctor suspects MS. You are very concerned as you know that she has three small children to care for and her husband is often away on business. You would like to help in a neighbourly way. Should you offer to do so?

A co-worker needs to type up a letter, but has forgotten her computer password. She asks if she can use your log-in for 10 minutes as she is in a hurry to catch the post and cannot spare the time to arrange for a new password. She says that the letter is confidential so you cannot type it for her. How would you respond to her request?

A married friend of yours had an affair with a man who is registered as a patient at your practice. Their relationship ended acrimoniously and now your friend has heard rumours that this man is HIV-positive. She confides to you that she is worried sick. You suggest that she gets herself tested, but she refuses, saying that she is too scared. She asks you to find out if the rumours are true by checking her ex-lover's medical records.

You discover that one of your colleagues has been gossiping about patients outside the surgery. What should you do about it? Would this person's status in relation to your own have a bearing on how you would act?

You receive a phone call from a patient's employer. He says that he is ringing to confirm that your patient attended for a consultation the previous day. Should you tell him that the patient has not been near the surgery for months?

Appendix 7.2: Risks associated with modern technology

- Mobile and cordless telephones – these use radio waves, and conversations can be overheard.
- Answering machines – place the machine where it cannot be overheard if someone is leaving a message or messages are being played back. Alternatively, turn the volume down. Remember that there may be cleaners and other non-medical personnel in the building after hours.
- Faxes – before faxing personal data, phone the recipient to make sure that someone is there to receive it, and to double-check their fax number. Always use a covering sheet with a confidentiality statement on it that says how many pages are in the fax. When sending the fax, stay with the machine until all of the pages have gone through – do not leave them unattended. If possible, anonymise the information by using the patient's NHS number in place of their name and address.
- Email – do not email confidential information about patients without their consent. Use encryption software. Send a test email to the recipient first to make sure that you have the correct email address. Use patients' NHS numbers rather than their names to identify them.
- Palm-tops – these are fantastic for home visits because you can download patients' records on to them. However, they are very appealing to opportunistic thieves, so please ensure that yours is password-protected and that you never leave it unattended. Treat it like your bag – either carry it on your person or lock it in the boot of your car when you are out and about. It is also a good idea to keep it in a locked drawer when you are in the practice.
- Computerised records – these are dealt with in detail in Chapter 9.

Appendix 7.3: Frequently asked questions

Can I disclose confidential information about a minor (e.g. to a parent) without the child's consent?
Once a child reaches the age of 16 years, you will need their consent before making any disclosures. If the child is under 16 years and is 'Gillick competent' (i.e. understands the implications), you must respect their wishes if they do not want you to disclose information about them, even to a parent.

Can I disclose confidential information to a patient's carer?
You may share sufficient information to enable the carer to provide healthcare for the patient, but no more than is necessary.

What if I suspect that a vulnerable patient (e.g. a child or an elderly person) is being abused or neglected?
You must act in the patient's best interests and bring your concerns to the attention of a person with the appropriate authority to investigate the circumstances. Document your reasons for sharing the information.

If the police ask me for details about a patient, should I tell them?
The police have no general right to confidential patient information. However, if they are investigating a serious crime such as murder, manslaughter, rape or child

molestation, you should provide enough information to help the enquiry. If the patient is at risk (e.g. is depressed and has gone missing), you should act in their best interests, so imparting a certain amount of information may be justified.

Should I tell a patient's partner if I know that they are HIV-positive?
You should do everything you can to encourage the patient to tell their partner. If, however, they refuse, you must then tell them that you have no choice but to do so yourself. Carefully document the salient points of your discussions with the patient.

What should I do if I receive a court order demanding a patient's records?
You must comply with the request. If the notes contain information about a third party, you may ask that these passages be omitted.

What should I do if a patient's employer asks me for details about a patient's illness and prognosis?
You would need the patient's consent before you could comply with the request.

If a patient is unfit to drive, must I report this?
First tell the patient that they are obliged by law to inform the DVLA that they have a medical condition that makes them unfit to drive. If the patient seems unwilling to do this, tell them that you will have no choice but to tell the DVLA yourself.

Do I need to obtain a patient's consent if I am asked to provide their medical records to an independent review panel?
Yes. Even if a patient has made a formal complaint that has led to the independent review panel, you still need to obtain their consent before making the medical records available to the panel.

Do I need a patients' consent before passing their personal details to the cancer registry?
No. The Secretary of State has made a temporary provision under section 60 of the Health and Social Care Act 2003 that allows you to supply this information to the registry.

Am I obliged to comply when a patient's solicitor writes to ask for a copy of the patient's medical records?
Yes, you are, so long as you are satisfied that the solicitor is acting on the patient's behalf.

Chapter 8

Communication and risk

Malcolm Thomas

Key learning points

- Communication between clinician and patient is a source of risk:
  - to the patient in terms of clinical outcomes
  - to the patient in terms of satisfaction
  - to the clinician in terms of being complained about or sued
  - to the clinician in terms of their psychological well-being.
- There is good evidence for all of this.
- We need to be clear which skills clinicians should aim to improve in order to achieve better outcomes in one or more of the above areas.
- Happily, the same suite of skills largely serves to secure improvement in *all* areas of risk – that is, the skills that are required to improve clinical outcomes also improve patient satisfaction, lower medico-legal risk and improve the psychological welfare of clinicians.

Introduction

All clinical risk ultimately arises from consultations between doctors and patients. The risk may arise either during the consultation (e.g. in diagnosis or prescription) or later on, as a consequence of the consultation (e.g. in the referral process or the ordering of investigations). Unsurprisingly, the evidence confirms that the process of the consultation of patients with doctors is a significant contributor to risk. Happily, the evidence also shows us ways to reduce this risk.

This chapter sets out some of the evidence concerning the main areas of risk in consultations, and Chapter 21 looks at some solutions.

Here we shall consider risk under the following four headings (and then look at a couple of special situations):

1 clinical effectiveness (i.e. doing a better job for patients)
2 medico – legal risk (i.e. risk of being complained about or sued)
3 risk to the welfare of the doctor (i.e. risk of burnout or dissatisfaction)
4 special communication situations (i.e. use of chaperones and interpreters).

Clinical effectiveness

Skills

The reporting of studies of effectiveness in relation to individual skills within consultations began in the 1960s. Egbert *et al.*[1] showed that pre-operative information given to patients was associated with less post-operative analgesia and a shorter hospital stay. This was the first study to link a communication behaviour with hard clinical outcomes. Then Korsch and colleagues published two papers[2,3] describing a study of 800 consultations in a paediatric walk-in centre in the USA. They used rigorous methods to link clinician behaviours to patient outcomes, and found increased satisfaction and/or compliance with the doctor's plan if doctors:

- were perceived as warm and friendly
- took patients' concerns and expectations into account
- avoided jargon
- gave clear explanations of *diagnosis* and *causation*.

Korsch and colleagues also discovered the size of the problem of ineffective doctor–patient communication (e.g. at only 24% of consultations was the mother's main worry mentioned to the doctor).

The pace of this research then increased. Byrne and Long[4] studied UK general practice, and the biggest problem they found was in doctors establishing the reason for the patient's attendance.

A study by Beckmann and Frankel[5] found that doctors interrupted patients' opening statements after an average of 18 seconds, whereas the average uninterrupted statement was just over 50 seconds long. Consequently, only a small proportion of opening statements were completed.

The Headache Study Group of Western Ontario[6] reported a prospective study of patients in family practice with a new diagnosis of headache. They found that the patients' perceptions of being able to discuss their headache and related issues fully at the initial consultation were the most important factor in symptom resolution at one year (symptoms were more than three times as likely to be resolved if these issues could be discussed fully at the initial consultation).

By 1995, two informative reviews[7,8] had been published of the evidence that links specific communication skills to 'hard' outcomes – that is, symptom reduction and/or improved physiological status, such as:

- lower blood pressure in patients with hypertension
- lower HbA_{1c} levels in diabetics
- improved functioning in patients with arthritis.

There is now considerable literature confirming these findings in other settings, and also linking evidence of specific communication behaviours and greater rates of the following:

- patient recall of information
- patients following the plan made during the consultation ('compliance' or 'concordance').

Some evidence now available shows the effects of the smallest differences in communication behaviour – that is, substituting single words. Bass and Cohen found that substituting the word 'concern' for 'worry' resulted in one-third of their patients disclosing concerns previously unrecognised by the physician.[9] Stone and colleagues came up with the entertaining concept of 'number needed to offend'[10] in a study of new neurology outpatients. They compared the acceptability to patients of various labels for symptoms that had no immediate medical explanation. In doing so they found that 'functional weakness' was the most acceptable label, rather than 'medically unexplained', with 'psychosomatic' and 'hysterical' predictably most likely to offend.

We also have evidence for the effect of the doctor's non-verbal behaviour on the outcome of the consultation. Many of us will have experienced patients complaining about a colleague along the lines of 'He was writing as I walked in and he never even took his eyes off his notes.' Studies have provided more concrete data on this topic. For example, DiMatteo and colleagues concluded from their study[11] that 'a modest but significant proportion of the variance in patients' satisfaction with their medical care was accounted for by the non-verbal communication of their physicians.'

Stewart and colleagues have recently produced a good overview.[12] The most comprehensive summary of this evidence can be found in *Skills for Communicating with Patients* by the Calgary–Cambridge collaborators.[13] For a far more detailed discussion of this literature, I recommend the reader to refer to this book.

Box 8.1 is a summary of the skill areas highlighted by the research base as being most influential to patient outcomes. A little reflection should convince you that these are in line with common sense. We also have a good idea of which 'microskills' matter within these areas. Chapter 21 addresses how to improve your skills in the most important of these categories. Most of these skills are self-explanatory, but the 'acceptance' response is a specific technique that will be explained in more detail in that chapter.

Box 8.1 Communications skills to improve outcomes for patients

---

- Openings
- Getting the full story, with the patient's perspective
- Demonstrating 'acceptance' and empathy
- Being explicit about the structure of the consultation
- Giving appropriate, timely explanations
- Involving the patient in explanation and planning
- Making an agreed final plan with follow-up and safety net

Models

Over the years a number of models have been proposed in which this evidence is presented in the form of a framework or checklist. Byrne and Long[4] started this, and the Calgary–Cambridge framework is the latest and most comprehensive model.[13]

In the UK we have a history of consultation analysis. Michael and Enid Balint are generally recognised as the originators of this approach.[14] Other highly influential texts include those by Pendleton *et al.*[15] and Neighbour.[16]

In North America, there has been more of an emphasis on promoting learner behaviour change. The *problem-based interviewing* approach, although British, owes its origin to North America.[17] This is a method of working with videotapes that starts with the learner's agenda and focuses on very small areas of skill.

The *four habits model* is another typical example.[18] This again concentrates on skill areas and proposes that one should:

* *invest in the beginning*
* elicit the patient's perspective
* demonstrate empathy
* *invest in the end.*

The Calgary–Cambridge framework[13] can be regarded as a synthesis of these two strands. There are other skills-based frameworks and programmes that are available or which have been published. The essential elements, which have been summarised in the Kalamazoo Consensus Statement,[19] are as follows.

* Build a relationship – the fundamental communication task.
* Open the discussion.
* Gather information.
* Understand the patient's perspective.
* Share information.
* Reach agreement on problems and plans.
* Provide closure.

This list repays study in relation to three fundamental changes that affect medicine everywhere and primary care in the UK in particular, namely:

* the move towards viewing doctor–patient relationships as partnerships[20]
* increasing fragmentation of care – reflected, for example, in the UK by the Government's emphasis on swift access to GPs,[21] which may further threaten continuity of care and make relationship building a matter of urgency in each consultation
* the increasing complexity of care – this is partly due to having older patients who have a greater number of active problems, with more interventions that can be offered. In the UK, there are also external demands on the consultation (e.g. meeting the requirements of the various NSFs and the new GP Contract).[22] The doctor's need to respond to these demands might reduce their attention to the problems with which the patient is presenting.

Medico-legal risk

Overview

The study of medico-legal risk in relation to communication has a shorter history. Much relevant material has been published in the last decade or so. The messages are becoming clearer and are consistent with the literature that links skills to better patient outcomes. The evidence is almost exclusively related to lawsuits, but we cannot find any reason to doubt that the risk of being complained about is subject to the same factors.

Typical of the emerging understanding were the findings of Shapiro et al.,[23] who documented considerable disagreement about the reason for the patient launching a lawsuit between three groups (patients who had sued, doctors who had been sued and doctors who had not been sued). Specifically, while more than 95% of suing patients judged there to have been negligence and/or error, only around 30% of doctors did so. In contrast, more than 50% of all three groups regarded unanticipated adverse outcomes as a major factor, the majority of which were judged to be unavoidable by the doctors.

Around two-thirds of all three groups rated improving doctor–patient communication as a significant factor contributing to future improvement, far more than for any other suggestion.

A very large study published in 1991 confirmed and extended these findings.[24,25] The Harvard Medical Practice Study was set up to determine the rate of significant adverse events in New York City hospitals. This rate was found to be around 4%, of which there was good evidence of negligence in around 25% of cases (i.e. around 1% of the total sample).

The researchers took the opportunity to investigate the link with malpractice lawsuits. It was found that only around one-third of the lawsuits were linked to clearly negligent cases. Another third were linked to cases with an adverse event but no documentation supporting negligence. This left a third of lawsuits started by patients who had not evidently experienced a significant adverse event.

Extrapolating from the sample to the whole of New York City, the researchers estimated that the number of lawsuits represented around 2–3% of the number of likely negligent cases. In other words, if you had been sued it is unlikely that you had made a mistake, and if you had made a mistake, it is unlikely that you had been sued.

A study of obstetricians in Florida[26] produced findings typical of the considerable subsequent literature. In this investigation, obstetricians' claims records for the period 1977–83 were compared with blinded assessment of the technical standard of their care in 1987, as judged by their medical records. On the basis of their claims record, they could be divided into four groups as follows:

- no claims
- one claim
- frequent claims
- high number of claims.

No difference was detected in any objective measure of clinical competence between the groups. *The conclusion from this (and similar) studies has to be that improving the individual technical excellence of doctors is unlikely to be helpful in reducing their risk of being sued.*

Bunting and colleagues have produced a useful summary of the relationship between communication and medico-legal risk.[27] In particular, they refer to the concept of separating the factors leading to a malpractice claim into two groups, namely precipitating and predisposing factors.

Precipitating factors (the technical factors typically targeted in risk management programmes and reported in the press in connection with sued doctors) include the following:

- adverse outcome
- iatrogenesis
- failure to provide adequate care
- mistakes or incorrect care
- system errors.

Predisposing factors are essentially interactional, and include the following:

- rudeness
- delay (especially if unacknowledged)
- inattentiveness
- miscommunication
- apathetic doctor
- no communication.

This review proposes (and our previous references support) the idea that *in the absence of predisposing factors*, a precipitating factor is unlikely to lead to a lawsuit.

Skills

So if two-thirds of all claims have their origin in communication behaviours, which skills keep complaints and lawsuits at bay?

A 1994 study suggests which communication areas to focus on.[28] Beckman and colleagues surveyed the records of malpractice claims made in the 1980s in a city in the USA. They proposed four behaviours that increased risk, namely:

- physician desertion (something went wrong and the doctor was suddenly unavailable)
- devaluing the views of the patient and/or relatives
- delivering information poorly (or not at all)
- failure to understand the perspective of the patient and/or relatives.

The literature now provides insight into the details from both positive and negative studies, three of which cover the ground.[29–31] The skills of malpractice claim prevention are summarised in Box 8.2.

Box 8.2 Communication behaviours to lower medico-legal risk

- Being available (returning phone calls, making and keeping appointments), especially if something has gone wrong
- Giving the perception of sufficient time (which can be done without taking up much extra time, and results from not giving out 'rushed' signals)
- Soliciting and understanding the patient's viewpoint
- Demonstrating empathy
- Demonstrating 'acceptance'
- Explaining the process of the consultation
- Giving explanations that are pitched at the patient's level

Fortunately, this list is compatible with the Kalamazoo Consensus Statement and other such frameworks, while emphasising some skills over others in the context of avoiding lawsuits.

Many doctors who are undergoing training in communication skills complain that useful behaviour change, in line with the above, is not possible without devoting increased time to their consultations. Furthermore, they feel that this is not possible within the constraints of their own particular workplaces.

The literature offers inconsistent guidance here. Some studies indicate that deploying certain skills carries no time penalty, while others show that longer consultations are associated with, for example, more time for patient concerns or more preventive medicine interventions. This literature is well reported in the review by Stewart *et al.*[12]

The only evidence specifically related to medico-legal risk comes from the paper by Levinson and colleagues,[30] which showed that longer primary care consultations were associated with a lower risk of malpractice claims against the doctors.

The following conclusions can be drawn:

- whatever the time you currently have available for your consultations, it can be used more effectively
- increasing the length of consultations *should* produce better outcomes, *but*
- only if the extra time is used effectively, for the deployment of increased communication skills.

Risk to the welfare of the doctor

From the above sections we can see that better outcomes for patients and lower medico-legal risk require a good understanding by the doctor of the patient and his or her perspective. Furthermore, the patient needs to appreciate that the doctor has achieved that understanding.

I trained as a doctor in an environment of 'not getting too involved'. Undoubtedly the motive for this advice was to help doctors to prevent the negative consequences assumed to arise from deeper identification with the patient.

To what extent is this prejudice valid and what remedies are available to deal with this risk to doctors?

There is some evidence that appears to back up the belief about 'not getting involved'. A recent study of new medical graduates in New South Wales, Australia is reported to show that older graduates and women experience more psychological distress on entering the medical workforce.[32] It is speculated that this is related to their more caring attitude.

However, there is apparent contradiction in other studies. For example, Ramirez and colleagues reported that clinicians who felt insufficiently trained in communication skills had a significantly increased rate of 'burnout'.[33] Three studies that reported similar findings, together with other useful material, are referenced in a recently published review.[34]

Closer reading of this evidence suggests that:

- doctors with a 'caring' personality are at increased risk (of 'burnout' and psychological distress)
- possession of better communication skills protects you, whatever your predisposition.

The essence is captured in the notion of the 'bogus' contract outlined by Smith[35] and reproduced in Box 8.3. It will be seen that moving to the new contract requires a redirection of patient expectations. If done well, this should improve outcomes for patients and doctors. This is likely to require enhanced communication skills.

Box 8.3 Doctors and patients: Redefining a bogus contract

The bogus contract: the patient's view
- Modern medicine can do remarkable things – it can solve many of my problems.
- You, the doctor, can see inside me and know what's wrong.
- You know everything it's necessary to know.
- You can solve my problems, even my social problems.
- So we give you high status and a good salary.

The bogus contract: the doctor's view
- Modern medicine has limited powers.
- Worse, it's dangerous.
- We can't begin to solve all problems, especially social ones.
- I don't know everything, but I do know how difficult many things are.
- The balance between doing good and harm is very fine.
- I'd better keep quiet about all this so as not to disappoint my patients and lose my status.

The new contract
Both patients and doctors know the following.
- Death, sickness and pain are part of life.
- Medicine has limited powers, particularly to solve social problems, and it is risky.
- Doctors don't know everything – they need decision-making and psychological support.
- We're in this together.
- Patients can't leave problems to doctors.
- Doctors should be open about their limitations.
- Politicians should refrain from making exaggerated promises and concentrate on reality.

Special communication situations

Chaperones

The issue of the use of chaperones appears at first sight to be straightforward. MPOs recommend the routine use of chaperones for all intimate examinations. On closer inspection, it will be found that turning this into a practical policy will involve some obstacles. The two main ones appear to be resource issues (presence of sufficient time and personnel) and which examinations should be considered 'intimate'. There is also the issue of whether it is in the doctor's or the patient's interest that the chaperone is present.

Studies from general practice in the UK in 1983 and 1993 obtained similar results.[36,37] Around two-thirds of male GPs never or rarely used chaperones during intimate examinations of members of the opposite sex. In the later study, around 95% of female GPs fell into this category. Furthermore, a substantial minority of chaperones were not professionals (i.e. nurses), and 25% of GPs reported using receptionists or other members of the non-clinical office staff.

Typical of the literature from the patient's point of view is a study from the USA,[38] in which the majority of all patient subgroups reported not requiring a chaperone. However, female patients in general, and teenage female patients in particular, reported a preference for a chaperone to be present during intimate examinations. The majority of patients rated a nurse as the appropriate chaperone, but teenagers preferred a family member.

The literature is reviewed in an editorial in the *British Medical Journal*.[39] The only other significant points to emerge are that male patients, especially younger ones, prefer not to have a female nurse present during genital examination, and that the majority of patients in relevant studies rate the presence of a female nurse as an acceptable part of a normal intimate examination, defined as examination of the genitalia, rectum or female breast.

As hinted at above, there are two considerations involved in having a chaperone to assist such examinations, namely the comfort of the patient (which can be both practical and psychological) and the protection of the doctor from allegations of impropriety. These have to mesh with the issue of patient preference. It would hardly be collaborative to impose a chaperone on a consenting patient who declined one.

We cannot better the current GMC guidance[40] as a summary (*see* Box 8.4). We would simply add that female doctors should follow this guidance in the same way as male doctors. The key points are as follows.

- Obtain informed consent for the examination.
- Routinely *offer* a chaperone.
- Bear in mind that some patients, especially younger female ones, will prefer a family member to be present.
- Delay the examination until the optimal conditions have been established, if this is clinically acceptable.
- Do not use office staff. Female nurses will usually be acceptable (but note the above caveat with regard to some (especially younger) male patients).

The guidance of the GMC is in fact in line with the recommendations of the MPOs in the UK.

> **Box 8.4** Intimate examinations: GMC advice (www.gmc-uk.org)
>
> The GMC regularly receives complaints from patients who feel that doctors have behaved inappropriately during an intimate examination. Intimate examinations – that is, examinations of the breast, genitalia or rectum – can be stressful and embarrassing for patients. When conducting intimate examinations you should follow the advice given below.
> * Explain to the patient why an examination is necessary, and give the patient an opportunity to ask questions.
> * Explain what the examination will involve, in a way that the patient can understand, so that they have a clear idea of what to expect, including any potential pain or discomfort (paragraph 13 of our booklet *Seeking Patients' Consent* gives further guidance on presenting information to patients).[40]
> * Obtain the patient's permission before the examination, and be prepared to discontinue the examination if the patient asks you to. You should record that permission has been obtained.
> * Keep the discussion relevant and avoid making unnecessary personal comments.
> * Offer a chaperone or invite the patient (in advance if possible) to have a relative or friend present. If the patient does not want a chaperone, you should record that the offer was made and declined. If a chaperone is present, you should record that fact and make a note of the chaperone's identity. If for justifiable practical reasons you cannot offer a chaperone, you should explain this to the patient and, if possible, offer to delay the examination until a later date. You should record the discussion and its outcome.
> * Give the patient privacy to undress and dress, and use drapes to maintain the patient's dignity. Do not assist the patient in removing clothing unless you have clarified with them that your assistance is required.

The Ayling Inquiry[41] reached similar conclusions and has suggested that trained chaperones be available to patients as widely as possible. This will certainly mean in GP surgeries.

Interpreters

In some ways, the issue of interpreter use mirrors that of chaperones. The counsel of perfection is to have a professional interpreter present in all relevant consultations. In practice, few healthcare organisations have access to the gold standard here, namely instant access to a variety of interpreters of both sexes who will be able to interpret for all the languages seen by the practice and who will also be culturally acceptable to the patients!

In the absence of this, let us see what the evidence shows and look for guidance. Trained interpreters are assumed to represent the gold standard. At best, with good training, they can provide the service of a confidential and accurate broker between doctor and patient. However, this relationship should not be assumed to be problem-free. A letter from Brafman reports a powerful anecdote in which the interpreter's prejudices were unhelpful.[42]

Conversely, it is often assumed that translation by family members is more problematic. Certainly it is reasonable to assume that a family member in the role of translator might have other motives in relation to their relative. This would be encountered in its most extreme form in the case of a husband translating for a wife who was the victim of his (domestic) violence.

Nevertheless, there are advantages to the use of relatives. First, they might know the patient well enough to contribute that perspective in the consultation. Secondly, this type of interpreter is often the most readily available. A recent qualitative study researched the views of young family members who had been used as interpreters.[43] This situation was chosen by the patients a significant proportion of the time. A perceived advantage was the opportunity for the young person to take on a responsible role for the family. It was found that poor communication by the doctors with the young interpreters was a factor leading to dissatisfaction some of the time. In particular, the doctor not looking at the young interpreter while talking or listening to him or her was rated very poorly.

A useful summary of the issues can be found in an article in the *British Medical Journal* from 1995.[44] This is a useful practical guide, and we recommend it to any reader looking for more detail. The main advantages and disadvantages of each type of interpreter were considered to be as follows:

- bilingual healthcare workers – ideal but rare
- trained interpreters – practically the ideal; good quality training is important. The issue of their personal prejudices is mentioned above
- friends or relatives – practically the most available. They are untrained and may possess variable skill in either the doctor's or the patient's language (or both!). They are considered to be more likely to have their own agenda in relation to the patient (and this could potentially be harmful; see above)
- untrained volunteers – less reliable than trained interpreters, but perhaps superior to family members, certainly in the case of the doctor who is harbouring doubt about relatives' motives.

Finally, we should remember that modest social fluency on behalf of a patient could mask a significant inability to follow the discourse of a medical consultation. If the doctor suspects this, an offer of an interpreter would seem appropriate.

The rule of consent applies again, with the following practical advice.

- Offer an interpreter in cases where this is judged to be necessary.
- Use bilingual professionals or trained interpreters if possible.
- Do not belittle family members in the interpreting role.
- In any event, treat all interpreters well. Pay attention to them when they are speaking and when you are addressing them.
- Be alert for the interpreter's own agenda, whether or not this person is a relative.

Summary

The evidence described above shows the scale of the communication task in doctor–patient encounters. We shall look at solutions in Chapter 21. Ian Kennedy chaired the public inquiry into paediatric cardiac surgery at the Bristol Royal Infirmary, and is Chair of the Healthcare Commission. A quote from him sums up the agenda as we see it:

> A mature culture will settle on sharing power and responsibility (*between doctors and patients*), on a subtle negotiation between professional and patient as to what each wants and what the other can deliver. This is the culture which we should work towards – helping each other as we go.[20]

References

1 Egbert LD, Batitt GE, Welch CE *et al.* (1964) Reduction of postoperative pain by encouragement and instruction of patients. *NEJM.* **270:** 825–7.

2 Korsch BM, Gozzi EK and Francis V (1968) Gaps in doctor–patient communication. *Pediatrics.* **42:** 855–71.

3 Francis V, Korsch B and Morris M (1969) Gaps in doctor–patient communication. *NEJM.* **280:** 535–40.

4 Byrne PS and Long BEL (1976) *Doctors Talking to Patients.* HMSO, London.

5 Beckman HB and Frankel RM (1984) The effect of physician behaviour on the collection of data. *Ann Intern Med.* **101:** 692–6.

6 The Headache Study Group of the University of Western Ontario (1986) Predictors of outcome in headache patients presenting to family physicians – a one-year prospective study. *Headache J.* **26:** 285–94.

7 Kaplan SH, Greenfield S and Ware JE (1989) Assessing the effects of physician–patient interactions on the outcomes of chronic disease. *Med Care.* **27:** S110–27.

8 Stewart MA, Belle Brown J, Wayne Weston W *et al.* (1995) *Patient-Centred Medicine: transforming the clinical method.* Sage, Thousand Oaks, CA.

9 Bass LW and Cohen RL (1982) Ostensible versus actual reasons for seeking pediatric attention: another look at the parental ticket of admission. *Pediatrics.* **70:** 870–4.

10 Stone J, Wojcik W, Durrance D *et al.* (2002) What should we say to patients with symptoms unexplained by disease? The 'number needed to offend'. *BMJ.* **325:** 1449–50.

11 DiMatteo RM, Taranta A, Friedman HS and Prince LM (1980) Predicting patient satisfaction from physicians' nonverbal communication skills. *Med Care.* **18:** 376–87.

12 Stewart M, Belle Brown J, Boon H *et al.* (1999) Evidence on patient–doctor communication. *Cancer Prev Control.* **3:** 25–30.

13 Silverman J, Kurtz S and Draper J (1998) *Skills for Communicating with Patients.* Radcliffe Medical Press, Oxford.

14 Balint M (1974) *The Doctor, his Patient and the Illness* (2e). Pitman Medical, London.

15 Pendleton D, Schofield T, Tate P *et al.* (1984) *The Consultation: an approach to learning and teaching.* Oxford University Press, Oxford.

16 Neighbour R (1987) *The Inner Consultation.* MTP Press. Dordrecht.

17 Gask L, Boardman J and Goldberg D (1991) Teaching communication skills: a problem-based approach. *Postgrad Educ Gen Pract.* **2:** 7–15.

18 Frankel RM and Stein T (2001) Getting the most out of the clinical encounter: the four habits model. *J Med Pract Manage.* **16**(4): 184–91.

19 Participants in the Bayer–Fetzer Conference on Physician–Patient Communication in Medical Education (2001) Essential elements of communication in medical encounters: the Kalamazoo Consensus Statement. *Acad Med.* **76:** 390–3.

20 Kennedy I (2003) Patients are experts in their own field. *BMJ.* **326:** 1276.

21 www.doh.gov.uk/pricare/improvedaccess.htm

22 www.doh.gov.uk/nsf

23 Shapiro RS, Simpson DE, Lawrence SL *et al.* (1989) A survey of sued and nonsued physicians and suing patients. *Arch Intern Med.* **149:** 2190–6.

24 Brennan TA, Leape LL, Laird NM *et al.* (1991) Incidence of adverse events and negligence in hospitalized patients: results of the Harvard Medical Practice Study I. *NEJM.* **324:** 370–6.

25 Localio AR, Lawthers AG, Brennan TA *et al.* (1991) Relationship between malpractice claims and adverse events due to negligence: results of the Harvard Medical Practice Study III. *NEJM.* **325:** 245–51.

26 Entmann SS, Glass CA, Hickson GB *et al.* (1994) The relationship between malpractice claims history and subsequent obstetric care. *JAMA.* **272:** 1588–91.

27 Bunting RF Jr, Benton J and Morgan WD (1998) Practical risk management principles for physicians. *J Healthcare Risk Manage.* **18:** 29–53.

28 Beckman HB, Markakis KM, Suchman AL and Frankel RM (1994) The doctor–patient relationship and malpractice. *Arch Intern Med.* **154:** 1365–70.

29 Hickson GB, Wright Clayton E, Entman SS *et al.* (1994) Obstetricians' prior malpractice experience and patients' satisfaction with care. *JAMA.* **272:** 1583–7.

30 Levinson W, Roter DL, Mullooly JP *et al.* (1997) Physician–patient communication: the relationship with malpractice claims among primary care physicians and surgeons. *JAMA* **277:** 553–9.

31 Mercer SW and Reynolds WJ (2002) Empathy and quality of care. *Br J Gen Pract.* **52(Suppl.):** S9–12.

32 Sweet M (2003) Being a caring doctor may be bad for you. *BMJ.* **326:** 355.

33 Ramirez AJ, Graham J, Richards MA *et al.* (1995) Burnout and psychiatric disorder amongst cancer clinicians. *Br J Cancer.* **71:** 1132–3.

34 Maguire P and Pitceathly C (2002) Key communication skills and how to acquire them. *BMJ.* **325:** 697–700.

35 Smith R (2001) Why are doctors so unhappy? *BMJ.* **322:** 1073–4.

36 Jones RH (1983) The use of chaperones by general practitioners. *J R Coll Gen Pract.* **33:** 25–6.

37 Speelman A, Savage J and Verburgh M (1993) Use of chaperones by general practitioners. *BMJ.* **307:** 986–7.

38 Penn MA and Bourguet CC (1992) Patients' attitudes regarding chaperones during physical examinations. *J Fam Pract.* **35:** 639–43.

39 Bignell CJ (1999) Chaperones for genital examination. *BMJ.* **319:** 137–8.

40 www.gmc-uk.org

41 Ayling Inquiry (2004) *Independent investigation into how the NHS handled allegations about the conduct of Clifford Ayling.* Chaired by Mrs Justice Pauffley. HMSO, London.

42 Brafman AH (1995) Beware of the distorting interpreter. *BMJ.* **311:** 1439.

43 Free C, Green J, Bhavnani V and Newman A (2003) Bilingual young people's experiences of interpreting in primary care: a qualitative study. *Br J Gen Pract.* **53:** 530–5.

44 Phelan M and Parkman S (1995) How to do it: work with an interpreter. *BMJ.* **311:** 555–7.

Chapter 9

The medical record in the electronic age

Nigel Watson

Key learning points

- The NHS increasingly uses computerised medical records as the sole source of clinical data relating to patients.
- GPs need to be aware of information technology (IT) developments in the NHS. If a practice does not develop the use of computers now, there will be a lot of catching up to do later.
- Good record keeping (written or computerised) is an essential component of safe medical care.
- There are risks with both written and electronic records.
- These risks can be reduced by using common sense, vigilance and some knowledge of the relevant law.
- There are proven benefits to electronic medical records.
- Careful planning is needed when moving from a paper-based to a computerised medical record system.
- Passwords need to be used by all members of staff, they should be unique to the individual and must be changed regularly.
- Breach of the Data Protection Act 1998 is a criminal offence. The Act covers manual *and* electronic records. All practices must have up-to-date registration.
- Email consultations are a risky substitute for face-to-face consultations.

The medical record in the electronic age

The use of computers in healthcare is not new (it has been around for some 20 years). However, it is only in the last five years that the NHS has introduced a more structured development process to try to secure the potential benefits that information technology offers.

Although information used in this chapter has been taken from documents produced by the General Practitioners Committee (GPC) and Local Medical Committees (LMCs), they reflect the author's views and do not necessarily reflect all the views of LMCs or the GPC.

Information for Health,[1] published in 1998, was the first major information strategy within the NHS to be introduced since the early 1990s. This was an attempt to focus IT use on clinical practice rather than merely using IT as an administrative or management tool. The document outlined the strategic direction for IT developments from 1998 to 2005.

In 2001, *Building the Information Core*[2] set out in detail the proposed implementation of NHS IT infrastructure and development, bringing together two major policy documents, *Information for Health*[1] and the *NHS Plan*.[3]

These policy documents indicated a direction of travel. A number of issues were raised and not resolved, many of which are addressed in this chapter.

High-quality medical records are important in providing a good standard of healthcare for patients. In the past, records were often kept by each professional group with little or no sharing of information. Medical records are now increasingly multi-professional, and this is of benefit to the patient.

Guidance written for doctors by the GMC in *Good Medical Practice*[4] states that 'medical records should be clear, accurate, legible and contemporaneous patient records that report the relevant clinical findings, the decisions made, the information given to patients and any drugs or other treatments prescribed'. This guidance also states that the medical records must keep colleagues well informed when sharing the care of a patient.

When faced with a serious complaint or litigation, many doctors wish that they had made more complete records. Complaints can be difficult to deal with when records are incomplete. Similarly, the successful defence of a claim may be seriously hampered by records that are illegible, inaccurate or incomplete (or indeed missing altogether).

It is essential therefore that doctors keep medical records to a high standard with complete information, both for the benefit of patient care and also to protect themselves.

What should good medical records contain?

The GMC guidance[4] is supplemented by that of the BMA[5] and the MPS.[6]

Good medical records should allow another medical practitioner to make a clear reconstruction of a consultation. They should be recorded in a logical way, whether they are written or computerised records.

The records should include the following:

- *history* – a summary of why the patient has presented, including details of symptoms, timescales, associated illnesses, allergies and relevant social history
- *examination* – record any important findings, both positive and negative. *Always* record details of measurements (e.g. 'blood pressure 140/80', *not* 'blood pressure normal')
- *diagnosis* – not only should a clear record of a diagnosis be made if possible, but also a record of how the diagnosis was reached. If several differential diagnoses are considered, record these and demonstrate why any were excluded
- *investigations* – record any that have been requested
- *patient information* – record what information has been given to the patient, including patient information leaflets. Any medical treatment of patients has risks and benefits, and these should be not only discussed with the patient but

also recorded. This is also relevant to the consent process, which is discussed in Chapter 12.

Some authorities also suggest recording the following:

1 when a patient has *declined information*
2 *specific questions asked by the patient* and the answers given

- *treatment* – it is essential to record specific details about treatment(s) recommended and, if this involves medication, details of dose, duration of treatment, and any advice or warning given about the treatment.

    It is also important to record any treatment that has been offered but declined

- *follow-up arrangements* – these include future appointments, follow-up investigations and any referrals made.

Occasionally every healthcare professional will have a consultation with a patient that does not go 'according to plan'. This can be due to a multitude of reasons, and may not necessarily be any one individual's fault. In these circumstances, it is important if at all possible to resolve any problems within the consultation. It is essential to record the consultation accurately, including details of any problems encountered and what attempts were made to resolve these.

Consider discussing the issues raised immediately with a colleague or, if appropriate, with the LMC or MPO. It may be useful to discuss these events at a significant event meeting. In these circumstances, consideration should be given to writing to the patient, setting out the issues and, on a positive note, discussing how these can be resolved. Never write a letter in anger. If this is done, always wait 24 hours, read the letter again and show it to a trusted colleague for an opinion before sending it.

Remember that a *telephone conversation* with a patient about their health is a consultation. The only thing that this consultation lacks is a physical examination – in all other respects it is as a face-to-face consultation would be. Therefore a comprehensive record of the consultation should be made as would be done for a face-to-face consultation.

Risks associated with written records

It is always interesting to review written medical notes and to see the different styles of keeping records. Very few would stand up to scrutiny as being comprehensive and complete.

Problems commonly seen in medical records, from the experience of both the author and the MPOs, include the following:

- poor handwriting and therefore illegible notes
- incomplete records (e.g. T Rx penv – it is assumed that the patient has tonsillitis and that a course of penicillin V has been prescribed, but this record would not be deemed acceptable by any professional body)
- lost records – It is common in both hospital and general practice for written records to go missing, and if there is no back-up copy these records are sometimes permanently lost.

Risks associated with electronic records

Some risks are the same as for written records (e.g. over-use of abbreviations or incomplete records), but computerisation has introduced a number of new risks.

- There has been much concern expressed that computerised records would be less comprehensive and contain more abbreviations. It is fair to say that the jury is still out on this issue. One recent study identified that paperless records compared favourably with manual records, with more paperless records being fully understandable and fully legible.[7] Yet another recent study concluded that the quality of individual consultation recording is highest in paper-only systems.[8]
- Misuse of codes – 'Read codes' are a clinical coding system that is used extensively in computerised health records to provide structure and allow complicated searches for specified codes. For example, a code for 'angina pectoris' could be added to a computerised medical record as a diagnosis, and if a practice patient database is searched for all patients with angina pectoris, this patient will be found. Consider the implications if a qualifying free-text entry of 'excluded' is made. The person making the record will believe that the diagnosis of angina has been excluded, but a search of all patients with angina pectoris will still detect this patient.

Benefits of electronic records

The benefits of electronic medical records could justify a whole chapter (or even a book). Here are just some of them.

Electronic medical records are legible and should be accurate. They are:

- safe, if basic advice is followed
- available when required
- rapidly retrieved
- readily analysed for audit, research and quality assurance.

Other potential benefits include the following:

- convenience
- integration of care – allowing multi-professional access to common clinical data
- improving clinical outcomes
- protection of privacy
- reinforcement of confidentiality
- accommodated decision support, such as the use of templates and PRODIGY
- they allow automatic reports
- they support email generation and electronic data interchange (EDI)
- they enable record transfer between healthcare professionals – GP–GP transfer of a patient's complete medical record should be available from 2004
- they enable record access where and when required
- they support selective retrieval of information
- they support CPD
- they can provide a comprehensive audit trail.

The real benefit is the development of an electronic health record (electronic patient record). It is estimated that up to 25% of a healthcare professional's time is spent either trying to access data held somewhere else in the NHS, or adding data to a medical record that is already available somewhere else.[1]

The potential benefits of electronic records are time saving and greater efficiency from less duplication and, in addition, greater sharing of information with a more comprehensive individual medical record.

The potential benefits to society are that research and meaningful audit are significantly easier to carry out, supporting 'evidence-based medicine'.

What is an electronic health record (EHR) and electronic patient record (EPR)

An *EHR* is defined as a lifelong patient health record.

An *EPR* is defined as a record to support clinical care through information management and technology. The EPR has six levels.

- *Level 1*. Clinical administrative data – this includes patient administration systems and independent department systems.
- *Level 2*. Integrated clinical diagnosis and treatment support – this allows a department to integrate in order to produce a common master index.
- *Level 3*. Clinical activity support – this is for everyday use by doctors and nurses, and it includes electronic test results, discharge letters, prescribing and care planning.
- *Level 4*. Clinical knowledge and decision support – this provides access to knowledge bases, embedded guidelines and electronic alert.
- *Level 5*. Information held on computer instead of paper – this would involve holding all information on computer, including X-rays, etc.
- *Level 6*. Telemedicine and multimedia – this would involve high-speed networks and multimedia for the benefit of patient care.

Potential risks and problems of dual systems

During the natural progression from using written clinical records to using electronic clinical records, records are kept in both the written and electronic format. For many who have made this journey, the period when dual records are being kept carries the *greatest risk.*

Time is crucial during a consultation, and the clinician has to make maximum use of it. Frequently in this situation when dual systems are being used, the information is inadequately recorded in both places to form a comprehensive record of the consultation. Another difficulty that is sometimes experienced in this situation is that one clinician records the clinical information in the written records almost exclusively, and the other uses the electronic records exclusively. Because medical care in general practice relies heavily on access to a comprehensive clinical record, difficulty is caused either by information not being recorded, or because two records need to be examined in order to obtain a comprehensive picture.

How to move to a paper-light system

Paperless systems were considered the ideal, but the reality is that the paper never disappears altogether and, realistically, 'paper-light' is a more accurate description.

The number of practices that believe they can reject the electronic clinical record and maintain solely written clinical records has decreased significantly over the last 10 years. The Department of Health conducted a survey in 2001 and concluded that over 99% of all GP practices in the UK had some form of computerised health record.

The NHS Executive announced in October 2000[9] that GPs were going to be permitted to maintain part or all of their patient medical records on a computer system. Prior to this date many GPs were doing exactly this and breaching their 'Terms of Service',[10] which required GPs to maintain patient medical records on specified paper. A change in the 'Terms of Service' was introduced and amendments were made to the regulations governing GP working in Personal Medical Services (PMS).

Health authorities were instructed to approve all requests for GPs to maintain EPRs if the following conditions were met.

1   The clinical computer system on which the EPRs were to be maintained must conform at least to the standards set out in *Requirements for Accreditation (RFA 99)*.[11]
2   The GP was aware of, and signed, an undertaking to have regard to the guidelines contained in the *Good Practice Guidelines for General Practice Electronic Patient Records*.[12]

The British Medical Association and the Royal College of General Practitioners produced Version 1 of the guidelines jointly in August 2000. Version 3 was published in September 2003, and is available on the website of the Primary Care Information Modernisation Programme.[13]

These guidelines cover the following:

• hardware requirements
• electronic record requirements
• security
• confidentiality
• training.

First steps to a paper-light surgery

Central processing unit (CPU) or clinical server

The essential part of any computer network is the CPU, sometimes called the 'server'. It is important that this has a fast processor, and also that it has sufficient capacity in terms of both hard disk and random-access memory (RAM). Generally it will need replacing every 3 to 4 years to ensure this.

In some practices the server is on site, while in others it is off site and managed by a third party.

The server must be protected by an uninterruptible power source (UPS) to provide protection in the event of power cuts or surges. All data must be backed up regularly, preferably daily (with the back-up being verified regularly to ensure that the process is working). The back-up tape (or equivalent) must be stored either off site in a secure place or, if it is stored in the practice, it must be placed in a fireproof safe.

The proposed back-up schedule is as follows.

- Perform back-up daily from Monday to Thursday, and store the back-up in a fireproof safe in the surgery.
- On Friday the back-up tape is taken off site and stored for 4 weeks.
- The first tape of the month is taken off site and should be kept for 6 months.
- Sufficient tapes, with spares, should be available to perform the agreed schedule.

Central servers

Some practices have moved away from having a server in the practice to having a 'central server' that is looked after by a third party at a different location. The third party maintains the server and ensures that regular back-ups are made. Most have a system whereby if the server 'crashes' then another will immediately take over. The third party adds all upgrades. This system is particularly attractive in situations where there is little or no IT expertise within the practice. Clear and robust contractual arrangements are needed to ensure quality control, etc.

The GPC of the British Medical Association (BMA) has produced some excellent guidance on 'central servers'.[14]

Many PCOs have been keen to perform this task on behalf of practices.

If a PCO hosts a practice's server, it should be understood that data should only be accessed by relevant practice staff. The following legislation applies:

- Data Protection Act 1998
- Access to Medical Records Act 1990.

Under the latter act, GPs are the custodians of the record. If they allowed PCTs to have access to named patient data, there is a good argument that this would breach the provisions of the act.

Local area network (LAN)

If one is not already in place, the practice will need to connect all computers via an LAN. This will require daily management and also a maintenance agreement allowing for rapid resolution of any problems. Workstations need to be positioned in places where staff will need access to the patient's EPR. Consideration must be given to protecting patient confidentiality (i.e. a workstation should not be placed in a position where it could be viewed by a third party). Printers are required for prescriptions, letters, patient information and reports. Increasingly, practices are using dual bin printers in consulting rooms (allowing prescriptions and plain paper to be printed without having to change the paper). Networked printers are useful, where several computers can share a printer. This can be cost-effective, allowing expensive and sophisticated printers to be used.

Agreed practice requirements for data entry

Currently, general practice uses a system of clinical codes called 'Read codes', which are essential to allow sharing of information between two computers. This is becoming increasingly important as EPRs are transmitted via NHSnet between two practices that use different computer systems.

All members of staff who are entering clinical data need to have an understanding of clinical coding.

Read codes

These include symptom codes (e.g. 'chest pain') and diagnostic codes (e.g. 'angina pectoris'). It is essential that if a patient has chest pain, prior to a diagnosis being made a symptom code should be used.

Doctors in some practices immediately add the code for angina and add free text *after* this. If the patient is subsequently found to have had indigestion, the free text is amended to 'not proven, indigestion'. If the diagnostic code for 'angina' has been used, this is now in error. If the symptom code for chest pain has been correctly used at the beginning and it is subsequently shown that the patient *does* have angina, then this diagnostic code should be added at that time.

The importance of the above will be apparent when the practice database is searched for patients with angina pectoris. The patient with the symptom code with the diagnosis in free text will not be identified, but the patient with a diagnostic code of angina with the free text of 'not proven, indigestion' will be identified as suffering from angina. This mistake will start to cost practices money following the introduction of the new GMS Contract in April 2004, whereby the quality and outcome framework will reward practices for delivering high-quality care. Incorrect coding will lead to incorrect data, and this will mean that targets are not met.

It is a useful exercise to look at key clinical areas such as coronary heart disease, and to agree on a standard set of codes to be used within the practice.

Essential steps for moving to EPRs

- Read the *Good Practice Guidelines for General Practice Electronic Patient Records.*
- Obtain the agreement of all GPs prior to the move. It only takes one who will not use EPRs to stop an effective migration.
- Discuss the migration from paper records to electronic records with the LMC and the PCO.
- Produce a practice plan and share this with the PCO.
- Identify additional resources that will be required and ensure that they are met by the PCO.
- Submit a formal application to move to EPRs to the PCO.

The migration needs to be planned and staged with clear written targets to be achieved before moving on.

The migration path should include the following.

- Register under the Data Protection Act – ensure the correct registration for keeping clinical records on computer.
- Inform the patients that the practice is moving from paper-based records to an electronic-based system (this is a requirement under the Data Protection Act).
- Use registration links to allow all registration details of patients to be exchanged electronically between the practice and the primary care organisation (now nearly 100% in the UK and Northern Ireland).
- Use item-of-service links.
- Use pathology links to enable the practice to receive pathology results electronically.
- Make all repeat prescribing electronic.
- Computerise all acute prescribing during a surgery consultation.
- Ensure that all prescribing during a home visit or out of hours is recorded on the EPR.
- Make the appointment system computer based.
- Add cervical cytology results to the EPR, with recall dates.
- Add vaccination and immunisation records to the EPR, with recall dates.
- Add all clinical measurements (e.g. heights, weights, body mass index (BMI), blood pressures) to the EPR.
- Add radiological investigations transmitted from hospital to the practice to the EPR.
- Add summaries of previous paper records to the EPR.
- Add disease-specific or chronic disease management data to the EPR.
- Add part of the consultation recorded electronically to the EPR.
- Record all of the consultation on the EPR.
- Add details of home visits to the EPR.
- Consider the use of associated electronic information sources and decision-support software.

The process described above would take a practice with little computerisation around two years to complete. If all GPs are not signed up to the process, it will be extremely difficult to make it succeed. To ensure that this process occurs seamlessly, it is essential to develop a comprehensive training programme that includes all individuals' needs.

Passwords

All clinical software programs require the entry of a unique identifier with an associated individual password. The password has many different functions.

- It limits access to authorised individuals only.
- It allows for different levels of access to information depending on the individual. For example, a medical practitioner may have access to all clinical information, but administrative staff may only have restricted access.
- The password identifies the individual who is accessing, altering or adding to the computerised medical records.

It is therefore essential that all members of staff have individual passwords, and that these are kept confidential and not shared by others. If temporary members of staff are employed (e.g. a sessional GP), they must be given an individual password and not be allowed to use another GP's password (which would record all entries as being made by the wrong person). This has significant medico-legal implications.

Passwords should be changed on a regular basis. Most clinical systems are programmed to make this happen automatically every 1–3 months.

When choosing a password try to avoid using your name, initials or date of birth. Many programs now require a mixture of characters and numbers – this makes it more difficult for the average person to guess a password.

Finally, do not allow another member of the practice staff to work at your terminal when you are the person logged on.

Encryption

Doctors have a duty to ensure that any information given to them by patients is kept securely and not shared with any person who is not entitled to access to it. The majority of information that is exchanged electronically (i.e. over the Internet or NHSnet) is handled by a third party during transmission and storage. The person who is sending and receiving the information has no control over who the third party might be or where this information is stored. It is therefore impossible to be certain that the information is being handled securely at all times and in all places during transmission from sender to receiver. BMA advice is that no patient-identifiable data should be transmitted over the Internet or NHSnet unless the message is encrypted.

Encryption is a method by which a message is 'scrambled' into a format that cannot be read. It is sent in this secure format and the receiver is then able to 'unscramble' the message. Although encryption has been BMA policy since the mid-1990s, it has only been with the advent of NHSmail that encryption has become widely available. It is now the case that any message sent between two NHSmail accounts is encrypted.

As part of the ongoing development of IT, hospitals are increasingly being 'connected' to general practices in order to allow the exchange of patient information electronically (e.g. pathology messaging, X-ray results, discharge summaries). This is to be encouraged, but only once a system is in place to ensure that the information can be transferred in a secure manner. At the moment, in many practices this is a source of risk with regard to loss of confidentiality.

If encryption is not available, any doctor who wishes to send patient information electronically can only do so with the patients' explicit and informed consent.

Online GP booking is now becoming widely available and is one of the IT targets of the NHS. This is being expanded in many sites to include online referrals. Many of the pilots use web-based technology. This essentially means that the GP accesses a 'server' in the hospital and then exchanges specific patient information. This alone is not secure, and is similar to accessing web-sites on the Internet. It can be made secure by using tools such as *secure socket layers (SSLs)*. When a secure website is accessed, a small padlock appears on the web browser. If you see this symbol, it usually indicates an SSL.

The advice that is provided may be flawed. For example, a hospital may tell a practice that this security is not necessary. If this occurs, consult the national policy of the National Health Service Information Authority (NHSIA).

Data Protection Act

The Data Protection Act 1998 came into effect on 1 March 2000 and replaced the 1984 Act.

Box 9.1 Summary of changes to the Data Protection Act

- Eight basic principles laid down in the 1984 Act have been revised and updated.
- The 1984 Act only covered computerised records, and the 1998 Act has been widened to cover both manual and computerised records.
- Safeguards have been introduced to cover the processing of sensitive data (e.g. ethnic origin, trade union membership and health). Thus storing on an individual's manual or computerised medical record that they are Roman Catholic, a member of the BMA (i.e. a trade union) and are heterosexual in poor health would be a breach of the 1998 Act unless the explicit and informed consent of the individual was obtained before storing and/or processing this data.

Failure to comply with the Data Protection Act is a criminal offence and is therefore subject to greater sanctions if an individual is found to have breached it.

Some practical advice for GPs and practices

- Ensure that the practice is registered under the Data Protection Act and that this registration is kept up to date.
- Any change in circumstances within the practice must be reflected in the registration.
- All doctors, nurses and practice staff should be made aware of the Data Protection Act 1998.
- All doctors, nurses and practice staff should be made aware that under the 1998 Act:
  - compensation may be paid to the data subject (i.e. the patient) if unlawful disclosure of information covered under the Act has occurred
  - data subjects have the right to view data that is held on them in both manual and computerised formats
  - data subjects have the right to have proven inaccurate or incorrect information about them corrected.
- All members of staff who have legitimate access to medical records must have an individual password so that any data entry or alteration can be attributed to an individual.

- Passwords should be changed regularly, at least every 3 months.
- All members of staff must sign a confidentiality agreement, and the Data Protection Act should be adhered to.
- Visual display units (VDUs) should be positioned so that members of the general public cannot view them accidentally.
- When leaving a computer unattended, make sure that the screen is secure – either log out of the patient's notes or activate the password-protected screensaver.
- When disposing of an old computer with patient information on the hard disk, do not assume that simply erasing files or formatting the disk will remove all files. An expert will still be able to access them. The only secure method is to destroy the hard disk with a hammer!
- If printouts of patient data are no longer needed, they must be shredded.

The practice should include a statement about the Data Protection Act in its practice leaflet and also on a prominent noticeboard in the patient waiting room.

Keep the information simple and easy to understand (*see* Box 9.2 for an example).

Box 9.2 Information to patients about the Data Protection Act 1998

Doctors and nurses in this practice use a computer to store all clinical information.

Practice staff use a computer and have access to clinical information only when required to perform their duties, for example when:

- issuing prescriptions
- making appointments
- adding clinical results to patient records
- typing referral letters to the hospital.

The practice is involved in teaching medical students and newly qualified doctors. Access to clinical information will be restricted to that which is essential.

The practice is involved in a number of research projects. Any clinical information supplied will be made anonymous wherever possible. Data required that could identify you will only be made available with your consent, which will be obtained prior to this information being used.

The Data Protection Act is poorly understood by many practices, and there is little case law involving general practice at present. It is well worth all practices reviewing their procedures on a regular basis to ensure that they comply with the Act. No one would want their practice to be the one to be the test case that makes case law in this area.

Email consultations: consulting in the modern world

Until recently a consultation usually meant a face-to-face meeting with a healthcare professional. During a consultation, the healthcare professional would take a clinical history and be able to examine the patient in order to make a full assessment of him or her.

The majority of consultations are face to face. However, consideration must be given to:

- telephone consultations
- telemedicine
- consultations via computer.

Telemedicine

Telemedicine is used to describe two distinct forms of consultation:

- real-time consultations
- delayed real-time consultations.

Real-time telemedicine is a live consultation where the healthcare professional and patient are communicating via a live audiovisual link. The quality of this consultation is directly related to the sophistication of the equipment used, both in terms of cameras and in terms of the speed of the Internet connection.

This form of consultation does not replace face-to-face consultations, and it has limitations (e.g. the healthcare professional is unable to examine the patient). However, it does have great benefits when remote areas need access to medical advice, and it has advantages over a telephone consultation.

'Delayed real-time' consultations allow a visual image to be transmitted electronically to a healthcare professional. Examples of this would be a digital picture of a rash transmitted to a dermatologist, or an audiovisual recording of an echocardiogram transmitted to a cardiologist.

Although this type of consultation was introduced with great enthusiasm, it has not expanded to the level that was initially predicted.

Consultations via computer

Live online consultations are those in which the healthcare professional and the patient are using a real-time electronic link. This form of consultation is limited to the exchange of text messages – in effect a personal medical chatroom. It has proved to be very useful in the outback of Australia, but there seems to be little benefit to be gained in the UK.

Text exchange of information is severely limited in capturing both the breadth and the depth of a consultation. Much can be deduced from speech – not just the words, but also in intonations and emphasis on certain words. In addition, text exchange is usually much slower than the spoken word.

Email consultations provide an exchange of text messages that are not live. Increasingly patients are discovering that each GP has a unique email address, and are attempting to bypass routine face-to-face consultations via this method. It is clear that there may be long delays in a healthcare professional accessing their emails due to holidays, etc. *Therefore this form of consultation should only be used for factual queries.* Guidance should perhaps be given to patients with regard to the nature and purpose (if any) of email consultation in a particular practice.

> Time-delayed email consultations are not safe enough for consultations. Providing authentication, security, interrogation and non-repudiation concerns are satisfied, they may be used for low-level, non-clinical communications with patients.[15]

Scanning of records and subsequent destruction of the original paper record

Many practices have struggled with the issues relating to scanning of documents, and also whether the original paper record can be destroyed once it has been scanned. There is a lack of definitive guidance, and sometimes conflicting advice is obtained from different sources.

Scanning of the record

Many organisations are finding the increase in paper records for storage a major problem. One method of dealing with this is to scan the image of the document in a format that can be stored electronically and retrieved easily.

The scanned document must be in a format that provides a 'photographic image' of the original which cannot be edited (the current acceptable format is TIFF 4 (Tag Image File Format) or the equivalent). Although it is possible to scan a document and then edit it before saving, this should not be done for storage of patient data.

The scanned recorded data must be stored safely and confidentially both in terms of access and also by providing regular back-up of the scanned documents. Reproduction to a high quality is essential, especially for medico-legal purposes.

Destruction of paper records once they have been scanned

The general advice given in the past has been to retain all medical records and not to destroy anything. In fact, some hospitals even have the policy that all 'Post-It'® notes which include patient information need to be retained.

Under their former 'Terms of Service' (TOS),[10] GPs were not prevented from shredding paper originals once they had been scanned into a computer.

GPs are required to send a full copy of a patient's records if that patient moves to a new practice. This would include a copy of the scanned document. So long as this is done, a GP will be deemed to have complied with his or her TOS requirements, as well as ensuring that a full medical record is transmitted for the benefit of the patient.

So what is the problem with shredding the original paper document?

- This is a legal problem rather than a medical one.
- Electronic records may not be admissible in court.

- The judge who is presiding over the case in which the record is required has to make that decision.
- However, it is increasingly the case that an unalterable electronic image is acceptable.
- Forensic tests on records (e.g. handwriting) cannot be performed on the electronic version or a printed copy, but can only be carried out on the original.
- Most correspondence is typed, and therefore the benefits of forensic tests are probably less. An exception to this is if a GP annotates the paper document with instructions, etc.

If a practice wishes to scan documents and shred the original paper documents, the following steps should be taken.

- Use a good-quality scanner.
- Ensure that the format used is TIFF 4 or the equivalent.
- Ensure that the image scanned cannot be altered in any way.
- Ensure that the documents scanned into a computer are backed up on a regular basis, preferably daily.
- Back-ups must be regularly verified.
- Back-up tapes should be kept for as long as there is a possibility of the information being required by the court.
- Documents should not be shredded on the day of scanning, to ensure that the scanned documents are backed up.
- An audit trail must be in place.
- If a patient leaves the practice, all scanned records must be passed on to the next GP or practice in either paper or electronic form.
- Under the Data Protection Act, the scanned document should be deleted after the patient has left the practice.

No case law currently exists in this area, which is why there is some uncertainty.

Caldicott Guardians

The Government established a committee to examine the protection and usage of patient-identifiable information. The committee was chaired by Dame Fiona Caldicott, and published its findings in December 1997.[16]

The committee published 16 recommendations, one of which established the Caldicott Guardian:

> *Recommendation 3*: A senior person, preferably a health professional, should be nominated in each health organisation to act as a guardian, responsible for safeguarding the confidentiality of patient information.

All NHS trusts and associated bodies are required to have a Caldicott Guardian. This includes general practice.

Access to medical records: guide and problems

All GPs, nurses and practice staff are aware of the sensitive nature of a patient's clinical details and will go some way towards protecting access to this information, but situations arise where there is some confusion as to who has the right of access to such information. The legislation covering this area includes:

- the Data Protection Act 1998
- the Access to Medical Records Act 1990
- Section 60 of the Health and Social Care Act 2001.

Patients

Any patient may apply for access to their medical records, and this must be allowed unless:

- it is likely to cause serious harm to the individual or a third party
- the records refer to a third party who has not given their consent, in which case this part of the record should be removed.

Letters from the mental health teams are increasingly causing problems. In many units these are routinely stamped with a statement that the contents of the letter may only be released to the individual to whom they refer, if the consent of the person who has sent the letter is sought and given. It could be argued that the patient must be granted access to this information under the Data Protection Act unless the two statements above are legally binding. The mental health units could argue that even if the above statements are not binding, disclosure of information may put the sender of the information at risk, and therefore release of the information must be restricted unless the consent of the sender is obtained.

Children

Access to a child's medical records is restricted to the parents unless the child is deemed competent to make this informed decision. It can become difficult if the parents have separated and conflicting demands are being made on the practice. The basic principle must always be that the interests of the child are paramount. Any significant uncertainty should be clarified by taking further advice from a medical protection organisation or the LMC (*see also* Chapters 12 and 16).

Other healthcare professionals

Practising medicine often requires teamwork and good communication. This can only be achieved in the best interests of the patient if all those involved in the care of an individual have access to the relevant clinical information. Unless the patient specifically states that they wish certain information to be withheld from other healthcare professionals, this is not usually a problem If such a preference is expressed by a patient, the GP should attempt to persuade the patient to accept the necessity for information sharing.

Relatives

Relatives (except parents, in the case of a child) have no rights of access to an individual's clinical records. This is sometimes very difficult in the elderly, especially where the patient is terminally ill. It may be that discussing some information will be detrimental to the individual's health. Patients have a right to know. Some do not wish to exercise that right but *do* wish their relatives to know, and vice versa. Doctors must always try to act in the best interest of the patient, and sometimes this may involve discussing information with the relatives.

Before sharing any information, make sure that, if challenged, this can be justified, and preferably make a note about the reasons at the time.

Solicitors

Any release of records to a solicitor must only be with the consent of the patient. Some solicitors try to gain access by stating that they are acting on behalf of the patient. They must demonstrate this with a valid consent form which proves that informed consent has been granted. Where this is not available, the onus is on the solicitor and not the GP practice to ensure that patient consent has been obtained for the release of records. Many practices, once they have received a request, choose to write to the patient clarifying the fact that the solicitor (and any person who is working on their case) will have full access to their health records, including much that will not be relevant. A significant proportion of patients will alter their consent under these circumstances.

If a solicitor informs the GP that they must release the records or they will obtain a court order, then they should be invited to obtain one.

If a doctor or nurse appears in court as a witness and is asked to breach patient confidentiality, they should initially decline to do so and explain the reasons for this. The judge may then order the release of this information.

Medical records may only be legally released without the informed consent of the patient if there is a direction to do so by a court.

Police

The police have no right of access to medical records unless valid consent has been obtained, failing which they must gain permission from the court.

Occasionally the public interest in disclosing information outweighs the individual's right to confidentiality – for example, drivers who are deemed unfit to drive but who continue to do so. Any patient with epilepsy who continues to have 'fits' but refuses to stop driving must be reported to the DVLA.

The GMC is clear in its guidance on these matters.

Difficulty may arise when a GP believes that a patient has committed a serious criminal offence. Should the police be informed? This situation is never simple, and advice from a MPO should be obtained as soon as possible.

Social services

Consent is required before giving information to social services. In the case of a child, in all but the most extreme circumstances (usually involving a significant risk to the child), consent to disclosure must be obtained from the parent. There are of course difficulties if the parents are not in agreement about disclosure. Then the GP may not release information unless the risk to the child is felt to be overwhelming. Careful records should be made of why any decisions were made to release information. Many practices are working more closely with social services and have social workers attached to the practice. The social workers must not have access to clinical records unless the patient has given consent. Social workers in child protection cases may suggest that the Children Act gives right to information, but this is only so if the GP feels that the risks justify not obtaining the parents' consent. Advice should be obtained in some of these circumstances (*see* Chapter 16).

Deceased patients

The duty of confidentiality does not end when the patient dies. Access to clinical records can only be given with the consent of the next of kin. Care must be taken to ensure that release of this information does not relate to a third party or cause any harm to other individuals. If the deceased person had indicated that they did not want details divulged even to the next of kin after their death then this restriction is binding.

Summary

Clinical risk management is an essential part of the logic of moving into the modern age of electronic medical records. The risks can be minimised by a knowledge of the issues covered above and by addressing these within organisations.

Postscript

The Freedom of Information Act 2000

Since this chapter was written full access rights under the Act became operative in January 2005. The Freedom of Information (FOI) Act was passed on 30 November 2000. It gives a general right of access to all types of recorded information held by public authorities, with full access granted from January 2005.

Under the Act all NHS organisations need to produce a publication scheme, which needed to be in place by October 2003. The schemes are aimed at informing the public how and when the NHS organisations (including GP practices) will make information available. The information can be provided in a variety of formats (e.g. by email, website or hard copy). To make it easier, information contained within a publication scheme is divided into classes. These classes provide categories of information (e.g. human resources) to help 'navigate' the scheme. Two useful websites are:

* www.foi.nhs.uk
* www.informationcommissioner.gov.uk/eventual.aspx?id=7303

References

1 NHS Executive (1998) *Information for Health: an information strategy for the modern NHS.* NHS Executive, Leeds.
2 NHS Executive (2001) *Building the Information Core: implementing the NHS Plan.* NHS Executive, Leeds.

3 Department of Health (2000) *NHS Plan: a plan for investment, a plan for reform.* Department of Health, London.

4 General Medical Council (2001) *Good Medical Practice.* General Medical Council, London.

5 British Medical Association (2004) *Medical Ethics Today: the BMA's handbook of ethics and law.* BMJ Books, London.

6 Medical Protection Society (2001) *Introducing Clinical Risk Management: a trainer's resource. Module 2. Patient records.* Medical Protection Society, London.

7 Hippisley-Cox J, Pringle M, Cater R *et al.* (2003) The electronic patient record in primary care – regression or progression? A cross-sectional study. *BMJ.* **326**: 1439–1443.

8 Hamilton WT, Round AP, Sharp D and Peters TJ (2003) The quality of record keeping in primary care: a comparison of computerised, paper and hybrid systems. *Br J Gen Pract.* **53**: 929–33.

9 NHS Executive Letter (2000) *Electronic patient medical records in primary care: changes to GP terms of service.* Ref PC – 01/10/00. NHS Executive, Leeds.

10 Department of Health (1989) *Terms of Service for Doctors in General Practice.* Department of Health, London.

11 Department of Health. *Requirements for Accreditation* (specifies a core set of requirements, which all GP computer systems should be capable of performing). www.dh.gov.uk/PolicyAndGuidance/OrganisationPolicy/PrimaryCare/PrimaryCareComputing/PrimaryCareComputingArticle/fs/en?CONTENT_ID=4062646&chk=Ugk95p

12 *Good Practice Guidelines for General Practice Electronic Patient Records*; www.bma.org.uk

13 *Primary Care Information Modernisation Programme*; www.pcimb.nhs.uk

14 *Remotely Held Records and Central Servers: guidance for GPs*; www.bma.org.uk

15 General Practitioners Committee of the British Medical Association (2001) *Consulting in the Modern World: guidance for GPs.* General Practitioners Committee of the British Medical Association, London.

16 Department of Health (1997) *The Caldicott Committee Report on the Review of Patient-Identifiable Information*; www.dh.gov.uk/assetRoot/04/06/84/04/04068404.pdf

Chapter 10

Results management

Paul Bowden

Key learning points

- Over 70% of general practices have identified results handling as a major risk area.
- GPs have a legal responsibility to inform patients of their results.
- Breaches in confidentiality regularly occur.
- Patients will assume that 'no news is good news'.

Introduction

When was the last time in your practice that a test result was lost, not conveyed to a patient, or done so incorrectly?

In over 200 practice CRSAs by the MPS, over 70% of practices identified result handling as a major risk area, but few of them had quantified the risk.

Accident and error analysts emphasise the need to structure systems in order to minimise risk,[1] in particular reducing the likelihood of human error. Although a great deal of information can be obtained by examining systems when they fail (*significant event audit*), there is also much to be gained from being proactive in this area. After all, prevention is better than cure, and it is also cheaper!

In this chapter we shall examine the process of result handling, identify risk areas and develop a system that will minimise risk.

Background

Despite the obvious risks associated with handling test results, there is little guidance for practices on how to ensure that their result management system is effective and safe. Without a robust system, GPs can find themselves liable for failing to ensure that all requested tests are performed, received and actioned as case law has indicated. In the case of Fredette v Wiebe,[2] the judge held that the referring doctor was *negligent* for failing to ensure that she had examined a pathology report.

It is clear that controversy and litigation are not unknown in this area, and certainly result-handling errors will account for a significant number of the 38 000 written complaints sent each year to general practice as estimated by the Department of Health.[3] Recent work by Sandars *et al.*[4] estimated that 0.8% of patient contacts (not just consultations) result in a significant error of some form, which represents 2 errors per week per average GP.

Perhaps the true scale of the problem will not be fully appreciated until the NRLS is fully functioning[5] and GPs have gained confidence in an anonymous reporting system for significant events.

The literature on this area is sparse. In 1996, Bhasale *et al.*[6] collected details of 500 incidents relating to results and analysed a sample of 56 incidents. Although this is a small sample, the distribution of errors and omissions was interesting in that they were fairly evenly spread throughout the different stages of the process, as follows:

• arranging test (e.g. labelling errors, sample lost in transit) – 26.9%
• testing process (e.g. wrong test performed, laboratory error) – 19.2%
• communication of test to GP (e.g. excessive delay or not sent at all) – 17.3%
• processing result (e.g. filed unseen, urgent test not shown to GP) – 15.4%
• communication to patient (e.g. GP forgot, patient given wrong result) – 21.2%.

Stephenson *et al.*[7] audited a system for dealing with results where, over a period of 2 weeks, tests were logged 'in and out' manually. This was found to be effective but too time consuming to be practicable, although the practice was not paperless at the time. This was also the experience in our practice when we tried to implement a similar system. Kelly *et al.*[8] surveyed their patients who had recently had tests performed, and found that only 61% knew their test results, and a significant number of abnormal results had not been communicated to the patient.

This study confirms that patients often assume that the doctor will contact them if their test is abnormal – that is, 'no news is good news'. This is a major risk area.

Systems

In Somerset Maugham's book *Then and Now*, Machiavelli tries to reassure the mother of his new companion with the words 'By observing the unfortunate consequences of my errors he will doubtless learn'. So it would seem that significant event analysis was alive and well in Renaissance Italy.

In the twenty-first century we observe both consequence and process, and this is best done with examples of real events.

Case Study 10.1

In 1993 a patient consulted her GP complaining of left iliac fossa pain. A full history was taken, abdominal and gynaecological examination was normal and a cervical smear was taken (the reason for this was unclear from the notes). The original symptoms appear to have resolved spontaneously, because it was some considerable time later (over 1 year) before the patient next saw the doctor and enquired about her smear result. In fact the smear was reported 'severe dysplasia – colposcopy recommended', and this came as a shock to the GP. There was no evidence in the notes as to when the result had been received, nor was there anything to confirm that the patient had been contacted or that any attempts had been made to do this.

In this case, there was no written practice protocol for dealing with abnormal results. In these circumstances you will appreciate that such cases are difficult to defend. Of course, 10 years on there are more fail-safes in place for cervical screening, but we can use this example to examine the process in more detail.

The process can be broken down simply as follows:

> Smear taken → sent to lab → test performed → result returned → action taken

It looks fairly simple and foolproof until you take into account the human factors:

> patient is sent appointment → patient attends → nurse takes smear → nurse labels sample and leaves it out for transport → samples are collected by hospital transport → sample reaches correct hospital department intact → laboratory receptionist processes sample → testing is performed by laboratory personnel → result is dictated → hospital secretary types report → report is signed off by consultant → report is sent to GP (electronically and/or manually) → report reaches correct practice → practice staff process report → doctor sees report → doctor indicates action (i.e. file/appointment/letter, etc.) → patient is contacted → appointment is made → patient attends.

There are at least ten different people involved in this process, so it is not difficult to imagine what the chances of error or omission are.

A fully computerised system would probably be safer, provided that enough safeguards are in place and, more importantly, that all members of the practice are working to an agreed system.

The process

There are four steps:

1 sampling
2 laboratory processing test
3 practice processing result
4 actioning

Sampling

The process by which samples are taken will vary from one practice to another. Some blood tests would be taken 'in-house' by either a nurse or a phlebotomist, but in some practices the patient is sent to the local hospital. In either case it may surprise you to know that it is the GP's responsibility to ensure that the test has been performed, not the patient's. In our experience, few practices have a system in place for 'tracking' tests in this way, although some will have a recall system for specific tests such as international normalised ratios (INRs) and glycosylated haemoglobin.

It is essential that the patient understands not only why the test is being performed but also the process that follows. It is generally accepted that the amount of information taken in by the patient during the consultation will vary, and recently it was found that up to 80% of this information will not be retained.[9] This is why I would recommend giving written instructions wherever possible. This has the added advantage that other information, such as which tests were performed and how to obtain the results, can be included (*see* Box 10.1).

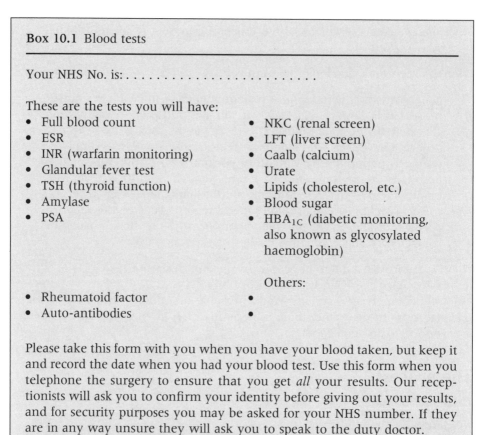

Box 10.1 Blood tests

Your NHS No. is: ....

These are the tests you will have:
- Full blood count
- ESR
- INR (warfarin monitoring)
- Glandular fever test
- TSH (thyroid function)
- Amylase
- PSA

- NKC (renal screen)
- LFT (liver screen)
- Caalb (calcium)
- Urate
- Lipids (cholesterol, etc.)
- Blood sugar
- HBA_{1C} (diabetic monitoring, also known as glycosylated haemoglobin)

Others:
- Rheumatoid factor
- Auto-antibodies

Please take this form with you when you have your blood taken, but keep it and record the date when you had your blood test. Use this form when you telephone the surgery to ensure that you get *all* your results. Our receptionists will ask you to confirm your identity before giving out your results, and for security purposes you may be asked for your NHS number. If they are in any way unsure they will ask you to speak to the duty doctor.

Your blood test results will usually be available after 5 working days (some require up to 2 weeks). Please telephone the surgery *after 3pm* and the receptionist will let you know the results and any instructions that your doctor has given. If you have any queries regarding your results, you can speak to your doctor by phone between 11.30 and 12.00 on weekday mornings, or you may prefer to make an appointment.

Once a test has been performed, the next step would be simply to send it off to the laboratory, but some practices record these tests and try to 'marry them up' with the results when they come in. This 'dual registry' of results is regarded as best practice, but in the busy primary care setting it is not always a practical option.

It is important that the information included on the request form is not only concise but also legible, as it may be the responsibility of one of your colleagues to act on the result. A good example of this type of risk would be the Friday-morning blood test.

> **Case study 10.2**
>
> _____
>
> An elderly woman presents to her GP on a Friday morning with a short history of fatigue and non-specific headache. Examination, including blood pressure, fundi and palpation of the temporal arteries, is normal and the GP records 'fatigue 2/52 o/e nad bp 140/80 for screening bloods and review'.
>
> The blood tests are taken by the nurse and the request form is marked 'fatigue'. As you might have guessed, the ESR is significantly raised. The result is phoned through by the laboratory that night and viewed by the duty doctor who, faced with a high ESR in an elderly woman with fatigue, assumes that any action can wait until Monday and does nothing further. In the mean time the patient is having a slight problem with her vision and is putting it down to old age, and besides she would never bother a doctor over the weekend with something so trivial . . .

It is a common mistake to simply record a symptom on a request form without a suspected diagnosis because the assumption is that the same doctor will see the result and remember the clinical scenario, but as the above example demonstrates, the consequences of omission can be catastrophic.

Looking at the above example what information on the request form would have alerted the duty doctor (apart from more comprehensive notes!)? Perhaps *'fatigue and headache'* or *'fatigue? TA.'*

If you examine the above example more closely, you might be critical of this fictitious doctor. If he suspected temporal arteritis, should he not have asked for an urgent ESR? If that were the case, would he not have alerted the duty doctor? Handover is an essential part of risk management in all forms of medicine.

There are certain clinical areas, in particular drug monitoring, which would benefit from standardised information written on request forms. Some examples include the following:

- disease-modifying anti-rheumatic drugs (DMARDs) and other cytotoxic drugs
- cardiac drugs (e.g. amiodarone, digoxin, ACE inhibitors, statins)
- aminophylline
- warfarin
- carbimazole
- lithium
- temporal arteritis/polymyalgia rheumatica (PMR)
- suspected neoplasia (e.g. mild anaemia in a patient with a change in bowel habit).

The task of prescribing specialist drugs is increasingly being delegated to general practice, but it is not just your budget that is at risk. Remember when you sign the prescription that you and you alone take full responsibility for what happens next, not the locum senior house officer in outpatients who recommended the drug in the first place.

Laboratory processing test

Despite having very little control over this part of the process the GP still retains responsibility for ensuring that the tests get done.[10] The laboratory does have a responsibility to communicate abnormal results,[11] but how they do this will vary according to their own protocols. Let us consider the example of the 'Friday ESR' in our patient with possible temporal arteritis. What if the result only became available later in the evening? How would the laboratory react if they phoned the surgery and found it closed? Would they fax the result or send it electronically? Would they have discharged their duty (this has yet to be tested in court!)? Some practices turn off their fax machines at night for this very reason, but it remains to be seen whether passing responsibility to the practice electronically will become acceptable.

One way of minimising risk is the handout (*see* Box 10.1) which indicates to the patient which tests have been taken and when to expect the results.

The new GP contract will end personal lists, and this will create problems for the laboratories in that they may have difficulty assigning the result to an individual GP, and it is likely that they will merely direct the results to the practice and let them sort them out.

Practice processing result

Manual systems vary, but in most cases results are 'stamped' and left in the relevant GP's in-tray. Some practices also record the results in individual result books in which the GP enters comments that can be communicated to the patient when they contact the surgery. In those practices with electronic lab links, results are sorted and then 'sent' to the individual GP's mailbox for the GP to read, but problems can develop when individual doctors are away and their results need action. A robust system for reallocating results to another partner rather than leaving them for a locum is always a sensible move, and once again it is helpful if this process is written down in the protocol. If there are no personal lists, staff must ensure that the result is sent to the doctor who ordered the test.

Results often arrive piecemeal, and there are risks involved when patients have multiple tests ordered since, unless you have a log-out/log-in system, neither you nor your partner may be aware that a certain test has ever been done. Remember that it is the GP's responsibility to check that the test has been done, not the lab's. The patient information leaflet (*see* Box 10.1) will help, but there is a need for a reconciliation process to be available electronically to replace the cumbersome manual system.

Sometimes a test will be returned because it was unlabelled, and it is quite easy for these to be overlooked. The practice staff should be aware of how these are dealt with, in particular recording any action taken.

Urgent results are usually communicated to the practice by phone, occasionally by fax but increasingly via electronic mail, and it is essential that every practice has a protocol for dealing with them. There is a natural tendency for hospital laboratories to delegate responsibility with regard to urgent results. This can cause problems when the surgery has closed. It would be unacceptable for the laboratory to fax the result to a closed surgery or to send it electronically on the assumption that it would be seen immediately. Likewise, it would be irresponsible for primary care not to have a system in place for dealing with such eventualities. Currently there are ad hoc arrangements with cooperatives and other out-of-hours services (OOHS), but when GPs have opted out of OOHS there could be serious problems, as they would no longer need to supply a contact number after 6.30pm. Given the limited information on request forms, it would be unlikely that the patient could be contacted without access to the practice's database. This issue and many others relating to 'handovers' will need to be addressed by the new providers of OOHS. The doctor is responsible for ensuring that urgent results are actioned promptly.

Actioning

A proactive system for dealing with abnormal results will dramatically minimise the risk of them being overlooked. Abnormal results are usually actioned before the patient telephones the practice, and the practice should make every effort to contact the patient (by letter if necessary), always remembering to record these attempts. It is advisable to send the letter by first-class post and to include your surgery address on the back in case the letter needs to be redirected, as patients may move house without telling you, especially if their new address is outside your practice area! When the patient has been contacted this should also be recorded in the notes, either on the computer record or as a manual entry on the result itself, which should also be dated. There should be a rule that no result is filed either electronically or manually unless it is marked as having been actioned.

In 1989, Maclean wrote that 'the duty to make disclosures (of information) is placed on the doctor',[12] which means that you have a legal obligation to inform the patient of *all* results but, taking a pragmatic view, this could be amended to 'results which would affect clinical outcome'. This is why even though you may feel that you have made every effort to contact a patient, it is still wise to include a recall date to ensure that action has been taken (this is sometimes done automatically when dealing with results electronically).

Forgetting to action results is not the only risk area in this part of the process – giving out results over the telephone is a confidentiality minefield. For this reason you should take all possible steps to ensure that you are giving the result to the appropriate person. Receptionists should be reminded not to give results to the patient's partner, employer, etc., as well as being mindful of 'sensitive results'.

There are of course high-risk areas, such as the following:

- pregnancy tests
- HIV results
- genito-urinary results
- DNA tests
- other tests specifically identified by the practice.

Staff should be on their guard when asked for these results, and should refer to the doctor if they are at all uncertain (*see* Box 10.1). It may be prudent to 'embargo' certain results to be dealt with by the GP alone.

The information that is given to patients should be clear and unambiguous. Phrases like 'OK-ish' and 'ish' or just simple ticks are unacceptable, and it is better to devise a standard set of actions which every patient and receptionist can understand. For this reason, any annotated text which you wish to be conveyed to the patient must be in a form that the receptionist can give to the patient verbatim.

Here are some suggestions.

- Tell the patient the result is normal and no further action is needed.
- Tell the patient the result is normal but that they need a routine follow-up appointment.
- The result is abnormal – ask the patient to telephone the doctor.
- The result is abnormal – a routine appointment is needed.

Of course the list is endless, but remember that it is not sufficient just to say 'normal' and leave the patient wondering what they should do next. Actioning means not just informing the patient but also telling them what action they need to take – even if it is nothing at all.

Holidays and ill health produce another risk, namely locums (*see* Chapter 18). In our experience some practices have developed a locum's handbook that details not just relevant practice procedures and protocols but also the responsibilities of the locum (e.g. to check all messages before leaving the surgery).

Another problem area is the result which arrives at the practice having been organised elsewhere (e.g. outpatients). Practices have reported that this behaviour is on the increase and may reflect the move towards 'one-stop clinics', reduced outpatient attendances in secondary care and shortened inpatient stays. Good examples of this are the abnormal MSU taken on the postnatal ward, the post-operative anaemia and an isolated raised ESR from outpatients. More recently our practice has noticed a dramatic increase in blood tests organised by specialist nurses in outpatients which are sent to the GP with very little clinical information. The major concern is that these tests may have been forwarded by non-clinical staff, and it is dangerous to assume that you are merely receiving a 'courtesy' copy. Although medico-legally it *may* not be your responsibility, it would be regarded as good practice if you ensured that the correct action had been taken. This may simply involve a phone call to the relevant consultant's secretary. The PCT does have a role in these situations, since it could be perceived as transfer of work from secondary to primary care, and the PCO will need to ensure that *all* doctors understand that they must take responsibility for dealing with the results of tests that they have ordered. In the USA, such 'duties of care' are well defined and open to litigation when breached.

Protocol

What makes a perfect protocol? The difference between a protocol and a guideline is that the former is inflexible and so not open to interpretation. It should also anticipate all eventualities and variables.

When designing a protocol, start with two questions.

1 Think of what might go wrong by starting your question with the words 'What if . . .'.
2 What has gone wrong before? Begin by looking at audits, significant event analyses and near misses.

So what usually goes wrong? It may be any of the following:

- an abnormal result filed inappropriately
- a patient not being informed
- a requested test not being performed
- a breach of confidentiality.

Having defined the risks, carefully examine the controls that you currently have in place and identify their weaknesses. How might they be improved?

There is no 'one size fits all' system, and it is up to each practice to devise their own protocol and to continue to review its systems regularly through audit and significant event analysis.

Any protocol should include the following key elements.

Testing

1 Inform the patient.
2 Complete a request form (legible and relevant clinical details).
3 Record the test performed.
4 Set a fail-safe recall date for important tests.

Processing the result

1 Reconcile the results with the tests ordered.
2 Record receipt of the result (electronically or manually).
3 Ensure that the result reaches the appropriate GP.
4 Have a system for allocating results when a doctor is on holiday.
5 Deal with urgent results.

Actioning

1 Record any action needed in unambiguous form.
2 Complete the filing process for normal results.
3 Record patient contact and action.
4 Complete the filing process for 'actioned' results.

Conclusion

No foolproof system exists, but the controls that you put in place will minimise risk by anticipating adverse events before they happen, and ultimately increase patient safety. If complaints do materialise or a significant adverse event occurs, it is always sensible to revise your protocol, making a note both of the changes and of the date on which they were made.

References

1 Leape L (1994) Error in medicine. *JAMA*. **272**: 1851–7.
2 *Fredette v Wiebe* [1986] 5W *WR* 222 (BCSC).
3 Department of Health (2000) *An Organisation With a Memory*. The Stationery Office, London.

4 Sandars J and Esmail A (2003) The frequency and nature of medical error in primary care: understanding the diversity across studies. *Fam Pract.* **20**: 231–6.

5 Wilson T and Sheikh A (2002) Enhancing public safety in primary care. *BMJ.* **324**: 584–7.

6 Bhasale A, Norton K and Britt H (1996) Tests and investigations. Indicators for better utilisation. *Aust Fam Physician.* **25**: 680–94.

7 Stephenson P (1993) Audit of a system for dealing with a practice's laboratory test results. *Br J Gen Pract.* **43**: 383–5.

8 Kelly MH and Barber JH (1988) Use of laboratory services and communication of results to patients in an urban practice: an audit. *J R Coll Gen Pract.* **38**: 64–6.

9 Kessels RPC (2003) Patients' memory for medical information. *J R Soc Med.* **96**: 219–22.

10 *Regina v Croydon Health Authority* [1998] *Lloyd's Rep Med.* 44.

11 *Holmes v Board of Hospital Trustees of City of London* [1977] 81 *DLR* (3d) 67 (Ont. HC).

12 Maclean S (1989) *A Patient's Right to Know.* Dartford Press, Aldershot.

Chapter 11

Prescribing

Mark Dinwoodie

Key learning points

- Medication errors are common and usually due to prescribing, dispensing or administration errors.
- Common specific examples include wrong dose, inappropriate medication and failure to monitor for toxicity or side-effects.
- High-risk groups include the elderly, patients in nursing or residential care, those on four or more drugs, patients with communication difficulties and patients with mental illness.
- Steroids and antibiotic allergies are the drugs most associated with claims.
- Adopt a systematic approach to prescribing any medication.
- A comprehensive and up-to-date repeat prescribing protocol is likely to reduce the risks associated with repeat prescribing.

Introduction

Medication has tremendous potential to assist in the treatment and management of patients, but equally it can cause considerable iatrogenic illness, which has a social cost in terms of resources and a personal cost in terms of morbidity and mortality. It does well to remember the axiom: 'First do no harm'. 1.3% of the population consult their GP every day[1] and of these approximately 50–60% will receive a prescription.[2,3] According to the recently published Department of Health document (2003) *Building a Safer NHS for Patients – Improving Medication Safety*,[4] GPs issue over 660 million prescriptions every year. This works out at approximately 1.8 million every day. While some medication errors are catastrophic and become headline news, e.g. the erroneous intra-thecal injection of *vincristine*,[5] these tend to be very rare (13 cases in 15 years). Conversely, less significant errors which don't attract publicity are much more frequent: one study gave a prescribing error rate in general practice of 7.46%.[6] It is these common medication errors that overall will cause the greatest morbidity and mortality and the most benefit is likely to be achieved by concentrating on these.

What is a medication error?

An 'adverse drug reaction' as defined by the World Health Organization includes 'any response to a drug which is noxious, unintended and occurs at doses used for prophylaxis, diagnosis or therapy'. A 'medication error' can be defined in a number of ways but is usefully defined by the US National Coordinating Council for Medication Error Reporting and Prevention as follows: 'A medication error is any preventable event that may cause or lead to inappropriate medication use or patient harm while the medication is in the control of the health professional, patient or consumer'.[7] An article on adverse drug reactions in the BMJ series *ABC of Allergies* reported a French study that showed 14.7% of adults aged 20–67, when attending a health centre, gave a reliable history of a systemic adverse reaction to one or more drugs.[8] Many of these are predictable and an accepted consequence of taking the medication. Others are idiosyncratic or unpredictable. Some, however, are caused by *medication errors*, which are preventable. Fortunately, not all medication errors cause harm.

How common are medication errors?

There is relatively little data on the frequency of medication errors in primary care. However, there are a few studies which demonstrate the scale of the problem and explain why the Department of Health in 2001, in its paper *Building a Safer NHS for Patients*,[9] set a target of reducing the number of serious errors involving prescribed medicines by 40% by 2005. It is likely that the number of reported errors represents only the tip of the iceberg of the number of errors actually occurring. It is suspected most doctors are unaware of how often they make prescribing errors.

- Dr Nick Silk at the MPS analysed 1000 consecutive claims and found that 19.3% were linked to medication and prescribing.[10]
- The Medical Defence Union reported that 25% of their claims were related to medication errors.[11]
- The Department of Health publication: *An Organisation with a Memory*,[12] claims that thousands of people report serious adverse events due to medication every year.
- In the USA it is estimated that 7000 deaths each year are caused by medication errors and that this number rose by over two-fold in 10 years.[13]
- An Australian study found that 0.8% of hospital admissions were associated with preventable medication errors.[14]
- Vincent found that a number of studies have shown rates for potential adverse drug reactions and/or prescribing errors for scripts issued in primary care and presented at community pharmacies as being in the range of 0.5–6%.[15]
- The NSF for Older People suggests that as many as half of all patients with chronic conditions end up using their medicines in a way that is not fully effective and that medication problems are associated with 5–17% of hospital admissions.[16]
- Medication errors have been estimated to cost the NHS £500 million a year in additional days spent in hospital, according to the Audit Commission.[17] It also suggested that medication errors account for about one-fifth (approximately 1200) of deaths due to all types of adverse events in hospital.
- A number of studies, including EUROASPIRE 1 and 11,[18] along with the NSF for Coronary Heart Disease demonstrate that many patients with coronary heart disease are not receiving medication from which they would benefit.

- Other information suggests that around 1% of patients on two or more medications are on a potentially hazardous combination.
- Medication errors are thought to contribute between 10% and 20% of all adverse events.[4]
- A study in Merseyside looking at 18 820 admissions to hospital, found that 1225 (6.5%) of these admissions were related to an adverse drug reaction (ADR), with the ADR directly leading to the admission in 80% of cases. ADRs were responsible for the death of 0.15% of all the patients admitted. Extrapolating the data to all English hospitals suggests that ADRs causing hospital admission are responsible for the death of 5700 patients every year. The authors' findings suggested that over 70% of these ADRs were either possibly or definitely avoidable.[19]
- A recent Department of Health document suggested that there was evidence to support the need for improvement in the management of medicines (non-compliance, large quantities of prescribed medicines returned to pharmacies, poor control of chronic conditions, unmet patient and carer need for high-quality information, lack of regular review to determine effectiveness and tolerability of medication).[20]

Box 11.1 Examples of medication errors

Example 1
A patient receiving lithium medication was issued a repeat prescription every two months. The practice did not have a system in place for reviewing repeat medication regularly. As a consequence he carried on receiving the medication for 18 months without attending the surgery and was finally admitted with lithium toxicity.

Example 2
A young female patient with epilepsy saw her GP requesting to start the oral contraceptive pill. She was prescribed the standard dose pill even though she was taking phenytoin, which increases the metabolism of the Pill and so reduces its effectiveness. She subsequently presented with an unplanned pregnancy.

Example 3
An elderly man was given the wrong prescription by a receptionist at his local GP practice. It was in fact for a patient with a similar name. He inadvertently took the wrong medication.

Example 4
A GP prescribed trimethoprim to a patient who was allergic to septrin (which contains trimethoprim). She had an unpleasant allergic reaction and complained to the GP, stating that it was documented in her medical records that this was the case from some years earlier. Although the written (manual) notes had an alert on the cover, the computer did not have an alert, as the notes had not been summarised onto the computer.

What are the most common medication errors?

The MPS in its publication *Common Problems: managing the risks in general practice* lists the four most common medication errors resulting in claims as:[21]

1   wrong dosage
2   inappropriate medication
3   failure to monitor treatment for side-effects and toxicity
4   communication failure between doctor and patient.

Other causes include:

• badly transcribed instructions
• illegible prescriptions
• miscalculation of dosage
• confusion between similar sounding drug names or similar looking packages
• prescribing contraindicated drugs
• not checking for potential drug interactions
• not reviewing repeat prescriptions
• failure to follow up/monitor.

Areas of risk

The NPSA, www.npsa.nhs.uk, considers the main areas of risk to be:

• primary/secondary care interface
• repeat prescribing
• over/under use
• monitoring of medication
• review of medication.

According to Dr Silk's work,[10] the most common drugs leading to claims, in descending order of frequency, are:

• steroids
• antibiotic allergy
• phenothiazines
• HRT
• contraception
• anti-epileptics
• opiates
• medication for children
• lithium
• anticoagulants
• NSAIDs

The Medical Defence Union in its 1996 publication *Problems in General Practice*[11] lists the following drugs in decreasing order of frequency of claims:

• steroids
• antibiotic allergy
• contraceptives
• anticoagulants
• NSAIDs
• opiates

How do medication errors occur?

Medication errors will be dependent on the actions of individuals, the systems and procedures that are in place, and the quality of the product itself. As in other areas of risk, medication errors are likely to occur where there is the combination of an *active failure* by an individual with vulnerable underlying or *latent conditions* of the organisation. Medication errors can be considered under the following categories.

Prescribing errors

A study carried out in the UK over a two-month period showed a prescribing error rate of 7.46% for over 37 000 items prescribed by 23 GPs. The incidence of serious error was low but in one in 2000 the wrong dose had been prescribed.[6] Over 50% of the errors relating to medication occur at the prescribing stage. Another study found that 0.066% of prescriptions presented to 23 community pharmacies in the UK had a serious or very serious error. This extrapolated to 280 000 potentially serious errors every year.[22] Prescribing errors include:

- lack of knowledge about the patient, e.g. relevant medical conditions (hepatic or renal impairment), other medications
- lack of knowledge about the drug, e.g. side-effects, interactions
- failure to utilise information already available about the patient and drug, e.g. known patient allergies, or failure to find out more information
- ignoring support systems or 'rules' to prevent error
- error in decision making, e.g. choosing the wrong drug or choosing to prescribe at all
- calculation errors, especially for paediatric doses
- illegible prescriptions
- confusion between drug names (*see* list below)
- use of abbreviations, zeros and decimal points
- incorrect dosage formulations, e.g. modified release medication. Medication with multiple dosage formulations, different doses for different routes of administration, difficult delivery systems and unusual frequencies of administration are more likely to be incorrectly prescribed[4]
- repeat prescribing, which will be discussed in more detail later in the chapter.

It is clear to see how easy it is to prescribe a drug of a similar name when offered a selection of similar drug names on a computer screen. While computers undoubtedly have many advantages when considering prescribing, they also have limitations. The following list from *In Safer Hands*[23] shows drugs most commonly prescribed incorrectly due to similar names:

1. carbamazepine and carbimazole
2. chlorpropamide and chlorpromazine
3. clobetasol and clobetasone
4. depo-medrone and depo-provera
5. fluoxetine and fluconazole
6. lamisil and lamictal
7. losec and lasix
8. noraday and norimin
9. penicillamine and penicillin.

Box 11.2

According to the Committee on the Safety of Medicines,[24] the drugs most likely to cause allergy that are commonly used in the community include:
1 amoxicillin
2 vaccines
3 trimethoprim
4 ciprofloxacin
5 lidocaine local anaesthetic.

Dispensing errors

Errors can occur at the interface between general practice and the community pharmacist. One study showed a community dispensing error rate of 0.26%.[25] There is little information regarding the frequency of dispensing errors. Errors that occur include:

* incorrect drug supplied
* wrong strength
* wrong warning or directions
* incorrect details on label
* incorrect containers
* out of date stock
* dispensed to wrong patient.

The single most commonest cause of error is similar sounding drugs. Misreading or transcription errors will be compounded by illegible prescriptions. Other errors may be due to drugs with similar looking packages.

Approximately two-thirds of errors seem to involve dispensing the wrong drug (either wrong dose or wrong product) and one-third relate to labelling errors. As with prescribing, errors are more likely to occur with unfamiliarity, inexperience and high workload.

The Department of Health's *Building a Safer NHS for Patients – Improving Medication Safety*[4] gives useful further details regarding the most common drugs involved in dispensing errors.

Patient concordance and compliance

Many patients are on a variety of medication and it is not surprising to find that there is often a considerable discrepancy between the intentions of the prescriber, and the treatment actually received by the patient. A recent editorial in the *British Medical Journal* stated that, 'While compliance describes the degree to which the patient follows the prescribed regimen of medicines, concordance describes an agreement between the patient and a healthcare professional about whether, when and how medicines are to be taken'.[26] A review by Giuffrida and Torgerson found studies showing that 6–20% of patients do not even redeem their prescriptions and that 30–50% delay or omit doses.[27] About half the medicines prescribed for patients with long-term conditions are not taken as prescribed.[16]

There is evidence to support the view that better compliance leads to better health outcomes[28] Many elderly patients find it difficult to comply with complex dosage regimes and some will stop taking medication due to side-effects but not tell their doctor and others will revert to previously prescribed medication. Other medication may be administered incorrectly by a relative, carer or nurse (*see* below). Many patients wish to have more involvement in their medication than they currently do.

Monitoring of treatment

See overleaf, under repeat prescribing.

Communication

In common with many areas of medicine good communication is vital. Areas where communication breakdown can lead to error include:

- primary/secondary care interface (*see* Chapter 13)
- general practice/community pharmacy interface
- health professional/patient interaction (*see* Chapter 8 on communication)

Administration of medication

Errors can occur due to the doctor, nurse, relative or carer administering the drug or due to problems with compliance and concordance from the patient's perspective (*see* above). For example:

- wrong patient
- wrong drug
- wrong dose
- wrong frequency/timing of dose
- incorrect method of administration
- incorrect formulation.

It is very easy to forget to take your medication or accidentally take it twice. People with impaired vision may struggle to choose the correct medication. As one patient remarked to his doctor 'I might as well have stuck those suppositories up my bottom for all the good they did me'!

Box 11.3 High-risk groups

- Elderly and housebound patients.
- Patients in nursing or residential care.
- Those on four or more drugs.
- Patients with disabilities or communication difficulties.
- Patients recently discharged from secondary care.
- Patients taking certain medications, e.g. NSAIDs, anticoagulation therapy.
- Patients with mental illness.

Repeat prescribing

A repeat prescription allows a patient to obtain medication they use on a regular basis without having to see their doctor. This is an area in which medication errors frequently occur and there is considerable waste (£100 million per year returned to community pharmacists).[29] There is a huge volume of repeat prescription requests being processed by an average sized practice every day. 587 million prescriptions were issued nationally in 2002 according to the NPSA. Repeat prescribing accounts for about 70–75% of these prescriptions and half of a practice's population will be receiving repeat prescriptions.[30] It works out at about 200 repeat prescriptions per GP per week. Concern has been expressed about the quality of the repeat prescribing process as suggested by McGavock *et al.* (1999)[31] who carried out a semi-structured questionnaire looking at 26 parameters to assess the quality of repeat prescribing in 60 GP practices in Northern Ireland. They found many serious deficiencies. A study in 1996 found that 66% of repeat prescriptions showed no evidence of authorisation and 72% showed no evidence of being reviewed in the preceding 15 months.[32]

Many practices have their own individual systems and in many ways the repeat prescribing system needs to be tailored to the individual practice. What matters is that the system is safe and effective. Having visited a number of practices to facilitate risk assessments, I am always surprised how few practices have a repeat prescribing protocol. An effective repeat prescribing system is a good way of improving the effectiveness and safety of medication. There are principles of good quality practice with regards to repeat prescribing that can be incorporated into individual protocols. Table 11.1 highlights potential risks and their possible solutions, which can be incorporated into any repeat prescribing protocol. When producing a protocol, it is important to involve all those involved in the process, e.g. doctors, nurses, pharmacists and administration staff. It can be helpful to map a patient's journey through the process of obtaining a repeat medication from the request being submitted to actually receiving the medication. It is important to update the protocol as new initiatives come along, and to regularly review it.

Following publication of *Pharmacy in the Future – Implementing the NHS Plan*,[29] pilots are under way looking at the process of *repeat dispensing* by pharmacists, where a patient can obtain repeat medications from their pharmacy in instalments, and *electronic transmission of prescriptions* systems, whereby a prescription can be sent electronically directly to a pharmacy. These are both exciting developments, which may help reduce some of the errors associated with repeat prescribing and enhance patient convenience.

Useful examples relating to the repeat prescribing process and guidance can be found via the National Prescribing Centre (GP Prescribing Support and Medicines Management) who produced the useful document *Saving Time, Helping Patients* in January 2004.[33]

For a repeat prescribing protocol to be successful, it is important that patients understand the process. It is helpful to outline this using a simple guide, on posters or in the practice leaflet.

It is important to involve patients and their carers regarding their repeat medication. There also needs to be a system of quality control, and regular audit of the process may be helpful. Defaulters need to be followed up under an agreed system.

Table 11.1 Risks and control mechanisms associated with repeat prescribing

Risk	Possible control mechanisms
Incorrect details supplied at time of **request** will lead to mistakes.	• Encourage patients to use tear-off repeat prescription request from previous prescription. Alternatively complete a request form asking for the appropriate details. • Inform patients about the preferred method of requesting. Most practices accept requests by post, fax and as above. Some will also accept e-mails. • It is generally felt that requests by phone lead to more errors and mistakes and in general should be avoided. • A list of equivalent proprietary and generic names should be available to staff to reduce confusion between the two.
Lack of clear system for **processing** requests will lead to errors and inconsistencies, particularly in regard to *additionally* requested items not on the patient's repeat medication list.	• Staff need to have protected time to carry out repeat prescribing. • Appoint someone to oversee and manage the process of repeat prescribing. • Regular staff training and updates need to be given. • Urgent and emergency requests from patients should be discouraged. • Consideration should be given as to whether any *additionally* requested medication should be added onto the patient's repeat medication list. • The clinician signing the repeat prescriptions needs to have access to the patient's medical record at the time of signing to assess: the suitability of additionally requested items, review dates and other issues flagged up by the administration process e.g. over-use.
A **delay** in processing a repeat prescription request may mean a patient will miss doses of their medication.	• Practices should aim to process all repeat prescriptions within 48 hours or 2 working days.
Differing **quantities of medication** for different items may lead to confusion for the patient, waste, over-ordering and increased work.	• Aim to synchronise all repeat items so that they last the same duration. • Most people recommend 28 or 56 days amount. Safer, less waste and possibly more efficient (28), against patient convenience (56). Consideration to the stability of the patient's condition should also be given.
Patient re-orders antidepressant for 1 year without being seen because it has been added as a repeat medication.	• Agree a practice policy as to what items are **unsuitable** to be put on as repeat medication. This will partly depend on how robust the system for reviewing medication is in the practice. • Most practices would avoid adding steroid eye drops, strong topical steroids or benzodiazepines as repeat medication. • Medication should only be added to the patient's repeat medication list when they are stable on the medication and by a clinician who has been involved in their care.

Continued

Table 11.1 *Continued*

Risk	Possible control mechanisms
Medication added incorrectly to repeat prescribing list.	• There needs to be an agreed system as to who adds medication to the repeat list and how this is done. If it is not done by the doctor, it needs to be on their instructions and checked closely by them afterwards. • Considerable care needs to be taken to ensure that all the details are correct and that it has been added to the correct patient!! • The condition for which the patient is taking the repeat medication should be clear from the medical record, e.g. hiatus hernia in the problem list for someone taking a proton-pump inhibitor.
• Patient obtains repeat prescriptions for several years of, for example, an ACE inhibitor without having his blood pressure or renal function checked due to lack of **medication review**	• Most practices have computerised repeat prescribing systems and these should include a **medication review date.** • It is important that all patients on repeat medication have their medication reviewed on a regular basis (6–12 monthly) to determine whether they are still on the appropriate medication, that it is safe, effective and in a suitable formulation. • Unwanted and unnecessary items can be removed. • A check can be made to ensure that appropriate monitoring is taking place and that clinical reviews of chronic diseases have occurred. • Quantities can be aligned and cost effectiveness reviewed. • Some practices take the opportunity of giving the patient a questionnaire at their annual medication review to assess their understanding, and allow them to indicate any side effects or difficulties with their medication (*see* below).
• Patient taking methotrexate developed neutropoenia and septicaemia due to **lack of monitoring.**	• Potentially toxic drugs such as lithium, warfarin, disease modifying agents such as methotrexate or azathiaprine, require regular monitoring with blood tests. • Ensure the patient is aware of this with an instruction leaflet. • Consider using a patient held record to encourage compliance and documentation of blood tests especially with 'shared care' medication. • Establish a safe audit system in the practice to ensure that all patients taking these medications have had the appropriate monitoring e.g. a search carried out every month asking for those patients taking lithium who have not had a lithium level carried out in the last 3 months. • Contact those who have not attended for the appropriate monitoring.
A patient **over-using** Salbutamol was admitted with an asthma attack due to poorly controlled asthma.	• There should be a feature within the repeat prescribing system to detect average over-use or under-use. Patients can then be called in for review. • Under-use may reflect poor compliance and may be particularly important in psychiatric illness.

Table 11.1 *Continued*

Risk	*Possible control mechanisms*
A patient was treated inappropriately as he reverted to his medication prior to admission to hospital even though it had been changed during his admission.	• The repeat medication list needs to be reviewed and **updated** whenever a patient is **discharged** from hospital or their medication is changed in **outpatients**. • A system needs to be in place to ensure that appropriate Read codes, allergies and medication changes are entered into the patient's medical record from any correspondence received about a patient, and that appropriate monitoring arrangements are established.
Confusion regarding dosage.	• Clear dosage instructions need to be on the repeat medication. Where possible avoid the instructions *as directed* as the patient may not remember what these are, or confuse them with another drug. If the drug is for, 'as required use', write for example, *b.d. as required.* Consider including what the medication is for under dosage instructions, e.g. one daily for angina.
Collecting prescriptions.	• Patient details should be requested before the prescription is given out to avoid problems with similar name patients and confidentiality issues. • A system should be in place to regularly review uncollected prescriptions as they might reflect under-use and poor compliance with possibly important consequences.

Close liaison with the community pharmacy is likely to be beneficial. General practices should advise on the safe disposal of unused or out-of-date medication, which usually involves advising patients to take them to their local pharmacist.

At the end of this chapter is the repeat prescribing protocol from my own practice. It is not perfect, but may act as a useful starting point. It reflects the fact that we use *EMIS* software for our computer system.

Medication review

All patients on repeat medication need to have their medication reviewed regularly. Opinion varies as to whether six- or 12-monthly is more appropriate. Those at greater risk (*see* above) or on more medication (four or more), need to have more frequent reviews, e.g. six-monthly. A balance clearly needs to be struck between the ideal and the practical. Some readers may be familiar with the 'Brown Bag review'[34] where a patient brings in all the medication that they are taking and goes through them all with the doctor.

Within the NSF for Older People, *Medicines for Older People*[35] provides a detailed guide on appropriate use and review of medication in the elderly. There is evidence to support pharmacist-conducted medication review.[36]

Medication reviews can take place at a number of levels from an ad hoc opportunistic review as part of another consultation, to a face–to-face review in a consultation dedicated to this purpose. It may not always be necessary to arrange a face-to-face review of repeat medication if the clinician is satisfied that a recent clinical consultation included the opportunity for discussion and review of repeat medication with the patient. In these circumstances the clinician can update the review date on the computer having reviewed the patient's medical record. Another option might be to telephone the patient with their medical record in front of you, while the patient has their medication in front of them.

The following are two useful websites: www.doh.gov.uk/nsf/pdfs/medicines-booklet.pdf and www.medicines-partnership.org/medication-review.

Issues to discuss at a medication review, as suggested by the Modernising Medicines Management, might include the following.

- Explanation and purpose of medication.
- Comparison of what is being taken and when, compared to what has been prescribed.
- Over-the-counter, herbal and homeopathic medication.
- Cost-effectiveness.
- Patient's and carer's understanding of their medication.
- Reviewing the appropriateness of medication.
- Assessing side-effects.
- Asking about alcohol intake.
- Reviewing whether relevant monitoring tests have been done.
- Reviewing practical aspects of obtaining medication.
- Reviewing any difficulties with compliance, e.g. opening containers, reading labels and whether a compliance aid would be appropriate.
- Discussing concordance, patients' wishes and any concerns (*see* www.concordance.org).

When reviewing each repeat prescription, consideration should be given to the following, as suggested by the NHS Executive in *GP Prescribing Support*.[37]

1 Is it safe?
2 Is it effective?
3 Is it necessary or still required?
4 Will the patient take it?
5 Is the present formulation appropriate?
6 Does it provide the most cost-effective treatment available?
7 Are all items prescribed in equivalent quantities?
8 Has the patient had a clinical review in the last 15 months?

Some clinicians provide the patient with a chart of their medication, detailing its strength, when to take it, its purpose, common side-effects and how long to take it for. Those involved in terminal care often find this useful.

Readers are referred to Chapter 25 for how to reduce the likelihood of medication errors and Chapter 13 for medication errors relating to the primary/secondary care interface.

Further resources

Along with the references and websites mentioned in the text, the reader may find the following resources useful:

- The *Drug Information Zone* is part of the NHS UK Medicines Information Agency (UKMI) and provides useful medicines information, www.druginfozone.org
- The *Prescriptions Prescribing Authority* provides PACT data, www.ppa.org.uk
- *Toxbase* gives useful information on overdoses and poisons, www.spib.axl. co.uk/
- The *National Teratology Information Service* provides information advice about all aspects of toxicity and drugs in pregnancy, www.nyrdtc.nhs.uk
- National Prescribing Centre (2004) *Saving Time, Helping Patients: a good practice guide to quality repeat prescribing*. NPC, Liverpool. www.npc.co.uk/repeat_prescribing/repeat_presc.htm
- Department of Health (2003) *Building a Safer NHS for Patients: improving medication safety*. DoH, London.
- *Dispensing Doctors Association*; www.dispensingdoctor.org/
- Naylor R (2002) *Medication Errors*. Radcliffe Medical Press, Oxford.
- *Electronic Medicines Compendium* (includes pharmaceutical patient information leaflets and Summaries of Product Characteristics); www.medicinesorg.uk

References

1 Office of Health Economics (2000) *The OHE Compendium of Health Statistics* (12e). OHE, London.
2 Britten N and Ukoumunne O (1997) The influences of patients' hopes of receiving a prescription on doctors' perceptions and the decision to prescribe: a questionnaire survey. *BMJ.* **315**: 1506–10.
3 National Prescribing Centre (2002) *Modernising Medicines Management: a guide to achieving benefits for patients, professionals and the NHS*. NPC, Liverpool, www.npc.co.uk.
4 Department of Health (2003) *Building a Safer NHS for Patients – Improving Medication Safety*. DoH, London, www.doh.gov.uk/buildsafenhs/medicationsafety/index.htm
5 Berwick D (2001) Not again! (editorial) *BMJ.* **322**: 247–8.
6 Nadeem S, Shah H, Aslam M and Avery A (2001) A survey of prescription errors in general practice. *Pharm J.* **267**: 860–2.
7 US National Coordinating Council for Medication Error Reporting and Prevention, www.nccmerp.org.
8 Vervloet D and Durham S (1998) ABC of Allergies: adverse reactions to drugs. *BMJ.* **316**: 1511–14.
9 Department of Health (2001) *Building a Safer NHS for Patients*. DoH, London, www.doh.gov.uk/buildsafenhs.
10 Silk N (2000) What went wrong in 1000 negligence claims. *Healthcare Risk Report.* **7**(3): 13–15.
11 Green S, Goodwin H and Moss J (1996) *Problems in General Practice. Medication errors*. Medical Defence Union, Manchester.
12 Department of Health (2000) *An Organisation with a Memory*. DoH, London, www.doh.gov.uk/orgmemreport/.
13 Phillips DP, Christenfeld N and Glynn LM (1998) Increase in US medication error deaths between 1983 and 1993. Research letter. *Lancet.* **351**: 643.

14 Wilson R McI, Runicman WB, Gibberd RW *et al.* (1995) The Quality in Australian Healthcare Study. *Med J Aust.* **163**: 458–71.

15 Vincent C (2001) *Clinical Risk Management: enhancing patient safety.* BMJ Books, London.

16 Department of Health (2001) *National Service Framework for Older People.* DoH, London, www.doh.gov.uk/nsf/olderpeople/index.htm.

17 Audit Commission (2001) *A Spoonful of Sugar: medicines management in NHS hospitals.* Audit Commission, London, www.audit-commission.gov.uk/.

18 EUROASPIRE 1 and 11 Group (2001) Clinical reality of coronary prevention guidelines: a comparison of EUROASPIRE 1 and 11 in nine countries. *Lancet.* **357**: 995–1001.

19 Pirmohamed M, James S, Meakin S *et al.* (2004) Adverse drug reactions as cause of admission to hospital: prospective analysis of 18 820 patients. *BMJ.* **329**: 15–19.

20 Department of Health (2004) *Management of Medicines: A resource to support implementation of the wider aspects of medicines management for the National Service Frameworks for Diabetes, Renal Services and Long-Term Conditions.* DoH, London, www.dh.gov.uk/assetRoot/04/08/87/55/04088755.pdf.

21 Medical Protection Society (2001) *Common Problems: managing the risks in general practice.* MPS, Leeds.

22 Greene R (1995) Survey of prescription anomalies in community pharmacies: (1) prescription monitoring. *Pharm J.* **254**: 476–81.

23 Royal College of General Practitioners and National Patient Safety Agency (2003) *In Safer Hands.* **2**. RCGP, NPSA, London.

24 Committee on the Safety of Medicines, www.mca.gov.uk/aboutagency/regframework/csm/csmhome.htm.

25 Quinlan P, Ashcroft D and Blenkinsopp A (2002) Medication errors: a baseline survey of dispensing errors reported in community pharmacies. *Int J Pharm Pract.* **10**(suppl): R68.

26 Marshall M and Shaw J (2003) Not to be taken as directed: patient concordance for taking medicines into practice. *BMJ.* **326**: 348–9.

27 Giuffrida A and Torgerson D (1997) Should we pay the patient? Review of financial incentives to enhance patient compliance. *BMJ.* **315**: 703–7.

28 Haynes R, McKibbon A and Kanani R (1996) Systematic review of randomised trials of interventions to assist patients to follow prescriptions for medications. *Lancet.* **348**: 383–6.

29 Department of Health (2000) *Pharmacy in the Future – Implementing the NHS Plan.* DoH, London, www.doh.gov.uk/pharmacyfuture/index.htm.

30 Harris C and Dajda R (1996) The scale of repeat prescribing. *Br J Gen Pract.* **46**: 649–53.

31 McGavock H, Wilson-Davis K and Connolly J (1999) Repeat prescribing management: a cause for concern. *Br J Gen Pract.* **49**: 343–7.

32 Zemansky AG (1996) Who controls repeats? *Br J Gen Pract.* **46**: 643–7.

33 National Prescribing Centre (2004) *Saving Time, Helping Patients: a good practice guide to quality repeat prescribing.* NPC, Liverpool. www.npc.co.uk/repeat_prescribing/repeat_presc.htm.

34 Nathan A, Goodyear L, Lovejoy A and Rashid A (1999) 'Brown Bag' medication reviews as a means of optimising patients' use of medication and identifying clinical problems. *Family Practice.* **16**: 278–82.

35 Department of Health (2001) *National Service Framework for Older People. Medicines for Older People.* DoH, London, www.doh.gov.uk/nsf/pdfs/medicinesbooklet.pdf.

36 Zermansky A, Petty D and Rarnor D (2002) Randomised controlled trial of clinical medication review by a pharmacist of elderly patients receiving repeat prescriptions in general practice. *Health Technology Assessment.* **6**: 20.

37 National Prescribing Centre and NHS Executive (1998) *GP Prescribing Support: a resource document and guide for the New NHS.* NPC, Liverpool and NHSE, Leeds, www.doh.gov.uk/nhsexec/gppres.htm.

Appendix 11.1
Repeat prescribing protocol

Fairfield Park Health Centre

1   **Requesting**: repeat prescriptions may be requested in writing by the following methods:
    - post
    - fax
    - by hand
    - e-mail.
        - Phone requests are not accepted routinely due to the risk of error.
        - Patients are encouraged to use the tear-off right-hand side of their previous prescription.
        - Emergency requests may be accepted by phone if approved by a Doctor.
        - Requests for repeat contraception should be advised to make an appointment with the sister. One month's emergency supply can be issued by attaching *'addition'* to the request, and passing it to the Doctor.
    - Patients should be informed about the process of repeat prescribing through the practice information leaflet.

2   **Processing**
    - Target: maximum of 48 hours to process.
    - Patients making emergency requests should be given a note with their prescription advising of the need for 48 hours' notice and of the disruption emergency requests cause.
    - The *addition slip* is used for patients requesting items not on their repeat medication list.
    - To issue a *repeat:*
        - PR-select appropriate patient
        - I for issue
        - select items requested; check strength, dose and quantity; press Return
        - P for print
        - enter destination, i.e. collection, post or chemist
        - add *attention, addition* or *review date* slip as necessary
        - fix SAE with a paper clip
        - check which doctors are in surgery next morning and divide equally.
    - Staff should be given protected time to carry out repeat prescribing.
    - Regular training and updates should be undertaken.
    - *Current/acute* prescriptions should be generated by a doctor or nurse only and signed by a doctor only.

3   **Generic/BANs and rINNs**
    - In principle, the practice prescribes generically. Patients may need informing regarding this.
    - Staff need to have a list of generic/trade equivalent names.
    - All prescribing should now occur using recommended International Names (rINNs) rather than British Approved Names (BANs). The computer has been adjusted and warnings are given.

4 **Quantity prescribed**
 * Currently two months in multiples of 28 unless pack size different, e.g. 30, then 2×30.
 * Scripts should be synchronised where possible to make the re-ordering easier for patients.
 * Pill and HRT can be prescribed for six months once established (three months initially) as an acute medication only.
 * New medication, e.g. anti-hypertensives, usually one month initially.
 * Patients in residential care and nursing homes, 28 days.
 * NSAIDs usually max. two weeks as an acute prescription.
 * Anti-histamines for hay fever, usually one month.
 * Inhalers, usually a maximum of two.

5 **Adding repeat medication**
 * Only Doctors should add repeat medication to the patient's medical record.
 * When adding a new medication, patients should be asked about over-the-counter remedies they are taking, known drug allergies and any herbal medication, e.g. St John's Wort.
 * Nurses adding medication as part of a protocol, e.g. starting a *statin*, should do so as an *acute medication*, advising the patient to request more as an addition to their usual repeats. They will need to check this with a Doctor and ask them to sign the prescription.
 * The Doctor can change it to a repeat at the next request and increase amount to two months.
 * The repeat medication list should be updated when *additional items* are requested to see whether these should be added as repeats.
 * Only a Doctor can sign a prescription (not a PRHO). There must be no pre-signed blank prescriptions, ever.
 * All prescription pads should be locked away safely and not left lying around consulting rooms. The first and last identification number should be recorded in the appropriate log book when removing prescription pads from the locked stationery cupboard.

6 **Review dates**
 * In general, should be updated every 12 months, by a Doctor only (elderly NSF suggests six-monthly for those on more than four medications).
 * Only Doctors are allowed to update review dates.
 * If overdue, the prescription is printed and a *review date* marker is attached to the prescription.
 * All medication should be reviewed and recently unused medication (longer than 18 months) removed.
 * In particular, all *acute medication* should be removed unless they are currently taking it, bearing in mind the length of the prescription.
 * Diagnoses justifying continuing repeat medication, e.g. *hiatus hernia,* should be updated on the *significant active problem* list and where possible linked to the relevant medication using *Shift F7 Problem Linker.*
 * Ensure appropriate review by practice nurse or Doctor has taken place and blood tests have been performed. If not, enclose a pre-printed letter with the prescription asking them to make an appointment with the sister for the appropriate check (e.g. diabetes, CHD). Document via an *additional*

consultation comment that this has been done. Do not update review date if this is the case.

- If patient fails to attend, a reminder will be sent via the chronic disease recall system.
- If necessary, phone the patient or arrange a telephone appointment to review repeat medication. Arrange a face-to-face consultation if inappropriate to update as above.
- If appropriate a district nurse should be asked to review a patient with a chronic disease, so that the review date can subsequently be updated by a doctor after discussion.
- Annual visits to residential homes and nursing homes are an appropriate time to update the review date.
- Issues to discuss at the medication review include: explanation of the purpose of the medication; comparison of what is being taken to what has been prescribed; over-the-counter and herbal medication; cost-effectiveness with reference to PCT formulary; patient concerns and questions; side-effects; relevant monitoring tests; practicalities of ordering and receiving medication; formulation of the medicines; compliance and allergies. It may be helpful to have a carer or relative in attendance.

7   **Inappropriate medication as a repeat**
The following are considered inappropriate to be added as repeat medications:
- very potent topical steroids
- oral steroids (those with *polymyalgia rheumatica* can be on repeat but with a three-month review date)
- steroid eye drops
- benzodiazepines (other than long-term existing patients, providing they have been counselled)
- anti-depressants (unless for uses other than depression or existing patients on long-term medication, who have been counselled re- long-term use).

8   **Potentially toxic drugs**
An audit system currently exists to ensure that patients receiving the following medication have had the appropriate recent blood tests performed:
- amiodarone
- lithium
- methotrexate
- azathioprine
- warfarin.

9   **Overuse/underuse**
- Underuse should be monitored at the review date.
- For overuse, only the *average* use is important. Ignore the *today's* use.
- If average use is more than 150% issue prescription but attach *attention* marker for Doctor to assess.
- If *average* underuse is less than 50% attach attention marker for Doctor to assess.

10   **Updating medication from hospital letters and discharge summaries**
- This should be done by the Doctor receiving the letter/discharge summary as a matter of routine.

11 **Dosage instructions**
   - Where possible these should be specific and *as directed* (ASD) avoided where possible.
   - If ASD is used, documentation of the instructions given should be recorded in the medical record.

12 **Collection of prescriptions and uncollected prescriptions**
   - These should be checked on a monthly basis, shown to a Doctor (in monthly rotation) to check any non-compliance of concern, e.g. *uncollected psychiatric medication*, and then shredded.
   - The person collecting the prescription should be asked for details of the patient such as address and date of birth and asked to check the prescription before leaving.

13 **Home visits**
   - Ensure any prescribed or altered medication is added to medical record when writing up visit.
   - When given option to print, press N, which will record that it has been issued, but won't print it.
   - Avoid having items with *no issue*.

14 **Dossett boxes**
   - Chemist normally requests 4–6 weeks' worth at a time.
   - The date will need to be changed for each one week prescription, i.e. 7th January followed by 14th January.
   - Once the sequence of prescriptions has been printed off ensure the date is reset to the current date.

15 **Controlled drugs**
   - Need to be written by hand, but ensure a record is made on computer as to what is given.
   - CD register must be completed for personally administered CDs.

16 **Prescriptions requested by a private Doctor**
   - Can be prescribed, providing satisfied that the patient has been appropriately counselled and that appropriate follow up, monitoring and review are in place.

17 **Prescribing requested by specialist**
   - Refer to Avon-Wide Traffic Light system, NICE guidelines and Bath RUH Drug Interface Group.
   - Shared care protocols now exist for some drugs when transferring from secondary to primary care prescribing.
   - Medico-legal responsibility lies with the person signing the prescription.
   - Ensure the patient has been appropriately counselled re- the medication and appropriate monitoring and follow up are in place.

18 **Patients going abroad**
   - In general, usual amount of repeat prescribing can be supplied (usually 2–3 months or 6+ months for *the pill*).
   - Ensure counselled re- effect of travel on medication, e.g. effectiveness and safety of *the pill*.
   - Patients requiring prescriptions for 'just in case medication' when abroad, should receive private prescriptions.
   - Anti-malarials should be prescribed privately. Some can be bought over-the-counter from pharmacists.

19 Health visitor prescribing
   - The health visitors are able to prescribe certain items. A list of these should be kept in the office.
   - All requests for these items such as *head lice treatment* and *Calpol* should be passed to them unless they are away.

20 Anticoagulant monitoring
   - All patients on anticoagulants (*warfarin*) should have a red anticoagulation card completed with start date, indication, duration of therapy, target INR and relevant medication/past medical history.
   - A daily list of all blood tests taken for INR monitoring should be kept at reception (including those taken at walk-in centre and by district nurses).
   - Late afternoon, these results are taken off the computer lab-links and written onto the red card. If necessary, the receptionist will phone the lab for the results.
   - The duty Doctor will write the recommended dose on the card and retest date.
   - The receptionist will then phone the patient informing them of the result, dosage and make the appropriate follow up appointment.
   - All patients should be fully counseled about the use of *warfarin* and the importance of regular monitoring.
   - All patients should have a hand-held *warfarin* booklet.
   - More frequent monitoring is necessary when patients are ill or taking a drug that might interact.
   - The current system will be updated when 'near-patient' testing starts.

(Updated December 2004)

Chapter 12

Consent and risk

Jane Cowan

The following quote serves as a summary of this chapter:

> It is a general legal and ethical principle that valid consent must be obtained before starting treatment or physical investigation, or providing personal care, for a patient. This principle reflects the right of patients to determine what happens to their own bodies, and is a fundamental part of good practice. A health professional who does not respect this principle may be liable both to legal action by the patient and action by their professional body. Employing bodies may also be liable for the actions of their staff.[1]

Key learning points

- When patients give consent they should be making an informed choice.
- The process of obtaining consent from your patients is an integral part of every doctor–patient interaction.
- In the majority of clinical encounters the consent process is straightforward.
- Doctors and other healthcare professionals need to be aware when further advice may be necessary to ensure that consent is valid.
- Healthcare professionals working in primary care should be as up to date with relevant legal and professional requirements as those working in secondary care.
- Training requirements should be addressed to ensure consistency of practice.

Introduction

Following commitments made by the Government in their plans for the NHS, the Department of Health in England established the Good Practice in Consent Advisory Group in 2000. The remit of the group was to review consent practice and make recommendations for change. A number of publications were produced for dissemination within the NHS. These include patient information leaflets as well as reference and guidance documents for staff.

The guidance documents produced by the Department of Health[1] should therefore be viewed as the framework documents for the modern consent movement and changes in practice in the NHS.

Although the Department of Health in England produced the initial documents, – they have been adopted with appropriate national amendments within the UK to reflect the law in practice within the separate countries. For example, the Welsh Assembly produced the Welsh version of the reference guide in April 2002.[2] In Northern Ireland, the Department of Health, Social Services and Public Safety produced their version in March 2003.[3]

The case law between the four countries is essentially similar, apart from the Incapacity Act in Scotland 2000,[4] which is dealt with briefly later in this chapter. Practitioners working outside England should be familiar with their own national guidelines.

The principles behind the guidance are based on common themes, professional codes of conduct and case law. The context of this chapter should be applicable to all four nations (except where specifically referred to).

Having established that valid (and fully informed) consent is necessary before every clinical interaction, each healthcare worker must be satisfied that they have sufficient knowledge of the appropriate legal and professional standards when obtaining that consent.

Ordinarily the practice of obtaining consent is relatively straightforward, assuming that the healthcare professionals understand the basics of relevant law and good practice requirements. Most doctors, nurses and professions allied to medicine (PAMS) have at least a reasonable grasp of the concepts. Some, although well versed in the complexities of the law in this area, are rarely required to apply it in their day-to-day clinical work. Conversely, and unfortunately, there are a few healthcare professionals who, while professing to have an understanding of the subject, fail to demonstrate that their consent practices are supportable at all times.

The subject of consent in clinical practice is vast – it is debated widely, and researched and written about extensively. Practitioners cannot be expected to have a working knowledge of consent to the level of those representing them. Nevertheless, there are some key concepts in the matter of consent that need to be fully understood and incorporated into everyday practice to protect both the patients and the professionals. All primary care organisations should ensure that their staff members have sufficient access to relevant material to enable them to remain up to date with current practice and legislation.

Assuming that most practitioners are familiar with the rudiments of consent, this chapter will attempt to deal briefly with the following important aspects of the consent process in primary care.

1 Consent principles and processes:
  * patient expectations
  * relevant key documents
  * relevant case law
  * competence and capacity
  * consent to examination and treatment
  * consent to recording, photography and video recording
  * consent to refer

- consent to share information
- consent to access and disclose information.

2 Policies and procedures:
- use of consent forms in primary care
- recording consent decisions
- developing a practice consent policy.

3 Children and young people
- childhood immunisations
- the young patient
- parental responsibility
- child protection.

4 The elderly patient.
5 Mental health and capacity problems.
6 Consent and prison medical services.
7 Developing and changing consent practice:
- developing a PCT consent policy
- consent training in primary care
- the new GMS contract and consent
- the CNST standard on consent and the PCT
- learning from lessons.

Consent principles and processes

Patient expectations

Within the modern NHS, care should be patient-centred, with the doctor and patient working together to reach the best solutions for care. This requires the patient (or parent) to be an active participant (wherever possible) in the decision-making process. The concept of GP decision making rather than informed choice is now seen as an anachronism. Realistically, for those who work in primary care, it is accepted that some patients abdicate the responsibility of making difficult decisions, leaving the healthcare professional to advise and guide them. In these situations, trust in the professional is the most significant contributor to the eventual decision.

Some of the early results from a major NHS consultation process that was conducted during 2003 have led to the publication of *Building on the Best: Choice, Responsiveness and Equity in the NHS*.[5] Several issues are addressed with respect to what patients say they want and need, and the following quote is highly relevant to the consent process:

> Almost 90% of respondents to the Choice Consultation Survey stated that they needed more information in order to make decisions and choices about their treatment or care.

These comments are wholly consistent with the principles of informed consent. Indeed patient consent, agreement or permission – whichever term is employed – is the linchpin of virtually all healthcare. There are, of course, exceptional circumstances, but these tend to be the minority of interactions in primary care.

For patients, parents and carers to participate effectively in healthcare decisions, they require information in a format that is accessible and appropriate. The

Department of Health has produced a selection of guidance booklets on consent. These are written for patients, parents, young people and carers, and should be widely available to the public through primary care centres as well as in the secondary care sector. The printed publications are available free from the Department of Health or can be accessed on their website.[1] The text can be reproduced for personal or in-house use without formal permission or charge.

The guidance booklets are written simply but logically in plain English, and they cover the main points and principles of consent, thus allowing the patient to understand their role in the process. The contents also empower patients, including young people, to question doctors if they feel that the information they have received is inadequate for the choices that they are being asked to make.

Language and cultural barriers can impede effective communication and the transfer of patient information. It is expected in those areas where specific ethnic groups regularly access a primary care service that appropriate steps will be taken to deal with these issues. This problem is also highlighted in child protection policies – with recommendations emerging from the Laming Report[6] (*see* Chapter 16).

The use of the patient leaflets should be encouraged to allow patients to contribute to care and treatment decisions. Written patient information is an addition to but not a substitute for proper discussion. It is also helpful if all staff members are conversant with the contents of the guidance leaflets, as this will start to address the training needs for all members of the primary care team.

Relevant key documents

To ensure consistency and to demonstrate that consent practice is taken seriously in the organisation, a compilation of a selection of relevant guidance and standards is useful.

As risk management and risk assessment develop and progress in the primary care sector, practices should begin to accumulate portfolios of evidence as these will assist with accreditation, re-accreditation, risk review, revalidation and appraisal.

Consent guidance fits in well with this approach, as there are simple, good-quality and easily digestible examples of best practice available from a number of different sources. In gathering the material, it may be useful as part of staff development to allow all members to contribute documents from their various professional and registering bodies, thereby maintaining a multi-disciplinary and comprehensive portfolio of standards.

Professional bodies such as the RCGP have a selection of guidance[7] on their websites which reinforce principles espoused by the GMC and debate issues of concern as they arise.

Unfortunately, a patient or relative may choose to make a complaint or bring a claim against the practice alleging problems with the consent process. In these circumstances, an organisation which is able to demonstrate that improving and maintaining consent practice and standards is part of their philosophy will be better placed than one that cannot do so.

Examples of consent documentation for the practice portfolio include the following:

- 12 key points on consent[1]
- good practice in consent – reference guide (depending on country)[1]

- good practice in consent – implementation guide[1]
- seeking consent – patient information leaflets[1]
- locally produced information leaflets
- information leaflets for patients who do not have English as their first language
- copies of consent forms used in the practice and the community
- GMC guidance[8]
- NMC guidance[9]
- RCGP guidance notes[7]
- MPS publications.[10]

Relevant case law

Common law based on case law in the UK determines the legal standards in consent against which healthcare professionals and organisations are judged. Numerous texts abound that debate and discuss the intricacies of case law set against the context of clinical care and the circumstances under which a doctor or other healthcare professional has been found or may be found wanting.

There are many well-publicised and often scandalous cases involving breach of trust, assault and lack of consent that occur in the primary care setting. Problems including unwelcome sexual advances or flagrant abuse of the doctor–patient relationship are cited as the reasons for bringing a case against the professional for what is deemed to be an assault. In fact, the allegation of an act of battery arising as a result of touching a patient without valid consent is rarely pursued as such.

Legal details are beyond the scope of this chapter, which is intended to address practical approaches to ensuring that consent practice is lawful.

The more relevant but less high-profile problems tend to relate to failure to adhere to the principles of consent. The patient may consider that the doctor has breached acceptable standards by failing to provide sufficient information or time for him or her to make an informed choice. This can relate to any aspect of care – examination, investigation, referral or disclosure. Cases brought against the doctor or PCT may be based on a claim of negligence if the patient has suffered harm as a result of poor or inadequate advice.

Breach of confidentiality and failure to obtain consent can often be tightly bound together. This is particularly so in the child protection arena, where obligations to the family have to be weighed up carefully to ensure that the child's interests are paramount. These situations may be hard to resolve even through legal channels, due to the complexity of the legal process and the necessity to adhere to the rights of all parties.

For the average GP, practice nurse or community physiotherapist, an overview of relevant case law is not specifically required, but the principles underpinning it are. The majority of doctors entering general practice have had virtually no formal teaching in the legal aspects of the consent process, nor have they undertaken any relevant background reading in medico-legal matters. Assimilation of legal principles tends to occur over time and, for some practitioners, by bitter experience. The legal principles are to a large extent mirrored by the good practice standards espoused by the professional bodies.

The Department of Health *Reference Guide*[1] contains a small but adequate legal reference section, which certainly suffices for the majority in clinical practice.

Case law in Scotland and Northern Ireland has some subtle differences, but relevant examples and references are easily available in each country. In particular, the Incapacity Act in Scotland 2000[4] has to be adhered to when dealing with those who lack capacity in Scotland.

Additional information about the Data Protection Act 1998[11] and the Human Rights Act 1998[12] and their relevance to everyday practice can be obtained through PCTs, MPOs and the Department of Health.

Legal advice can also be readily obtained both during and outside working hours. Most PCTs have a contractual arrangement with an experienced firm of solicitors specialising in healthcare. All doctors who belong to a protection organisation have access to 24-hour helplines for support and advice.

Box 12.1 Relevant case law: key points

- The law is complex and constantly evolving.
- The basics of the law relating to consent can be easily accessed.
- Always seek advice in more complex situations.
- Advice is available on a 24-hour basis.

Competence and capacity

Box 12.2 Valid consent

For consent to be valid, it must be given voluntarily by an appropriately informed person (the patient or, where relevant, someone with parental responsibility for a patient under the age of 18) who has the capacity to consent to the intervention in question. Acquiescence where the person does not know what the intervention entails is not 'consent'.[1]

Competence can be defined in a number of ways depending on the circumstances, and is a term frequently used in the context of consent.

Dictionary definitions of competence and capacity from the *New Oxford Dictionary of English* are given in Box 12.3.

Box 12.3 Definitions of competence and capacity

Competence – the ability to do something successfully or efficiently, the scope of a person's knowledge or ability.
Capacity – the ability or power to do, experience or understand something.

When considering capacity in decisions relating to consent, the patient needs to be able to process information in such a way that they:

- comprehend information that is presented to them clearly
- believe it
- retain it long enough to consider it and make a decision.

All those working in the healthcare environment are aware of the many factors that affect or appear to affect a patient's capacity and competence. These factors include *age, mental health, physical health, fear, language* and *cultural barriers*. These should be borne in mind by the doctor who is attempting to ascertain whether he or she has consent to undertake a particular task or procedure.

Within primary care, many GPs will find themselves in a situation where healthcare processes are under way when consent has not been appropriately obtained due to lack of capacity. In most cases, the care given is appropriate, as the doctor has relied on his or her previous knowledge of the patient, their wishes when capable and their current circumstances.

Decisions about capacity and competence are often poorly documented. Other practitioners reading the records may be unable to ascertain what, if any, assessments have been made. *Review within the practice as to how assessments of capacity and competence are recorded may be useful. This enables the healthcare professionals to make appropriate judgements about interventions that are required or recommended in the care and management of the patient with limited or no capacity.*

Again the Department of Health guidance is worth reviewing.[1]

Consent to examination and treatment

Box 12.4 Consent to examination and treatment: key points

- The examination and/or treatment of a patient – by any healthcare professional – always requires consent.
- Every patient should have an opportunity (circumstances permitting) to agree or contest what is proposed.
- The use of a chaperone may not always be possible, but consent to proceed is mandatory in all circumstances.
- What is seen as intrusive by one patient may not affect another.
- All members of the healthcare team should abide by consent principles when dealing with patients.
- Review the Department of Health *Reference Guide*.[1]

Based on principles of good practice, GPs and other primary care health professionals should be fully aware of the need to obtain appropriate consent before proceeding with any examination or intervention.

The differences between implied and explicit consent are explored in virtually all texts on consent. *Explicit consent* is a process of discussion between the doctor and the patient. *Implied consent* is the assumption by the doctor that the patient's behaviour signifies consent. Where any doubt exists, it is prudent to make consent explicit.

The assumptions that are occasionally made under the pretext of implied consent can create unnecessarily difficult situations for patients and doctors. We advise against relying on this concept. It is far better to explain to all patients:

- what you are intending to do
- the nature and purpose of it
- what will happen afterwards.

In this way you can avoid precipitating a misunderstanding that could destroy the trust that is so crucial for the successful doctor–patient relationship.

Concerns about intimate examinations have again led to the production of guidance from a number of sources. Some of the simplest and most practical guidance is available from the GMC, and will be a useful addition to the consent documentation that is held in the practice.[13]

It is important to remember that *any patient can withdraw or refuse consent at any time*.

Once consent has been given, it only remains valid for as long as the competent person continues to engage in the healthcare process to which they consented. Patients can for their own reasons choose to withdraw consent at any time. While this may on occasion seem illogical or irrational, the healthcare professional must respect the decision unless the patient's capacity is in doubt. In the latter circumstance, decisions in the best interests of the patient would prevail.

Consent refusal includes the following:

- refusing to allow an examination or intervention to proceed
- insisting that the examination or intervention is terminated
- refusing to take treatment
- refusing to accept referral or investigation.

Withdrawal of consent must always be appropriately documented.

If a patient withdraws consent, you should try to find out why. There may be serious underlying factors that prevent the patient from accessing treatment or investigation that is in their best interests. However, the patient's choice remains the priority.

Consent to recording, photography and video recording

The majority of primary care consultations do not involve the regular use of recording or photographic equipment, and patients attending are aware that clinical details are recorded either purely electronically or using a combination of paper and electronic records. If a practice chooses to record certain consultations, either as part of the teaching process or as an agreed part of the consultation for other therapeutic purposes, then the patient needs to be in full agreement with the process. In addition to this, doctors may be required to video record consultations for professional examinations.

In 2002 the GMC produced guidance with respect to photographic and other recordings, and this can be found on the GMC website.[14] The message is extremely clear – no video recordings or other recordings of patients are to be taken without their proper permission. The guidance is written with great clarity, and as part of any review of policy and practice in a surgery the staff should be encouraged to access this guidance. Indeed, it may be helpful to retain a copy in the policy files relating to consent and confidentiality. Similarly, if appropriate, particularly in a teaching practice, the practice leaflet should make reference to this policy.

Box 12.5 GMC basic principles, taken from *Making and Using Visual and Audio Recordings of Patients, 2002*[14]

1 When making recordings you must take particular care to respect patients' autonomy and privacy, since individuals may be identifiable to those who know them from minor details that you may overlook. The following general principles apply to most recordings (exceptions are explained in the GMC guidance).
   - Seek permission to make the recording, and obtain consent for any use or disclosure.
   - Give the patient adequate information about the purpose of the recording when seeking their permission.
   - Ensure that the patient is under no pressure to give their permission for the recording to be made.
   - Stop the recording if the patient asks you to do so, or if the recording is having an adverse effect on the consultation or treatment.
   - Do not participate in any recording that is made against a patient's wishes.
   - Ensure that the recording does not compromise the patient's privacy and dignity.
   - Do not use recordings for purposes outside the scope of the original consent for use, without obtaining further consent.
   - Make appropriate secure arrangements for the storage of recordings.
2 If children who lack the understanding to give their permission are to be recorded, you must obtain permission to record them from a parent or guardian. Children under 16 years of age who have the capacity and understanding to give permission for a recording to be made may do so. You should make a note of the factors that were taken into account in assessing the child's capacity.
3 If a mental disability or mental or physical illness prevents the patient from giving their permission, you must obtain agreement to recording from a close relative or carer. In Scotland you must seek agreement from any person appointed under the Adults with Incapacity (Scotland) Act 2000 who has an interest in the welfare of the patient.
4 People who agree to recordings being made on behalf of others must be given the same rights and information as patients acting on their own behalf.

The RCGP has produced a model consent form to use when video recordings are being made for the purposes of examination. A copy of this would be useful if kept in the practice consent file so that GP trainers can satisfy themselves that appropriate consent is obtained at all times. The consent form can be downloaded from the RCGP website.[15]

The standard NHS form for consent to examination or treatment is less suitable for the documentation of video and other recordings, and practices may have already developed their own forms for this purpose if the recordings are made other than for examination assessment purposes.

Consent to refer

The referral of patients from the primary care setting to other healthcare providers or agencies should only occur with the consent of the patient, as the process is discussed and agreed during the consultation.

There are circumstances when referral to another agency or organisation is prompted by additional information that is received but not necessarily discussed with the patient. Even if the referral has been generated with the patient's interests in mind, it is unsafe to assume that the patient will have no objection. A complaint is the most likely outcome if the patient or their relevant carers raise any objections. This is an avoidable upset.

Vulnerable patients are often at greatest risk of breach of consent principles. If the patient's needs appear to be great, and their ability to choose, decide or indeed cope is limited due to (or contributed to) by the condition that requires referral, the healthcare professional may choose to involve others without appropriate discussion with and agreement from the patient. If the doctor makes a decision that the patient is unable to make or incapable of making, this must be mentioned in the documentation.

Similarly, in a situation where safeguarding children is the priority, the healthcare professional must satisfy him- or herself, taking advice as necessary, as to what referrals can be made to other agencies or individuals without obtaining consent from those with parental responsibility. Decisions leading to and actions arising from this should also be documented.

Consent to share information

The principles in the previous section apply equally to the sharing and ultimate disclosure of clinical and personal information (*see* Chapter 9).

Consent to access and disclose information

A practice policy on disclosure should be included in the consent policy portfolio of a general practice. This can take account of the relevant consent processes required to satisfy statutory requirements. Practice information on disclosure should be available for patients so that appropriate decisions can be made about how information is used and shared. This allows the patient the opportunity to withdraw their authority if necessary.

Policies and procedures

Use of consent forms in primary care

Guidance in this area, is far from clear and practice is less than consistent. Some GPs rarely take written consent, while others use consent forms in specific and agreed clinical circumstances.

In revising the NHS consent forms, the Department of Health produced four separate consent forms for use, copies of which are available on their website.[1] The emphasis in the guidance has been slanted towards secondary care, and there is minimal advice about the use of consent forms in primary care.

Of the four forms produced, Form 3 (copied in Appendix 12.1 at the end of this chapter) is most suitable for use in primary care. It is intended for procedures during which consciousness is not impaired, and is therefore appropriate for minor surgery.

Many primary care practitioners argue that the use of a specific consent form is not necessary for the limited range and nature of procedures that are undertaken in the surgery. This would be a valid point if the routine documentation that accompanied these interventions was regularly completed to an acceptable standard. However, reviews of primary care records when procedures have been undertaken rarely allow one to ascertain the nature of any discussion that occurred prior to consent being obtained, and what the patient had actually consented to.

Interestingly, for minor surgery procedures undertaken in a day-surgery unit in secondary care (e.g. excision of ingrowing toe nails), a written consent form would be completed, almost certainly complying with the standard form advocated by the Department of Health.

A limited review (undertaken by the author) of consent forms in use across primary care organisations in different geographical areas produced a bewildering array of paperwork. Overall the standard appeared to fall short of what could reasonably be expected, given the production of guidance in 2001. It was notable that in some practices consent forms were in use that have not been seen in secondary care since the early 1990s. Some practices have more comprehensive forms, but these are also in need of revision. The use of such forms with limited if any clinical information detailing discussion and relevant side-effects, risks or benefits is difficult to justify today. Practices with poor written consent procedures are not in a stronger position than those that have opted not to take written consent.

Conversely, some practices have adopted the Department of Health's Form 3 with some minor amendments, and use accompanying patient information to support the consent process. Examples are given in Appendix 12.2 (courtesy of Ashfield and Mansfield District PCT).

It would appear that in those practices where written consent is taken, the use of forms largely reflects the minor surgical procedures for which payments are made. It is notable that in order for payment to be made there is no requirement for specific agreements about how information is recorded, or indeed how it is provided to the patient. It is assumed that in those practices which undertake these procedures under the new GMS contract,[16] additional rigour will be applied to the recording of consent, as will be discussed later in this chapter.

> **Box 12.6** Examples of minor surgical procedures for which written consent is obtained
>
> • Joint injections
> • Joint aspirations
> • Incisions
> • Excisions
> • Some cryocautery.

Recording consent decisions

For many practitioners, the only time when their written (and/or electronic) clinical records come under scrutiny is when the notes are disclosed to patients or their representatives. Access is not usually requested in order to call their GP's care into question. However, there are times when patients request copy records in order to ascertain whether their own medical care has been of an adequate standard.

Under these circumstances, healthcare professionals often realise that their record keeping was far from exemplary. It is to the detriment of both the patient and the healthcare professional if the clinical records are found wanting.

Within primary care, by virtue of the different clinical services that are offered, the recording of consent decisions has not always reflected the level of discussions that occurred before the patient opted for one approach over another. The trigger factors for the patient who wishes to review their records usually occur when the procedure has gone wrong or when an unexpected complication has arisen. The consent process is not always the motivating factor, but when it becomes apparent that there is no evidence that the untoward outcome was anticipated or discussed, the consent process and documentation will be thoroughly dissected.

We recommend that organisations review their current policy and practice for the recording of consent. It is possible to record this electronically using Read codes. However, in the absence of any other supporting evidence in the records this process is of little value. We recommend that this is explored further within individual primary care organisations in order to establish a consistent approach.

Developing a practice consent policy

The introduction of a practice policy on consent is likely to be of value to most practices.

The policy does not need to be totally comprehensive or a treatise on the current law on consent. However, it does need to be practical, relevant and accessible.

Some practices may already have consent policies that they are willing to share within a PCT to prevent unnecessary duplication of work. The Department of

Health model consent policy can be adapted to a certain extent, but will need considerable customisation for many practices.

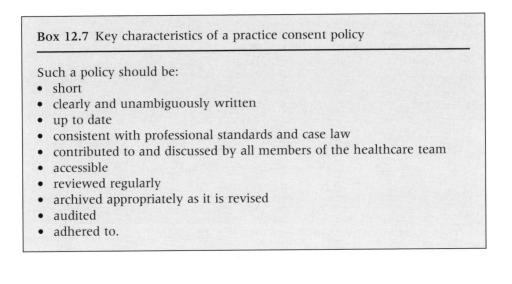

> **Box 12.7** Key characteristics of a practice consent policy
>
> Such a policy should be:
> * short
> * clearly and unambiguously written
> * up to date
> * consistent with professional standards and case law
> * contributed to and discussed by all members of the healthcare team
> * accessible
> * reviewed regularly
> * archived appropriately as it is revised
> * audited
> * adhered to.

Children and young people

Childhood immunisations

The recording of consent for immunisations varies between practices and between PCTs. Some clarity is required to ensure that a similar approach is adopted within geographical areas. Ultimately it is to be hoped that there is greater consistency of practice nationally to ensure that the occasional problem cases which arise as a result of poor information sharing are reduced.

The guidance and policy that already exist are clear, namely that *consent for immunisations must be obtained at the time of each immunisation*. There has been a degree of confusion in the past about the value and purpose of the consent form that parents sign when they register for surveillance and immunisation after the birth of a new baby.

Parents consent initially to have their child *included* on the immunisation and surveillance programme only, with all that entails (e.g. appointments, notification and recording of information about surveillance and immunisation status). This initial consent does not give any healthcare professional the right to give any child any vaccine as part of the routine immunisation programme without obtaining consent at each visit. Whether the consent is written at each immunisation attendance is a matter for practice and PCT policy.

The manner in which consent is recorded varies between practices. PCTs may well address this as part of the consent development under the CNST standards.[17]

The RCGP gives some direction under the Quality Practice Awards (QPA) and Quality Team Development (QTD) standards.[18] Consent and the recording of it are integral parts of any quality programme. Good-quality parental information is a significant part of this process.

Box 12.8 Immunisation: key points

- Ensure that practice policy on immunisation consent is reviewed.
- Clarify the difference between inclusion on the programme and obtaining specific consent for each immunisation.
- Ensure that parental information is widely available and up to date.
- Agree on methods of recording consent for each immunisation undertaken.
- Ensure that all members of the healthcare team are aware of the requirements.

The young patient

Many enquiries are received by medical protection organisations in relation to seeing, treating and examining young patients. All published guidance about the rights of the young person establishes the conditions under which young people are able to actively participate in healthcare decisions. There are certain (and indeed many) situations where the young person can lawfully consent to examinations or treatment. The Department of Health *Reference Guide* has a relatively large section on children and young people, and is worth reading – not least because the relevant sections can usefully be included in the local consent policies.

There are several cases where the wishes of the young person have been overridden initially by the parents and subsequently by the courts. In the majority of situations where there is a discrepancy of opinion, it is unusual to require legal input as the matter is eventually resolved within the family. However, it is important that local policy confirms that young people are entitled to refuse to be examined or treated. This decision must be respected unless it is evident that refusal may lead to serious harm. Various situations can arise during the care of the young person when there are clear differences of opinion between the parents, the young person and the healthcare professional. If an immediate solution is not vital for the health and well-being of the young person, the decision can be delayed until such time as a resolution can be found.

Conversely, situations will be encountered in primary care where the decision taken by the young person does not appear to be in their best interests. The doctor should then seek external advice as soon as possible to ensure that, where necessary, additional support can be obtained. It may be helpful to establish who else should be involved in the management of the young person if the situation becomes more challenging.

The concept of Gillick competence (taken from the Gillick case in 1985)[19] principles in the case of the minor is very much a feature of primary care practice. The *Fraser Guidelines* adapted from the judgement in the Gillick case are largely applied to the prescribing of contraceptives in the under-16s. The more general application of the principles to care of the under-16s is a regular occurrence. The importance of good-quality documentation under these circumstances cannot be over-emphasised – it is essential.

Within the primary care team, staff can attach different interpretations to the guidance, and this may lead to confusion for the young patient as they encounter alternative approaches within the practice. It is useful as part of continuing education to ensure that all healthcare professionals are fully conversant with the concept of the 'competent minor' and how they should be dealt with. The use of the Department of Health *Reference Guide* will assist with this at a basic level.[1]

Inclusion of children in the consent process is to be encouraged. There is a Department of Health consent form specifically designed for children and young people that they are able to sign as well as their parent(s). This is available on the Department of Health website.[1] It is unlikely that this would be used to any great extent in primary care. However, a review of the rights of the child and how they apply may be of benefit for the practice.

Parental responsibility

Within primary care teams, confusion can often exist about the precise definition of parental responsibility and its relevance to the treatment of the child or young person. Due to societal changes in the structure of the family, it is often the case that the father figure in a household (if present) does not have parental responsibility for the children in the true legal sense. The situation can also arise where children reside with their natural father (assuming he was married to their mother at the time of their conception) and a new female partner is the 'mother' in the household. Neither the new 'father' nor the new 'mother' have rights of parental responsibility for children who are not theirs under these circumstances. These new partners are therefore unable to lawfully give consent for medical examinations, procedures, immunisations, etc.

Many practitioners will be aware of the existence of the Children Act 1989. This Act specifies the definitions of parental responsibility, which include the rights, duties, powers, responsibilities and the authorities that a parent has in relation to a child and his or her property. Those working in primary care should be aware of the basic premises so that decisions about children are lawfully taken.

Recent changes in legislation have occurred in England by virtue of the Adoption and Children Act 2002. Likewise, changes are occurring in Northern Ireland and Scotland. These will allow unmarried fathers to assume parental responsibility for their children if their name is given on the birth certificate.

We recommend that all staff are given some training about the rights of parents and the current and proposed changes to the system. Specific advice for practices should be available from the PCT, their legal advisers, medical protection organisations or local social services.

Child protection

Specific problems with regard to consent practice when safeguarding children are dealt with in Chapter 16.

All practitioners who are faced with dilemmas in relation to consent and confidentiality must at all times place the interests and welfare of the child first. This is likely to lead to conflicts in some situations, especially where there is pressure to release information on a 'need-to-know' basis.

Having established that the child will not come to any harm in the interim, staff are advised to check local guidelines for sources of advice and to seek external support as necessary. This is dealt with in more detail in Chapter 16.

The elderly patient

> It should *never* be assumed that people are not able to make their own decisions simply because of their age or frailty.[1]

The elderly patient is of specific interest in relation to consent. A significant proportion of the primary care workload is taken up by the elderly, many of whom have complex and chronic conditions and may have interactions with several other healthcare professionals.

Assessments of capacity in this group of people are increasingly required. This demands skills and patience in settings where time is often a limited commodity.

The guidance document *Seeking Consent: Working With Older People* (available from Department of Health publications and off their website[1]) is particularly valuable in emphasising the difficult and sensitive tasks and problems that have to be undertaken or overcome in order to assess and assist the older patient. In particular, it is also worth considering the following:

> Capacity should not be confused with your assessment of the reasonableness of the person's decision.[1]

The guidance mentioned above considers the problems that can arise with regard to consent in patients who are having difficulty communicating and those who lack capacity. It also provides some basic advice about withdrawing and withholding life-prolonging treatment.

The advice in the booklet may be particularly helpful for those doctors who undertake work and provide services in some of the elderly care homes, where capacity and communication problems can at times impede healthcare interventions.

Mental health and capacity problems

The patient with mental health problems must be treated with respect and dignity at all times. The impact that a serious mental health problem has on the decision-making process should not be underestimated in the consent process.

There are clear legislative requirements for appropriate care and treatment under the Mental Health Act, and GPs should be familiar with the parts of this act that are relevant to primary care practice.

In addition to mental health problems that may need separate management under the Mental Health Act, patients can present with a range of other health problems. They should be dealt with in as similar a fashion as possible to other patients. Information and choice are necessary for the patient to make the correct decision with regard to the treatment, investigation or management of their healthcare problems.

The Department of Health's *Reference Guide*[1] again provides a useful overview of how to deal with patients when capacity may be in doubt.

The patient with learning disabilities, dementia or other problems that may impede decision making can, in certain circumstances, consent to limited healthcare interventions, and as such is able to give their consent. These issues are explored in greater depth in the guidance booklets[1] as follows:

- *Seeking Consent: Working With People With Learning Disabilities*
- *Consent: What You Have a Right to Expect – a Guide for Relatives and Carers*
- *Consent: What You Have a Right to Expect – a Guide for People With Learning Disabilities.*

These are recommended for review within practices. All members of staff involved in the care of those with limited capacity should be familiar with these texts.

In current English law, no one can lawfully give consent for an adult to receive medical treatment or interventions.

In Scotland, the situation changed with the introduction of the Adults with Incapacity (Scotland) Act 2000. The medical part of this act came into force in 2002.[20]

A draft bill under consideration in England is the *Mental Incapacity Bill*. When this is introduced (within the next three years) it will dramatically change the position on consent to medical treatment in certain circumstances, and will require a review of consent policy in healthcare.

Consent and prison medical services

The Department of Health, the Prison Service and the Welsh Assembly Government, in recognising the special needs of the prison population, have produced specific guidance for obtaining consent from patients who are receiving custodial sentences.

These patients have rights as individuals irrespective of their position as prisoners, and doctors are encouraged to ensure that consent processes in the prison service are of the same standard that would be reasonably expected for any other patient.

The management of primary care services for prisons has been under the control and care of the PCTs since April 2004, and standards for the provision of these services should come under the usual governance arrangements. Therefore development of and adherence to a policy on consent are to be expected.

The text of the leaflet can be found on the Department of Health website.[21]

Developing and changing consent practice

Developing a PCT consent policy

During 2003, many PCTs were developing and reviewing consent policies. Several known to the writer have undertaken an audit of current practice. This has produced interesting results in some areas, and has confirmed the variations in approach within practices, within professions and across all employees.

Some areas of concern have already been highlighted earlier in this chapter. Considerable effort will be necessary to produce workable policies that will suit the range of skills and practices working across any one PCT.

Unfortunately, wholesale adoption of the model consent policy produced by the Department of Health is not the answer for most PCTs, as the policy is geared towards secondary care provision. Although the principles are transferable, the language will need to be modified. New policies should reflect the actual work undertaken.

There are several PCTs in which consent policies have been introduced without adequate discussion with the GP body, leading to misinterpretations and a failure to engage clinicians in a vital piece of work. We recommend that input from the GPs is essential to shape and produce a primary care consent policy that will be relevant for modern clinical practice.

A simple policy that reflects the nature of the clinical situation in primary care can easily be prepared and implemented. This should take into account the various healthcare professionals employed in the community, all of whom need to engage in consent decisions and processes with their patients/clients.

Consent training in primary care

There are few primary care teams to date in which formal training and updating in consent have been a regular part of practice development. There is no doubt that the skills and understanding of different members of the healthcare team can be variable across a whole range of topics, and consent is no exception to this.

It is reasonable for a patient to expect that at all stages of their interaction with the primary care team, the various team members understand the basic premises underpinning the consent processes in healthcare. The attention to detail that one member of the primary care team may show in relation to consent will not protect the others from practice that is generally seen to be outdated and inappropriate.

When considering the training requirements of the practice, the current level of knowledge and awareness should be assessed, based on some of the themes discussed in this chapter. A clinical audit project would be a valuable baseline by which standards could be assessed and training requirements clarified.

Consent training can be easily linked into several other practice development approaches in the implementation of the new GMS contract. PCTs may also be willing to consider hosting events to debate some of the areas of local controversy. External advice/input can often be provided to meet educational needs. Training events may act as catalysts for change if new policies are necessary or existing ones need review.

Once a training programme that is appropriate for the different staff groups has been agreed, we recommend that it be included in induction programmes to ensure that all new staff comply with accepted practice policy. Updates should be planned from time to time (at the very least, when changes in the law occur or new professional guidelines are issued).

The new GMS contract and consent

With the publication of the new GMS contract,[16] systems changes will be occurring in all practices and PCTs. There is a limited emphasis in the new contract with regard to consent. However, there are several defined areas where consent practice is inextricably linked with other processes and should be reviewed as changes and improvements are made.

Examples (taken from the competency framework) where assessment of consent practice should be considered as part of the process of clinical audit, managing risk, etc., are shown in Box 12.9.

Box 12.9 Competency framework for practice management (GMS contract):[16] relevant sections for consideration

---

Practice operation and Development
    Clinical audit
    Organisational audit
    Professional development

Risk management
    Risk assessment
    Significant event audit
    Confidentiality
    Ethics

Partnership issues
    CPD requirements

Patient and community services
    Information
    Patient protection
    Social services

Human resources
    Induction training

IM & T (information management and technology)
    Patient records
    Data management
    Data security
    Data interpretation

The CNST standard on consent and the PCT

PCTs now belong to the CNST,[17] details of which can be found on the NHSLA website.

Independent practitioners are not included in the indemnity arrangements of the NHSLA or the formal CNST assessment process of implementation of the risk management standards. However, since April 2004 the PCT's management of independent contractors has formed part of the assessment. Progress towards the implementation of appropriate consent policies and procedures will be reviewed under this system.

Of the 12 criteria in the standards that were published in May 2004, criterion 8 is concerned with the consent process.

The CNST 2004 version of risk management criterion 8 for primary care and relevant to consent is set out in Box 12.10 below:

Box 12.10 Criterion 8: clinical care, competence and communication[17]

From April 2005

1A 8.1   Consent procedures recognise the central importance of the rights of each person.

1A 8.1.1 The PCT's consent policy and all forms for investigation and treatment used comply with Department of Health guidelines for design and use.

1B 8.5   Appropriate information is provided to practices on the risks and benefits of the proposed treatment or investigation and the alternatives available.

1B 8.5.2 The PCT has a robust, documented process for the development and updating of patient information leaflets.

In preparing for a CNST assessment, the PCT will review current policy and the quality of patient information available within the PCT. This will include information that is used by non-medical practitioners who are employed by the PCT to provide patient services.

It would not be unreasonable for others involved in patient care to review the literature and information available to patients and to assess what, if any, needs reviewing.

It is also important to ensure that any updated patient information is clearly dated, and that examples which have been replaced have been archived properly. This applies to the PCT as well as the individual practice.

Learning from lessons

Occasionally complaints and claims arise from poor consent practice in primary care. These are infrequent compared with the number of healthcare interactions that occur every day. Careful analysis of complaints and claims may demonstrate problems with consent practice.

Misunderstandings of intentions can easily occur, and may be brushed off by the healthcare professional without an objective review of how and why the misunderstanding took place.

However, these problems merit debate among members of the team, as there may be issues that have not previously surfaced that are relevant to clinical practice and behaviour. This is particularly important in a training practice, where opportunities exist to analyse and develop clinical skills that can ultimately shape a lifetime's work.

Consultations with 'difficult' patients are worthy of discussion in the appropriate learning environment in order to minimise problems in the future. Intimate examinations undertaken by clinicians who may adopt a more brusque approach to clinical consultations and examinations may likewise be the subject of complaints. The feelings and sensitivities of the patients must be considered at all times, and it is often only when they feel able to register a complaint that the patient's views actually surface (intimate examinations and relevant guidance are discussed in Chapter 8).

Finally, detailed documentation and meticulous recording of any healthcare encounter that seems to have led to a loss of rapport as a result of misunderstandings is always advisable.

Conclusion

Good practice with regard to consent is a professional, ethical and legal requirement. The majority of clinicians understand the basic principles underpinning the consent process and are increasingly aware of the pivotal role of the patient in all healthcare decisions.

Maintaining a high standard of consent practice is a prerequisite for modern medicine – information is widely available and we have given the clinician suitable references for accessing it. Similarly, in the more complex clinical situation where the rights of the patient may be difficult to establish, the doctor must not hesitate to seek appropriate and timely advice.

References

1 Department of Health (2001) *Reference Guide to Consent for Examination or Treatment.* (Various) Department of Health, London; www.dh.gov.uk/Home/fs/en and www.dh.gov.uk/PolicyAndGuidance/HealthAndSocialCareTopics/Consent/ConsentGeneral Information/fs/en
2 www.wales.gov.uk/subihealth/content/keypubs/pdf/refguide-e.pdf and www.wales.gov.uk/subihealth/topics-e.htm#NHS
3 www.dhsspsni.gov.uk
4 www.scotland.gov.uk/health/cmo/incapacity_act_toc.asp
5 Department of Health (2003) *Building on the Best: choice, responsiveness and equity in the NHS.* Department of Health, London.
6 *The Victoria Climbié Inquiry, January 2003*; www.victoria-climbie-inquiry.org.uk
7 www.rcgp.org.uk/corporate/position/confidentiality/conf2.asp
8 www.gmc-uk.org/standards/default.htm
9 www.nmc-uk.org/nmc/main/publications/$allpublications
10 www.medicalprotection.org/medical/united_kingdom/publications/booklets/default.aspx – MPS guidance on consent
11 Data Protection Act 1998 (chapter 29)
12 Human Rights Act 1998 (chapter 42)
13 www.gmc-uk.org/standards/INTIMATE.HTM
14 General Medical Council (2002) *Making and Using Visual and Audio Recordings of Patients*; www.gmc-uk.org/standards/AUD_VID.HTM
15 www.rcgp.org.uk/exam/forms/patconsent.doc
16 Department of Health and British Medical Association General Practitioners Committee (2004) *Standard General Medical Services Contract*; www.dh.gov.uk/assetRoot/04/07/51/59/04075159.pdf
17 *CNST Standards*; www.nhsla.com/Welcome_to_NHSLA.htm
18 www.rcgp.org.uk/external/standards/topics.asp?alpha=Immunisation
19 *Gillick v Wisbech and West Norfolk AHA* [1985] 3 *All ER* 402.
20 www.scotland.gov.uk/health/cmo/incapacity_act_toc.asp
21 www.dh.gov.uk/PublicationsAndStatistics/Publications/PublicationsPolicyAnd Guidance/PublicationsPolicyAndGuidanceArticle/fs/en?CONTENT_ID=4008751&chk=5D2Uc1

Appendix 12.1

Patient identifier/label

[NHS organisation name] consent form 3

Patient/parental agreement to investigation or treatment
(procedures where consciousness not impaired)

Name of procedure (include brief explanation if medical term not clear)
....
....

Statement of health professional (to be filled in by health professional with appropriate knowledge of proposed procedure, as specified in consent policy)

I have explained the procedure to the patient/parent. In particular, I have explained:
The intended benefits ....
....
....
Serious or frequently occurring risks:...
....
....

I have also discussed what the procedure is likely to involve, the benefits and risks of any available alternative treatments (including no treatment) and any particular concerns of those involved.

☐ The following leaflet/tape has been provided ....

Signed: ....   Date ....
Name (PRINT) ....   Job title ....

Statement of interpreter (where appropriate)
I have interpreted the information above to the patient/parent to the best of my ability and in a way in which I believe s/he/they can understand.

Signed ....Date....................Name (PRINT).....................................

Statement of patient/person with parental responsibility for patient
I agree to the procedure described above.

I understand that you cannot give me a guarantee that a particular person will perform the procedure. The person will, however, have appropriate experience.

I understand that the procedure will/will not involve local anaesthesia.

Signature ....   Date ....
Name (PRINT) ....   Relationship to patient ....

Confirmation of consent (to be completed by a health professional when the patient is admitted for the procedure, if the patient/parent has signed the form in advance)

I have confirmed that the patient/parent has no further questions and wishes the procedure to go ahead.

Signed: ....   Date ....
Name (PRINT) ....   Job title ....

Top copy accepted by patient: yes/no (please ring)

Guidance to health professionals (to be read in conjunction with consent policy)

This form
This form documents the patient's agreement (or that of a person with parental responsibility for the patient) to go ahead with the investigation or treatment you have proposed. **It is only designed for procedures where the patient is expected to remain alert throughout and where an anaesthetist is not involved in their care: for example for drug therapy where written consent is deemed appropriate.** In other circumstances you should use either form 1 (for adults/competent children) or form 2 (parental consent for children/young people) as appropriate.

Consent forms are not legal waivers – if patients, for example, do not receive enough information on which to base their decision, then the consent may not be valid, even though the form has been signed. Patients also have every right to change their mind after signing the form.

Who can give consent
Everyone aged 16 or more is presumed to be competent to give consent for themselves, unless the opposite is demonstrated. If a child under the age of 16 has "sufficient understanding and intelligence to enable him or her to understand fully what is proposed", then he or she will be competent to give consent for himself or herself. Young people aged 16 and 17, and legally 'competent' younger children, may therefore sign this form for themselves, if they wish. If the child is not able to give consent for himself or herself, some-one with parental responsibility may do so on their behalf. Even where a child is able to give consent for himself or herself, you should always involve those with parental responsibility in the child's care, unless the child specifically asks you not to do so. If a patient is mentally competent to give consent but is physically unable to sign a form, you should complete this form as usual, and ask an independent witness to confirm that the patient has given consent orally or non-verbally.

When NOT to use this form (see also 'This form' above)
If the patient is 18 or over and is not legally competent to give consent, you should use form 4 (form for adults who are unable to consent to investigation or treatment) instead of this form. A patient will not be legally competent to give consent if:
- they are unable to comprehend and retain information material to the decision and/or
- they are unable to weigh and use this information in coming to a decision.

You should always take all reasonable steps (for example involving more specialist colleagues) to support a patient in making their own decision, before concluding that they are unable to do so. Relatives **cannot** be asked to sign this form on behalf of an adult who is not legally competent to consent for himself or herself.

Information
Information about what the treatment will involve, its benefits and risks (including side-effects and complications) and the alternatives to the particular procedure proposed, is crucial for patients when making up their minds about treatment. The courts have stated that patients should be told about 'significant risks which would affect the judgement of a reasonable patient'. 'Significant' has not been legally defined, but the GMC requires doctors to tell patients about 'serious or frequently occurring' risks. In addition if patients make clear they have particular concerns about certain kinds of risk, you should make sure they are informed about these risks, even if they are very small or rare. You should always answer questions honestly. Sometimes, patients may make it clear that they do not want to have any information about the options, but want you to decide on their behalf. In such circumstances, you should do your best to ensure that the patient receives at least very basic information about what is proposed. Where information is refused, you should document this overleaf or in the patient's notes.

The law on consent
See the Department of Health's *Reference guide to consent for examination or treatment* for a comprehensive summary of the law on consent (also available at www.doh.gov.uk/consent).

Appendix 12.2

These forms are reproduced here with the kind permission of Ashfield and Mansfield District PCT.

Patient consent form (agreement to undergo treatment/procedure)

Form 1
Patient name: . . . .

Date of birth:. . . . .

Responsible health professional:. . . . .

Proposed treatment/procedure: . . . .

. . . .

. . . .

Statement of health professional (to be completed only by a health professional with appropriate knowledge of proposed procedure/treatment)

I have explained the procedure to the patient. In particular, I have explained:

The intended benefits:. . . . .

Serious or frequently occurring risks/side-effects: . . . .

I have discussed what the procedure is likely to involve and any particular concerns raised by the patient.

In the case of the patient being aged 16 years or under, I confirm them to be Fraser–Gillick competent in my opinion.

Signature (health professional): . . . . Date: . . . .

Statement of patient
I agree to undergo the procedure/treatment as it has been explained to me and documented above.

I understand that the procedure/treatment will be carried out by a health professional with appropriate training and experience.

Signature (patient):. Date:. . . . .

A witness should sign below if the patient is unable to sign but has indicated their consent and is legally competent to do so.

Minors who are Fraser–Gillick competent may sign their own consent, but where possible it is good practice to ask a parent or legal guardian to countersign below.

Name of witness and stated relationship to patient:. . . . .

Signature (witness):. Date: . . . .

Patient consent form for children and adolescents who are not Fraser–Gillick competent (agreement to undergo treatment/procedure)

Form-3

Patient name: . . . .

Date of birth:. . . . .

Responsible health professional:. . . . .

Proposed treatment/procedure: . . . .

. . . .

. . . .

Statement of health professional (to be completed only by a health professional with appropriate knowledge of proposed procedure/treatment)

I have explained the procedure to the patient. In particular, I have explained:

The intended benefits: . . . .

Serious or frequently occurring risks/side-effects: . . . .

I have discussed what the procedure is likely to involve and any particular concerns raised by the patient or their parent/guardian.

Signature (health professional): . . . .   Date: . . . .

Statement of parent/legal guardian

I agree to my child undergoing the procedure/treatment as it has been explained to me and documented above.

I understand that the procedure/treatment will be carried out by a health professional with appropriate training and expertise.

Signature (parent/legal guardian): . . . .   Date: . . . .

Chapter 13

The primary/secondary care interface

Mark Dinwoodie

Key learning points

- Errors at the primary/secondary care interface are common.
- Specific areas include prescribing, admissions, discharges, results, referrals and 'Did Not Attend' (DNAs).
- Communication and an appreciation of responsibility are fundamental principles.
- Electronic communication could become an important mechanism for reducing risk in this area.
- Safe and efficient systems need to be established across the interface, involving key personnel.
- Local working groups established across the primary/secondary care interface could tackle the various areas of concern.

Introduction

The primary/secondary care interface offers an ideal opportunity for things to go wrong. These are two large workforces with a blurred boundary of responsibility. There is often a feeling from within one sector that those in the other sector are unappreciative of the difficulties involved for those not working in their sector. There have traditionally been criticisms raised by secondary care that they receive inappropriate or delayed referrals and inadequate correspondence. Primary care, on the other hand, complains about the lack or delay of discharge summaries, patients being discharged too early, long waits for treatment, the 'offloading' of work, and having to act as the 'safety-net' for secondary care. It is sometimes helpful to consider a patient's progress between the various health sectors as a journey, which should be made as smooth and seamless as possible.

Common themes associated with risk at the primary/secondary care interface

These include the following:

- communication
- responsibility
- lack of adequate systems, and failure to follow existing systems.

Communication

This is dealt with in more detail throughout the chapter. Good communication by whatever means is the cornerstone of reducing risk at the primary/secondary care interface.

There are now increasing numbers of ways to communicate (face to face or by telephone, post, email, fax or 'text'), so there is little excuse for poor communication. The main issue seems to relate to perceiving the need to communicate in a given situation. It is always worth putting yourself in someone else's position in order to appreciate how they would manage without adequate communication from you. Breakdown of communication seems to occur:

- between the community and the hospital on admission
- between the hospital and the community at discharge
- between healthcare professionals and patients.

Communication at a more strategic level needs to occur between primary and secondary care. This might take the form of a GP users group or GP forum. Cross-sector groups need to be established to optimise patients' care, such as *integrated care pathways* for chronic diseases, or drug interface groups (see below). There are many examples of clinical interface agreements between primary and secondary care – for example, the Camden and Islington Interface group in Adult Mental Health (www.londondevelopmentcentre.org/resource/local/docs/C&IInterface.DOC). The Audit Commission reported on the success of introducing a diabetes educator practitioner to improve the interface between primary and secondary care for diabetes in West Norfolk (www.diabetes.audit-commission.gov.uk/casestudies/examples/westnorfolk/printable.htm). Locally, in Bath we have been running an integrated care pathway for coronary heart disease, which includes a whole range of healthcare professionals from primary and secondary care.

Similarly, groups need to work on the systems and administrative issues that cross the sectors such as information management and technology. The Whittington Hospital and local PCTs established the Whittington Primary Care Interface Group (www.whittington.nhs.uk/default.asp?c=1423&t=1,154) in 2002 with the aim of providing a high-level forum that would integrate the following aims across the three local PCTs:

- primary care liaison
- service developments
- clinical projects across the primary and secondary interface
- two-way communication
- a modernisation agenda
- linking to commissioning and performance issues.

The Rapid Response or Discharge Facilitation team is one of the primary care interface services which aims to facilitate a safe discharge for those patients who are medically fit to be discharged, but where there may be difficulties with social circumstances or who, with additional nursing and community support, might be managed at home.

Better systems for communication include the increased use of electronic communication, which is likely to be quicker, more reliable, easier to distribute and possibly more inclusive. Concerns have been raised about issues of confidentiality, but these problems can be overcome by suitable encryption, confidentiality protocols and adherence to the Data Protection Act.

Some departments and disciplines have used *patient-held records* for some time (e.g. *maternity notes* for antenatal care, and *parent-held records* (usually a *red book*) for child health). These act as a shared-care record and allow the contribution of several healthcare professionals while ensuring that the information accompanies the patient and is readily available. Concerns about patients or parents losing their notes seem to have been largely unfounded, although parents do not always remember to bring their child's 'red book'.

Diabetes UK (www.diabetes.org.uk) is often asked about providing a template for a 'standard' patient-held record, following the success of various diabetes patient-held records (www.diabetes.org.uk/infocentre/carerec/patient_records.doc). While appreciating that they need to take into account local needs and priorities, they list a number of features that they feel should be included (*see* Box 13.1).

Box 13.1 Suggested contents of a patient-held record

- Patient's and relevant professional's contact details
- Patient's medical details
- Explanatory notes
- Treatment
- Instructions for emergencies
- Education checklist
- Details of regular check-ups
- Details of annual reviews
- Space for patient's own notes
- Glossary of medical terms
- Educational notes

Patients often have a self-monitoring book for conditions such as diabetes or asthma, and the idea of holding their own records seems to be very acceptable to them. The use of diabetes self-held records has been shown to improve diabetic patients' quality of care.[1] Locally, we have developed a patient-held record for coronary heart disease to facilitate communication following admission with a heart attack or angina. This gives details of the event, tests, medication, future plans, etc.

Plans are well under way for the introduction of an *electronic patient record* as outlined in the Department of Health's document *Information for Health: an Information Strategy for the Modern NHS, 1998–2005*,[2] published in 1998 and updated with *Building the Information Core: Implementing the NHS Plan*[3] in 2001. The main proposals for the development of electronic records include the following.

- Organisational records documenting treatment of a patient will become electronic and known as *EPRs*, and a subset of them will contribute to a lifelong record of a patient's healthcare, namely the *EHR*.

- There will be increased availability of medical information about a patient to relevant healthcare professionals.
- It should enhance the process of *medicines management*, out-of-hours and emergency management of patients, as well as avoiding duplication and improving audit.
- There will be patient involvement in their EHR.

The EPR should improve communication at the primary/secondary interface and hopefully reduce some of the risks currently associated with this domain.

The electronic record development and implementation programme run by the NHS Information Authority has now closed, but the website contains a wealth of information from pilot projects and lessons learned in developing EPRs along with an evaluation. It is a useful resource for anyone developing or implementing electronic records (www.nhsia.nhs.uk/erdip/pages).

Other possibilities include the use of 'smart cards', or other forms of patient-held electronic data.

Communication of information between general practices is also currently a problem, and can lead to inadequate patient information being held on GP computers. At present there is no electronic means of transferring patient records between GP practices, so this has to occur through a paper process. This is partly due to a variety of GP software systems. Incomplete GP records may lead to incomplete information being passed to secondary care at times of referral or admission. Pilot studies are currently under way that are looking at the electronic transfer of patient records between practices, and hopefully this will become the standard process in the near future.

Availability of professional colleagues

There are occasions when it is helpful for patient care for healthcare professionals from one sector to be able to quickly contact their colleagues in the other sector. The hospital sector has facilitated this for junior staff through the use of a pager or bleeper system. However, it is often difficult to get past the receptionists at a GP practice or the secretaries at a hospital. Mobile phones have helped a little, but both sectors need to have an efficient system for passing messages on, so that valuable time is not wasted returning calls back and forth as healthcare professionals try to get hold of each other. Electronic communication may well help further in this respect.

Responsibility

There is a danger that when a patient falls between two sectors of the health service, each sector will assume that the other has taken responsibility, with the net result that neither does so adequately, and the patient suffers as a consequence. A good example of this is the following up of test results arranged in, say, secondary care with the results arriving in primary care, where it is assumed that secondary care will sort it out (who don't, thinking that as the results have gone to primary care, they will sort it out). The same problem can occur between primary care and tertiary care centres following a specialist procedure, where GPs might incorrectly assume that everything related to that procedure will be sorted out by the tertiary centre, even though the patient has been discharged home.

Exactly who has responsibility for particular aspects of patient care, and when, needs to be clearly established through systems and protocols rather than by informal ad hoc arrangements (*see* Figure 13.1).

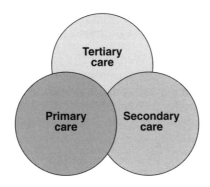

Figure 13.1 Areas of overlap of responsibility.

Lack of adequate systems, and failure to follow existing systems

The area of the primary/secondary care interface has historically been neglected with regard to protocols and systems to ensure that a patient has a smooth journey and seamless medical care when progressing from one sector to another. In other cases, the protocols or systems that are in place are often overridden or ignored, increasing the likelihood of error.

The main areas of risk at the primary/secondary interface are as follows:

1 prescribing and medication
2 discharge from hospital
3 admission to hospital
4 referrals to hospital
5 results
6 'Did Not Attend' (DNAs).

Prescribing

Issues relating to medication errors and prescribing in primary care are dealt with in Chapters 11 and 25. This section will deal with medication errors arising from problems at the primary/secondary care interface. GPs are often asked to prescribe medication at the request of their secondary care colleagues, and to provide further repeat medication. The legal responsibility for a prescription lies with the person who signs the prescription. In 1991 the Department of Health published an Executive Letter[4] recommending that a transfer from hospital of drug therapies with which GPs would not be familiar should not take place without full local agreement and the dissemination of sufficient information to individual GPs. The Department of Health had previously published a Health Notice[5] stating that 'The duty of prescribing rests with the doctor who at the time has clinical responsibility for the patient's treatment, so that where a hospital doctor bears the clinical responsibility for a patient having a course of investigation or treatment as an outpatient, he should prescribe for the patient's needs. When the hospital doctor decides to return the patient to the care of his general practitioner, the responsibility for prescribing will thereafter rest with the latter.' The decision as to which doctor has clinical responsibility at any given time is clearly a very grey area. Many hospital clinicians feel that it is impractical for them to be issuing repeat prescriptions on an ongoing basis. Inevitably the issue of cost and budgets has an influence on this debate. However, legal responsibility lies with the doctor who signs the prescription.

Box 13.2 Examples of medication errors that arise at the primary/secondary care interface

---

Example 1
A GP was asked to prescribe a medication by a hospital consultant, who wrote to the GP confirming the details. The patient was told to phone his surgery to collect a prescription. The GP issued a prescription as requested. The patient suffered unpleasant side-effects and complained that he had not been warned about any potential side-effects by either the GP or the hospital consultant.

Example 2
A patient was discharged with changed medication and requested a repeat prescription, but was given her old medication that she had been taking prior to admission. Her condition deteriorated and she had to be readmitted. The patient's repeat medication list had not been updated by the GP on receipt of the discharge letter.

Example 3
A confused patient was admitted and found to have lithium toxicity. The GP had assumed that the hospital was carrying out the monitoring, while the hospital thought that they had devolved this responsibility to the GP.

Example 4
An elderly woman was discharged on warfarin, but was unable to read the doses on the bottles and took the wrong amount. This resulted in her having a haemorrhagic stroke.

Potential prescribing problems at the primary/secondary care interface

- *Inadequate patient counselling.* Patients need to be counselled about any medication that they take, with reference to its advantages and disadvantages, dose, frequency, method of administration, potential side-effects, monitoring requirements and follow-up arrangements. Consent by the patient to take the medication needs to be informed. Therefore GPs should not write a prescription at the request of secondary care colleagues unless they are satisfied that patient consent is informed, or are able to counsel the patient themselves.

- *Interactions*. The majority of prescribing for any patient will occur in primary care. Doctors in secondary care may not be aware of all the medication that the patient is taking, as the patient may be uncertain him- or herself, the correspondence may be inaccurate, or the medication may have changed since the time of referral. A drug that interacts with other medication could therefore be prescribed inadvertently.
- *Lack of monitoring*. Certain potentially toxic medication requires monitoring (e.g. rheumatic disease-modifying drugs such as methotrexate, and lithium) while other drugs require monitoring for therapeutic effect (e.g. thyroxine and warfarin). Unless clear instructions are given to the patient and arrangements are made with the GP, it is possible that the appropriate monitoring will not occur. The GP needs to ensure that appropriate action is taken following correspondence from the hospital, in order to be certain that monitoring occurs on a regular basis, confirmed by regular audits. National guidelines are available regarding the appropriate monitoring of disease-modifying drugs from the British Society for Rheumatology.[6]
- *Specialist drugs*. Hospital specialists are by their very nature more likely to prescribe newer or more specialised drugs. A GP may be very unfamiliar with a specialised drug, and may therefore not be able to monitor the therapeutic response, adjust the dose, detect side-effects or counsel the patient adequately.
- *Delay*. There will inevitably be a delay between the time when the patient sees the hospital specialist and the arrival of the correspondence recommending the new medication. Patients are often keen to get started on treatment, especially if it is likely to alleviate their symptoms. This can lead to frustration or sometimes the temptation to initiate treatment on the basis of what the patient tells the GP. This is clearly a risky thing to do. The problem is sometimes overcome by giving a handwritten note to the patient. Unfortunately, these are sometimes illegible, give insufficient detail or do not indicate whether the patient has been appropriately counselled and consideration given to interactions and contraindications.
- *Problems with continuity of medication supplies when moving from one care setting to another*. A patient may well be discharged from hospital with different medication to that with which they were admitted. Failure to update the repeat prescribing list in general practice will result in the possibility of the patient being prescribed their pre-admission medication. The patient may not question or even realise this. General practices therefore need to have a robust system for ensuring that a patient's repeat prescribing list is updated following that patient's discharge, along with changes following attendance at outpatient clinics. Outpatient letters must also be readily available for the next GP consultation, whether in paper or electronic format.

  One of the difficulties on discharge is that patients are currently sometimes only given 7 days' supply of medication (this is commonly in standard plastic containers that all look the same, but with different writing on the labels). The patient may find it difficult to see their GP within the next few days, perhaps because they are still recovering or have difficulty getting an appointment at short notice. Most hospitals are now discharging patients with 28 days' supply of medication.
- *Conflict of drug formularies between primary and secondary care*. Hospitals tend to have quite restricted drug formularies, partly dictated by cost. Drugs may be

relatively cheaper in secondary care than in primary care and so formularies may differ. This sometimes results in patients being switched from one type of drug to another in the same class for cost reasons. At one time, some pharmaceutical companies appeared to operate a 'loss-leader' approach with the intention of discounting drugs to secondary care so that patients were initiated on a particular brand, in the hope that the patient would be continued on the same drug in primary care, but at a much higher price. Healthcare communities need to establish a group that combines professionals from both sectors in order to resolve these issues and develop care pathways, joint treatment guidelines and joint formularies.

• *Problems with patient compliance and concordance following discharge.* Many patients are not involved in decisions about their treatment and medication. Others, or their carers, are confused about the purpose of their medication and so these patients may not take it as intended.

Reducing the risks related to prescribing at the primary/secondary interface

1 There needs to be a *local strategy and policy* involving PCTs and local hospitals with regard to prescribing and medication. Inevitably cost will be high on the agenda but, overall, medicines management should be the leading issue. There is a need to adopt formularies and treatment guidelines across a locality irrespective of whether the patient is in primary or secondary care. The introduction of NSFs and the publications by NICE have helped to set standards for prescribing in certain conditions that are equally applicable to primary and secondary care (www.nice.org.uk and www.doh.gov.uk/nsf/ nsfhome.htm).

   In addition the Department of Health has recently published a useful document with regard to the medicines management of patients with chronic diseases, *Management of Medicines.*[7]

2 There are a number of programmes and initiatives established nationally and being piloted locally that aim to improve medicines management across primary and secondary care. These include the following.

   • *Modernising Medicines Management: A Guide to Achieving Benefits for Patients, Professionals and the NHS,*[8] produced by the National Prescribing Centre (NPC) and the National Primary Care Research Centre, along with the *National Collaborative Medicines Management Services Program* for primary care (for further information, visit www.npc.co.uk/mms) (*see* Chapter 25 for more details).

   • The *Pharmaceutical Services Negotiating Committee (PSNC)* along with four other national pharmaceutical organisations is piloting the provision of a structured medicines management service within community pharmacies in England (for further information, visit www.psnc.org.uk).

   • The *Task Force on Medicines Partnership* based at the RPSGB is a two-year study looking at the issues of concordance (for further information, www.concordance.org).

   • In 2001, the *Association of Scottish Trust Chief Pharmacists* produced a very useful report about improving medicines management across the primary/secondary/tertiary care interface.[9] They make a number of recommendations.

- – The patient's own medicines are used throughout the patient journey.
- – One-stop dispensing – that is, sufficient medicine is supplied during the patient's hospital stay to cover both inpatient and discharge requirements.
- – The patient should receive medication in a form and quantity that ensure continuity of care (e.g. original packs).
- – Ensure that the patient receives written and, where appropriate, verbal information consistent with their needs.
- – Identify which groups of patients are able to take responsibility for administering their own medicines in hospital.
- – Shared-care protocols should be developed for specialist medication.
- – Improve communication by integrating medical records and improving technology.
- – There should be 24-hour access to pharmaceutical services by patients and members of the public. (An issue addressed in a recent DoH report.)[10]

3 *Good communication, information flow and effective systems* are the key factors that reduce risks in this area. These factors will be discussed further in the sections on admission and discharge. Better and swifter communication should become possible as technological advances translate into practical working solutions for the NHS. Electronic communication will probably soon become the norm.

4 Many PCTs and local hospitals have established *drug interface groups* or similar committees of relevant personnel (e.g. pharmacists, hospital clinicians and GPs) to agree medications which are suitable for prescribing by primary care (or not). Examples of this are the Effective Shared Care Agreements (ESCA) set up in the West Midlands by the Midland Therapeutic Review and Advisory Committee (MTRAC),[11] www.keele.ac.uk/depts/mm/MTRAC/. A multi-disciplinary group discusses products at each meeting and assigns them to one of three categories, similar to the list below:

- • medication that is only suitable for prescription by a specialist
- • medication that can be prescribed in primary care under shared-care arrangements and protocols
- • medication that can be prescribed by primary care (i.e. medication other than that in groups 1 and 2).

MTRAC has developed templates for developing or negotiating a shared-care agreement for a number of suitable new drugs. They recommend that ESCAs should be patient specific; used when the condition is stable or predictable, with the willing consent of patients, carers and doctors; have clear identification of areas of responsibility; have an established communication network for problems including out-of-hours; be accompanied by a clinical summary; are accompanied by identification and provision of any training needs in primary care; and that funding issues are resolved.

Clearly the list needs to be updated regularly in the light of increased knowledge and experience of a particular drug. Practices need to have a clear record of those drugs that are prescribed solely in secondary care, so that if they prescribe any additional medication they can consider any potential interactions.

It is possible that the hospital-prescribed medication will not be on the GP computer database.

- There is a move towards discharging patients with *28 days' supply in original packs*. This will aid compliance with and continuity of medication, and patients will recognise the original packs with which they are familiar. There are considerable advantages, including patient acceptability, compliance, security, child resistance, medicine stability, hygiene, stock control, labelling, traceability and accountability, patient information, reduction in errors and improved efficiency.[12] Four key organisations – Pharmaceutical Services Negotiating Committee, Guild of Healthcare Pharmacists, Primary Care Pharmacists Association and the Royal Pharmaceutical Society of Great Britain – commissioned the development of guidance with regard to patients' discharge medication.[13]
- Similarly, at the time of admission to hospital the Accident and Emergency department or the acute admissions ward may not have unusual medication easily available, and the patient may miss doses. One solution is to *use the patient's own drugs* while they are in hospital. The advantages of this, as suggested by the NPC's *Modernising Medicines Management* (www.npc.co.uk/mms/index.htm) and adapted from an article in *Hospital Pharmacist*,[14] are as follows.
  - It allows patients to continue with familiar medication during their admission.
  - It enables a more accurate drug history to be taken, as the patient has their existing medication with them.
  - It avoids duplication of therapy.
  - It avoids waste, as previously medicines that patients brought with them into hospital were destroyed.
  - Out-of-date, inappropriate or poorly stored medication can be discarded, removing the risks associated with these drugs.
  - Discontinued medicines are removed in order to prevent them from being inadvertently restarted by the patient on discharge.
  - It may reduce some of the delay in providing medicines at the time of admission or discharge.
- According to the Department of Health's publication *Pharmacy in the Future: Implementing the NHS Plan*,[15] the intention is for there to be *repeat dispensing* by community pharmacists and *e-pharmacy* where prescriptions can all be processed electronically. These developments may well improve communication between primary and secondary care in the field of medication.
- The *pharmacist* has a key role in reducing risk. Several studies and pilot projects have looked at the role of the pharmacist in facilitating the prescribing process at the primary/secondary care interface and providing seamless care. One mechanism by which this occurs involves sending the community pharmacist a copy of the discharge and medication summary.[16] Another is for there to be direct communication between community and hospital pharmacists with regard to complex patients such as the elderly, those on numerous medications, patients with frequent admissions, the mentally ill or those with learning difficulties. In Harrogate, a pharmacy discharge letter scheme has been developed in which each patient's medication is reviewed prior to discharge,

and an electronic discharge letter is produced citing the reasons for any changes, with copies sent to the patient/carer, GP and community pharmacist.[17] The Royal Pharmaceutical Society has produced some useful admission and discharge checklists.[18] The hospital pharmacist is in an ideal position to assess particular needs of the patient prior to discharge (e.g. whether a compliance aid is needed, or to check inhaler technique). Further information and examples can be found in the Health Executive's document *GP Prescribing Support* (available on their website at www.doh.gov.uk/nhsexec/gppres.htm).

Other possibilities with regard to facilitating medicines management across the primary/secondary care interface include the following.

- *Healthcare professionals with a specific role to facilitate seamless care across the primary/secondary care interface.* This could involve either individuals such as a pharmacist, or a team incorporating a nurse, pharmacist, social worker, etc. Some hospitals already have *discharge facilitation teams* or *rapid assessment teams* that act in this way.
- *Using the patient's knowledge about their own condition and medication.* It is probably in everyone's interests that patients are well informed about their medication and involved in the decision-making process with regard to prescribing, a process known as Medicines Partnership (aimed at putting the principles of concordance into practice) (www.medicines-partnership.org). The Expert Patients Programme aims to ensure that patients with chronic conditions will be in a position to manage aspects of their condition, including medication use (www.doh.gov.uk/cmo/progress/expertpatient and www. expertpatients.nhs.uk/index.shtml). To a certain extent this already happens for patients with diabetes who adjust their insulin dose, and for asthmatics who alter their inhalers when unwell. Self-monitoring and adjustment of dose is, for those patients who want to be involved, an important part of *feeling in control* of their condition.[7] Some hospices carefully write out a list of all medication that a patient is taking, along with the purpose and potential side-effects and a chart showing what medication to take when – a medicines reminder chart.
- *Availability of information about medication.* There is a need for easy-to-access information about medication. This might be through the community pharmacist, improved patient information leaflets, useful telephone advice lines such as *NHS Direct*, or specific websites. The latter include:
  - NHS Direct Online (www.nhsdirect.nhs.uk)
  - the National electronic Library for Health (www.nelh.nhs.uk)
  - patient information (www.patient.co.uk/)
  - patient information leaflets regarding medication and conditions (www.doctoronline.nhs.uk)
  - treatment notes (www.which.net/health/dtb/treatment.html).

Other developments include *NHS Direct Information Points*, which are touchscreen information points, and *NHS Digital*, which is exploring the potential of digital television for providing heath information and advice.

- *Education and training* for healthcare professionals are issues that will always need to be considered.
- *Local examples* of some of the above initiatives are available through the Medicines Management Services (MMS) at the NPC (www.npc.co.uk/mms).

Admissions to hospital

Admission of patients to hospital usually occurs at a time when they are seriously ill and need fairly urgent treatment. Their optimal management may depend on accurate and useful information supplied by the patient, their relatives or carers and their GP. This information includes the patient's past medical history, drug history, allergies, history of presenting complaint and social history. Some patients may be able to supply all of this information themselves, but others may be too ill, confused or distressed to do so.

Again, good communication is paramount. Traditionally this has been in the format of an admission letter accompanying the patient. With the advent of fax and email there is little justification for a patient arriving in the Accident and Emergency department or medical admissions unit without a letter. Some GPs use a printout of part of the patient's computer record to help improve speed and accuracy, particularly if the patient has an extensive past medical history or medication list. It is often helpful to encourage a relative, close friend or carer to attend with the patient when they are admitted to hospital, as they may well be able to offer useful information. Ask the patient to take all of their current medication with them. Some GP out-of-hours co-operatives and surgeries use a standard admission letter with sections that prompt for the appropriate information. Others use a computer pro forma, which extracts data from the computer record and inserts it into a letter which can include the last consultation, with the GP only having to fill in a few gaps. Clearly this is not always a practical option, but as more information becomes transmitted via email, admission letters will probably increasingly become computer generated and be emailed to the hospital.

A good quality admission letter should contain the following:

- patient details including DoB, address, hospital or NHS number
- GP practice details including phone number
- date and time patient seen
- history of presenting complaint and treatment so far
- past medical history
- drug history and allergies
- social history and occupation
- family history if relevant
- any known details regarding patient's wishes, e.g. advance directives
- relevant examination findings
- results of any relevant tests or investigations, e.g. blood, urine and radiology
- provisional or differential diagnosis
- purpose of admission or assessment
- what the patient has been told (where relevant).

Discharges from hospital

In comparison with the clinical state on admission, the patient is hopefully somewhat better on discharge, which allows the possibility of a more planned transfer from secondary to primary care. Communication and planning are the key issues with regard to discharge. Some of the problems which can arise around the time of discharge are listed below.

- *Lack of or delay in providing a discharge summary.*

Box 13.3 Example of lack of a discharge summary

A patient with chest pain was discharged and was unclear about his diagnosis. He re-presented 3 days later with the same complaint (i.e. chest pain at rest). There was no discharge summary to indicate the diagnosis and investigations that had taken place or the future management plan. The patient had been given medication for angina and was already on treatment for gastro-oesophageal reflux. The GP had little option but to readmit the patient, whereas if the information on a discharge summary had been available this might not have been necessary.

- *Lack of liaison.* Patients often have complex medical, psychological and social problems.

Box 13.4 Example of lack of liaison

A vulnerable patient who lived alone was sent home on a Friday afternoon having just been started on warfarin. She was fairly immobile due to her deep vein thrombosis. Social services were unable to offer support until the following Monday. Along with the practical difficulties of trying to monitor warfarin in the community at the weekend, the patient was unable to support herself at home over the weekend.

- *Further investigations and hospital follow-up.* Patients will often need further investigations or follow-up after an admission.

Box 13.5 Example of need for further investigations and follow-up

A discharge letter from the cardiology team that had admitted the patient stated 'patient needs endoscopy and follow-up with gastroenterologist: to be arranged'. The discharged summary was sent 6 weeks after admission, so there was already a delay, and the GP assumed that the hospital would make the appointment for endoscopy and the follow-up with a gastro-enterologist, and reassured the patient that this would be the case. When the patient had still not heard after a further 3 months, the GP chased up the appointments only to find that the hospital had assumed that the GP would arrange them.

Reducing the risks associated with discharges

- Many hospitals have introduced a multi-professional discharge team who start to plan the patient's discharge well before the discharge takes place.
- Patients and their carers need to be actively involved in decisions about their discharge.
- Good communication with members of the primary healthcare team (e.g. GP and district nurse) is vital, especially if any immediate action is needed on discharge (e.g. in the case of dressings or anticoagulant monitoring).
- Consider the timing of the discharge and whether it puts the patient at increased risk.
- Involve social services early on where appropriate.
- Timely and detailed discharge letters are needed. My personal opinion is that discharge letters are as important as the medication with which the patient is sent home. As in the case of their medication, I do not think the patient should be allowed to leave hospital without one.
- Copies of the discharge summary should be given to the patient, the GP, the community pharmacist and the district nurse where appropriate.
- Consider the use of patient-held records or the introduction of electronic communication for discharge summaries.

Box 13.6 Information to be included in a good discharge summary

---

- Patient details, including date of birth, address and hospital/NHS number
- Date of admission and discharge
- Main diagnosis and subsidiary diagnoses
- Results of major investigations
- Abnormal results of minor investigations
- Progress during admission
- Details of any operative procedures performed
- Treatment given
- Discharge medication
- What the patient has been told (where relevant)
- Any further investigations needed, and whether these have been arranged
- Action needed by GP/district nurse/health visitor
- Advice about further management
- Other agencies involved
- Follow-up arrangements

Results

The results of most investigations will be held on hospital computers, and so the results of tests carried out in primary care may well be available to secondary care.

Exceptions to this will include cases where patients are admitted to a different hospital from that which performed the tests, such as a community hospital or different district general hospital. It is important therefore that details of results and investigations performed are included with referral or admission letters. It is very frustrating, a waste of resources and puts patients at risk to needlessly repeat investigations.

Although many GP practices now receive the results of tests that have been initiated in primary care via a process referred to as *Lablinks,* most practices do not have access to all tests performed by their secondary care providers, unless they specifically phone the relevant department.

Investigations that are initiated in secondary care are sometimes *copied to* primary care. What then becomes unclear is whose responsibility it is to *action* any abnormal result. Although the person who initiates an investigation should find out and action the result, once a GP becomes aware of an abnormal result from hospital they have an obligation to ensure that any further management required is in hand. This can present a difficult situation, as the following case study demonstrates.

Case study 13.1

A GP received a copy of the histology report from a biopsy of the cervix taken at the colposcopy clinic a few weeks earlier showing invasive cancer. He contacted the hospital but was unable to find out whether the patient had a follow-up appointment. He therefore phoned the patient to ask her if she had a follow-up appointment, which she did. Not surprisingly, she asked about her biopsy result and the GP found himself having to break the bad news over the phone in far less than ideal circumstances. She asked about specific treatment and the GP felt that he was not the best person to discuss this. Both the GP and the patient felt very unsatisfied with the way in which the result had been handled.

There needs to be a clear local agreement about which results should be routinely copied to primary care. In addition, if a test is arranged in outpatients or during an admission that is appropriate for follow-up in primary care, then a clear agreement needs to be reached with the individual GP that they *will* follow up the result, rather than the current situation of *assuming* that the GP will deal with the result. Similarly, from a GP perspective, where a letter states that a result will be sent or copied to the GP, the GP practice needs to have a system for ensuring that these results are chased up. A further complication is that some electronic *Lablinks* systems are unable to deal with results *copied to* primary care by secondary care, so the GP never receives them!

Several pilot projects are currently being undertaken to look at *bar-coding* all blood test requests accompanying the blood sample to improve accuracy when they arrive at the hospital. Ideally, the GP software system needs to match all investigations that are sent to hospital against results that return to the practice. In this way any outstanding or 'lost' results can be chased up. This process is often referred to as *matching 'ins' and 'outs'*.

Referrals

The main areas of risk with regard to referrals are:

*   failure to refer
*   lost referrals
*   inadequate referral letters
*   suspected-cancer urgent referrals
*   outpatient waiting times.

Failure to refer

There are many reasons why GPs fail to refer. The referral process is often very idiosyncratic to the individual or their GP practice. In general, the longer the delay from the decision to refer to the actual referral letter being produced, the more likely it is that the referral will be overlooked. This may be because the notes have been removed for another purpose, or because the prompt to remind the GP to refer has disappeared. Practices need to have a safe and efficient system. Some practices put a Read code or other marker on the computer so that a search can be done on the computer at the end of each month for a list of patients who should have been referred. This can be compared against a list of letters or referrals generated. Some doctors actually dictate their referral letter in front of the patient, which helps to improve the accuracy of the referral and reduces the likelihood of it being overlooked. It is also fits in well with a patient-centred approach to consulting. It is more difficult with complicated referrals or those that involve certain conditions, such as possible malignancy or psychiatric conditions.

Lost referrals

There are plenty of opportunities for referrals to get lost – within the practice, in the post to the hospital, and within the hospital. Many practices have to rely on a fairly unsatisfactory safety-net of saying to the patient that if they have not heard by a given time, they should contact the practice to chase up the referral. This is not very consistent with the modern age of electronic communication. The NHS Plan[19] states that by the end of 2005, waiting lists for hospital appointments will be abolished and replaced with booking systems. The main national initiative is the *National Booking Programme: Access, Booking and Choice*, which sits within the Service Improvement Team of the Department of Health's Modernisation Agency (for further information visit www.doh.gov.uk/waitingbookingchoice and www.modern.nhs.uk/scripts/default.asp?site_id=21).

The plan is for the following:

*   an electronic booking service that incorporates information about waiting times and other data provided by local health communities
*   a bookings management service whereby patients can make and change appointments
*   the use of booking guidance and clinical protocols.

For further information, a useful website is: www.doh.gov.uk/nhsplanbooking systems.

Many localities have pilot projects in place that are already achieving some of these aims. At our local district general hospital most of our referrals are sent electronically, sometimes using standard referral forms (e.g. for rectal bleeding). This helps our secondary care colleagues to prioritise the referral appropriately. The patient can be given a phone number to ring and can book their appointment at a time that is convenient to them. This *electronic bookings* website lists waiting times and provides guidelines. The process allows confirmation that the referral has been received, read and *actioned* by the hospital. In addition, the appointment date can be included, and whether the patient attended.

There are many potential advantages to this system, including increased efficiency and less time spent chasing hospital appointments.

A variation of this scheme is a *partial booking system*, in which the patient is contacted once the referral has been received by the hospital informing them to this effect, along with the approximate waiting time and confirmation that they will be sent a definite appointment nearer the time.

Inadequate referral letters

In a similar way to admission letters, referral letters need to contain adequate detail and information. In particular, it is important that the reason for the referral is included, to try to ensure that this is addressed.

Suspected-cancer urgent referrals

GPs need to be aware of the symptoms and signs that merit urgent '2-week referrals' for suspected cancer. This information is available on www.doh.gov.uk/cancer/referral.htm.

There needs to be a secure fax or electronic system to ensure that this process is reliable. The practice also needs to ensure that the referrals have been received by the hospital.

Outpatient waiting times

In some areas and specialties there are long waiting times to be seen in outpatients. It is important that GPs do not assume that once they have sent off a referral, their responsibility for that particular illness of their patient has ended. It is often appropriate to arrange to review the patient after a suitable time period to see whether:

- the patient's condition has worsened, requiring the appointment to be expedited
- the patient's condition has improved or resolved, possibly allowing the appointment to be cancelled
- additional treatment or investigations are appropriate prior to the patient being seen in outpatients.

Practices might like to consider auditing their referrals from a clinical governance perspective. This might help to improve the quality, appropriateness and priority of referrals. It was the Government's aim for all clinic letters to be copied to patients from 2004. Further details are available from the DoH publication *Copying*

Letters to Patients: Good practice guidelines[20] and their website, www.doh.gov.uk/patientletters/issues.htm. The DoH has acknowledged that this has not been achieved and that it is a challenging target, but is continuing to work with local organisations to try and implement it further. This might help the communication process and add another layer to the defence against things going wrong. However, there is some concern that it will restrict what is said in such letters. For example, a mention of the possibility of malignant disease might alarm a patient if included, but it could be important for a fellow healthcare professional to have this information.

Did not attend (DNAs)

A number of patients will have moved and not managed to inform either the hospital or their general practice. A *change of patient details* is probably the commonest reason for patients not attending their outpatient appointment. When a referral is made, it is an ideal opportunity to check the patient's details and to remind them that, should they move, they should inform both the practice and the hospital.

When a patient fails to attend an outpatient appointment, the letters *DNA* (**D**id **N**ot **A**ttend) are entered in the notes, and a letter is written to the GP informing them of this. The secondary care clinician needs to make a decision, based on clinical need as to whether a further appointment needs to be sent, and should inform the GP of this in the letter.

On receipt of the DNA letter from the hospital, the GP practice should check the patient details, and then the GP who made the referral should decide whether to re-refer or review the patient, depending on the nature of the referral. This is particularly important for those referrals where there was some concern about a possible underlying serious illness. Otherwise there is a danger that important referrals will be overlooked or delayed.

Summary

There is considerable potential to improve the patient's journey from one healthcare sector to another with the goal of achieving true seamless care. Healthcare workers from all health communities have a responsibility to work together to reduce the risks at these interfaces. There are good examples from around the UK where substantial improvements have been made, and information about these is available from the references listed in this chapter.

References

1 Davies M and Quinn M (2001) Patient-held diabetes record promotes seamless shared care. *Guidelines Pract.* **4**: 54–62.
2 Department of Health (1998) *Information for Health: an information strategy for the modern NHS, 1998–2005. A national strategy for local implementation*; www.nhsia.nhs.uk/def/pages/info4health/contents.asp
3 Department of Health (2001) *Building the Information Core: implementing the NHS plan*; www.nhsia.nhs.uk/def/pages/info_core/overview.asp

4 NHS Executive (1991) *Responsibility for Prescribing Between Hospitals and GPs*. Department of Health, London.

5 Department of Health (1976) *Health Notice HN(76) 69*. Department of Health, London.

6 British Society for Rheumatology (2000) *National Guidelines for the Monitoring of Second Line Drugs*; www.rheumatology.org.uk

7 Department of Health (2004) *Management of Medicines: A resource to support implementation of the wider aspects of medicines management for the National Service Frameworks for Diabetes, Renal Services and Long-Term Conditions*; www.dh.gov.uk/assetRoot/04/08/87/55/04088755.pdf

8 National Prescribing Centre (2002) *Modernising Medicines Management: a guide to achieving benefits for patients, professionals and the NHS*; www.npc.co.uk/mms

9 Association of Scottish Trust Chief Pharmacists (2001) *Improving Pharmaceutical Care and the Patient Journey: redesign of medicines management across the primary/secondary/tertiary care interface*; www.show.scot.nhs.uk

10 Department of Health (2004) *Delivering the Out-of-hours Review: Securing proper access to medicines in the out-of-hours period*; www.out-of-hours.info/downloads/short_medicines_guidance.pdf

11 Jones B and Clark W (2003) Shared care agreements – how to overcome the blank page. *Pharm J*. **270**: 165–6.

12 Roberts K and Sharp J (1988) Original packs – what do patients think? *Pharm J*. **240**: 382–4.

13 Royal Pharmaceutical Society of Great Britain (2003) *Medicines Management During Patient Discharge*; www.rpsgb.org.uk/pdfs/medsmanpatdisguid.pdf

14 Dua S (2000) Establishment and audit of a patient's own drug scheme. *Hosp Pharm*. 7: 196–8.

15 Department of Health (2000) *Pharmacy in the Future: implementing the NHS Plan*; www.doh.gov.uk/pharmacyfuture/

16 Duggan C, Feldman R, Hough J and Bates I (1998) Reducing adverse prescribing discrepancies following hospital discharge. *Int J Pharm Pract*. **6**: 77–82.

17 McAdam K and Norris C (2002) The pharmacy discharge service. *J Guild Healthcare Pharm*. **Feb**: 12.

18 Royal Pharmaceutical Society of Great Britain (1993) *Admission and Discharge Checklists*; www.rpsgb.org.uk

19 Department of Health (2000) *The NHS Plan: a plan for investment, a plan for reform*; www.nhs.uk/nhsplan

20 Department of Health (2003) *Copying Letters to Patients: Good practice guidelines*; www.dh.gov.uk/assetRoot/04/08/60/54/04086054.pdf

Chapter 14

Complaints

Mike Deavin

Key learning points

- The nature of modern healthcare delivery is such that complaints from dissatisfied patients and their relatives are inevitable. While it is true that complaints bring difficulties that add to the workload, they also bring very important messages and sometimes illuminate a view of service delivery that would otherwise go unnoticed simply because we are standing too close.
- Complaints are more likely to be well managed in circumstances where:
  - the practice philosophy is one that is open, receptive and responsive to comment or criticism
  - a complaints policy is not only in place but is genuinely used as a day-to-day work tool
  - issues raised during complaint investigations are valued as a significant contribution to the clinical governance agenda
  - all members of staff believe that they will be well supported if they are unreasonably accused, or abused.

Background: an overview

A formalised NHS complaints procedure, *Complaints, Listening, Acting . . . Improving*,[1] was introduced in 1996 following the publication of Professor Alan Wilson's report *'Being Heard'*[2] in May 1994. The procedure identifies a two-stage process for the resolution of complaints, and retains the possibility of referral to the Health Service Ombudsman if the two stages fail to resolve substantial issues of concern.

The two stages, namely *local resolution* and *independent review*, have been the subject of much criticism, and in 2000 a formal study of the process was commenced. The research brief was to 'provide an evaluation of how the new complaints procedures are operating across all parts of the NHS and to meet the needs of policy makers and managers concerned with the future development of the system'. An executive summary of recommendations made as a result was published in March 2001, and *NHS Complaints Reform: making things right*[3] was published in February 2003.

This document left much of the practical part of local resolution procedures unchanged, but placed new and robust emphasis on dialogue, openness and mediation. In addition, it endorsed the valuable contribution to complaints resolution made by Patient Advice and Liaison Services (PALS) and patient involvement groups.

The majority of changes were seen in the second stage *independent review* process. The *'listening exercise'*[4] completed in October 2001 identified that true independence was neither achieved nor seen to be achieved by staff and complainants alike. It was clear that all parties to the process had very little confidence that it was sufficiently robust or objective.

The substantive changes proposed for the local resolution stage were as follows.

- The Board of every NHS organisation would be held accountable for the performance of the organisation in handling complaints.
- The complaints procedure would be integrated into the clinical governance/ quality framework of the organisation.
- The same principles and process would apply to all parts of the NHS.
- The complex nature of multi-agency complaints would be recognised.
- Time limits for consideration of complaints and for the preparation of responses would be lengthened.
- PCT Boards would receive appropriate information at least quarterly on the causes of complaints and the action taken.
- Front-line staff would receive training in complaints handling.
- Criteria for granting an independent review would be published and applied consistently throughout the NHS.

The second stage (independent review) would no longer be in the gift of the *complaints convenor* (who was usually a non-executive member of the Trust Board). The Healthcare Commission (formerly the Commission for Health Audit and Inspection, CHAI) and the Commission for Social Care Inspection (CSCI) would assume responsibility for managing the independent review stage of the NHS and social services complaints procedure.

In December 2003, the Department of Health launched a consultation on the draft regulatory framework[5] that would underpin the reformed complaints procedure. The consultation period ended on 31 March 2004. The DoH later published the Complaints Regulations[6] and the changes took effect from 30 July 2004. Some of the more radical changes were deleted from the final draft leaving the following as the most significant.

- The complaints procedure should apply to all NHS bodies (including PCTs).
- Primary care complaints can be addressed to the practitioner *or* the relevant PCT.
- Explicit recognition that complaints can be raised with any member of staff.
- Independent Complaints Advisory Service (ICAS) information must be given to complainants.
- NHS organisations must designate a Board member or similarly senior person to ensure that complaints receive full consideration and that action is taken as a result of complaint investigations.
- A person who is affected by or *likely to be affected by* the action, omission or decision of the NHS body can bring a complaint.
- Representatives who may make a complaint on behalf of a patient are identified.

This is not the end of the process. Parliament has indicated that it will look very seriously at any recommendations that are made following the conclusion of the Shipman Inquiry. At the moment the guidance provided to support the implementation of the new procedure makes it clear that the guidance booklets from 1996 for Family Health Services Practitioners have not been amended. Those who operate practice-based local resolution complaints procedures will need to understand the new arrangements that apply to the second stage of the process. It would seem logical to assume that in the fullness of time all parts of the NHS will operate a common complaints policy that is easily understood by patients who do not necessarily make distinctions between primary and secondary care, particularly when they feel they have a grievance that needs resolving.

Complaints management in practice

It is perhaps a little naive to assume that all complaints will be received with open arms and acknowledged as learning opportunities. However, it is important to subject all complaints to a standard process to ensure that:

- you comply with the complaints procedure
- you identify any learning opportunities so that changes can be put in place.

The following is offered as a practical guide to working through the process.

1   The first task of course is to decide whether you have received a complaint, an enquiry or notice of a legal claim. Clearly a degree of subjectivity is involved, but a definition of a complaint as *an expression of discontent that requires a formal response* should differentiate important issues from minor queries. A word of caution – 'important' means *important from the complainant's point of view.*
2   Complaints are usually received very soon after the incident occurred. *NHS Complaints Reform: making things right*[3] suggests 6 months as a reasonable time for complainants to make their dissatisfaction known, and identifies that it is unreasonable for staff to be subject to the threat of complaint indefinitely. The report goes on to say 'Subject to the exercise of discretion in appropriate cases, the existing time limit of 6 months should be retained'. The regulations that apply from 30 July 2004 endorsed six months as appropriate and go on to explain that in situations where the complainant had *good reason* for delay or where it remains possible to investigate *effectively* and *efficiently*, the complaints manager may choose to waive the time limit.
3   A major factor in handling complaints well is to have an administration system that prompts good practice. The demands made by the timescales imposed and the need for investigation and detailed information from hard-pressed colleagues makes it very easy to lose track of what needs to be done when.
    Dedicated IT software complaints-handling packages are available, but are perhaps excessive for all but the largest practices. A diary system that is marked up in advance once a complaint has been received will be a real help as the process unwinds.
4   Complainants may well refer to their intention to go to a lawyer in their pursuit of justice, and of course they have every right to do so. The only circumstance in which a complaint investigation is inappropriate is where you have clear evidence that a damages claim has commenced, and you form the

view that an investigation would compromise or prejudice the damages claim. Lawyers often advise their clients to pursue matters through the complaints procedure, and may well assist them as the investigation unfolds. A lawyer's involvement will often help in that they provide an objective and unemotional contribution to what can be a subjective and emotive problem.

5 Complaints received directly from the patient do not raise consent issues. However, complaints received from third parties (partners or other relatives, the MP, care home proprietors, etc.) require careful consideration in terms of the release of information. If the patient has capacity, their signed consent to release medical details to a third party is necessary. If the patient lacks capacity, a representative should be involved.

   If the patient is deceased or is unable by reason of physical or mental capacity, the representative must be a relative or a person who (in the opinion of the complaints manager) has *sufficient* interest in the patient's welfare and who is *suitable*. If the patient is a child the representative must be a parent, guardian or other person who has care of the child. If the child is in local authority care the representative must be a person authorised by that local authority. One interesting duty now placed on complaints managers is to decide on the suitability of representatives. If he/she deems a person suitable then the complaints process continues, if unsuitable then the complaints manager must write to the person explaining why they appear unsuitable.

A host of organisations may be involved in supporting or assisting complainants.

• PALS personnel are now employed directly by PCTs and acute trusts. Although their primary remit is to advise patients when organisational issues arise, they may well point patients at and support them through the complaints procedure.
• The Independent Complaints Advisory Service (ICAS) was established with funding from strategic health authorities to take on the complaints support function from the now dissolving Community Health Councils.
• The Citizens Advice Bureau (CAB) plays an active role in NHS complaints in some areas.
• AvMA is more commonly involved in medico-legal claims, but may assist with complaints.

The involvement of these organisations can assist greatly and should be welcomed, particularly in circumstances where the issues are highly emotive. Developing a straightforward and open relationship with staff whose task is to facilitate the process can be very helpful.

Why do patients complain?

It may help to consider at this point why people complain and what outcome they seek.

   Patients complain for precisely the same reason that you might complain about poor service or substandard goods. The realisation that expectation has not been matched by the reality of experience has the potential to prompt all of us into a concerted effort to gather information, seek redress and perhaps effect change (the expectation–reality gap and strategies designed to reduce that gap are discussed later in this chapter).

Complaints that are made in a spirit of constructive criticism with a genuine wish to effect change for the benefit of others are more easily dealt with from an emotional point of view than those made in anger by patients who are motivated by a wish for retribution. The impact of complaints on staff must not be underestimated. Every year staff leaving the service cite increasing numbers of complaints as a factor that contributed to their decision to go. It can be very difficult, particularly in small practices, for staff to access the degree of support necessary to remain objective and relaxed while under fire from dissatisfied patients. It is an issue that could be considered proactively and mechanisms put in place before a problem develops.

Acknowledging the complaint

Once a complaint has been received, it should be acknowledged in writing within 2 working days. The acknowledgement should contain a copy of the practice complaint policy leaflet identifying how the process works and the timescales involved. It must also contain information about how to access the local Independent Complaints Advisory Service.

For example, the acknowledgement letter could read as follows:

> I write to acknowledge receipt of your letter dated 10 January. I am both sorry and concerned that you are dissatisfied with the service provided. I will ensure that the problems you mention are thoroughly investigated and I will write again with information once my investigations are completed.
>
> Enclosed please find a copy of the practice complaints leaflet that identifies how the NHS complaints procedure operates and the timescales involved.

If issues concerning consent are identified, they can be explained in the acknowledgement letter. A request that the patient signs a copy of the letter is often the quickest and easiest way of establishing consent and making progress.

Investigating the complaint

The nature of the investigation will be entirely dependent on the nature and seriousness of the complaint received. At one end of the scale the complaint can be quickly and simply resolved. At the other, police involvement, legal help and staff disciplinary action may all be necessary. Complaint letters are highly likely to contain a mixture of fact, emotion and misunderstanding. On receipt of the letter:

1　read it at least three times, on the last occasion with a highlighter pen to identify the issues that require investigation
2　note what information you require and, importantly, who needs to provide it
3　set a deadline for information gathering (10 days is probably about right, given that you may need to contact a number of colleagues, all of whom may be able to provide one part of the response jigsaw)

4 the formal requirement is that the complainant should receive a written response within 20 working days or as soon as is reasonably practicable. If this cannot be achieved, the complainant should receive a rationale for the delay and regular updates on progress.

The complaint response

It is difficult to be prescriptive about the style of the response. A regular criticism is that the response fails to address all of the issues, apologies seem hollow rather than heartfelt, and insufficient information is provided about the extent to which change has been implemented. Responding to a complaint or criticism can be an emotive issue. Good practice suggests that objectivity is more likely if the investigator and author of the response are not directly involved in the circumstances of the complaint. (The only reason why full-time complaints managers are not permanently in the consulting room is that they have the luxury of dealing with complaints that are not usually about them!) Of course this is difficult to achieve in smaller practices, but in medium-sized and larger practices the non-medical practice manager is ideally placed to oversee the whole process.

The quality of the response received by the complainant is the factor most likely to determine the success or failure of local resolution. The complaints procedure dictates timescales, but the style of response is completely dependent on the individual who deals with the complaint investigation.

Consider two potential responses to a complaint that the doctor failed to visit as quickly as the patient's family thought was appropriate:

> Thank you for your letter concerning what you allege to be a delayed home visit. While I am sorry you feel the doctor did not come as quickly as she could, my information is that other ill patients took priority and she came as quickly as she could have done in the circumstances.

This is short, providing no real information, a hollow apology, and is highly likely to antagonise. Now consider the following:

> I am now able to respond to your letter of 1 January. I do of course realise what a worrying time you must have had waiting for Dr Jones to call after your mother was taken ill last Tuesday. When I received your letter I contacted Dr Jones and Mrs Brown, who is our new receptionist, in an attempt to discover the background to this incident. Mrs Brown tells me that when she received your call at approximately 12.30pm she made a note of the symptoms you described and put the message on top of the list of notes Dr Jones had prepared for her afternoon visits.
>
> Dr Jones tells me that as soon as she finished with her last patient at lunchtime she collected her list of notes and went off to start her visits. It was at 2.45pm when she phoned in to the surgery that she spoke to Mrs Brown and realised that your call should have been added to the 'urgent' calls she had on that day. She did come as soon as she realised the problem, and I am very pleased she was able to arrange help for your mother very soon after she got to you.

Both Dr Jones and I are very sorry this error on our part caused such concern. Clearly we need to look at our procedures to ensure that a similar error does not occur again, and once we have decided what changes are necessary I will contact you and let you know.

Can I send my best wishes to your mother and thank you for bringing this matter to my attention?

Of course the second response takes more time and effort, but it is far less likely to result in protracted correspondence. Importantly, the risk issues become much clearer when a full investigation takes place, and the likelihood of a repeat with major consequences is greatly reduced. The Complaints Regulations in force since 30 July 2004 require that a final response letter contains a notification of the complainant's right to refer the complaint to the Healthcare Commission.

A response drafted in haste or through the red mist of anger is unlikely to be truly objective! Share your draft with practice colleagues and invite their advice and comment. You should also involve those who are directly involved in the complaint, as they may be able to provide the detail that is central to the whole problem.

A concern that is often expressed relates to the 'legal status' of a statement in a response letter that something has gone wrong. If your investigation reveals that an error was made, it is quite appropriate to say so. An apology in these circumstances is very different from a formal admission of liability, and economy with the truth is both unnecessary and, more importantly, unreasonable.

It is highly likely that once a well-drafted and detailed response has been made, the correspondence will cease. An optimist will say that the complainant is now entirely satisfied with the explanation and understands the problem from a different perspective. A realist will recognise that in some cases, at least, the complainant has simply run out of energy or feels that nothing is to be gained from prolonged pursuit of the problem. It is vital that this is not seen as the end of the process.

Complaints and their management are an integral part of the overall clinical governance process and need to be afforded high priority in governance terms. Clearly there is a link between complaints and significant or untoward incident management. In practices where robust systems are in place, not only are complaint numbers low but also other governance processes give advance warning that a complaint is on its way.

Learning from the complaint

From a patient's point of view, a complaints procedure is in place to provide information and explanation. From the healthcare provider's point of view it allows an opportunity to review and learn. This process is not complete until the following questions have been answered in detail.

- What are you going to change?
- How will you implement that change?
- How will you convince your colleagues that change is necessary?
- Who needs to know about this episode?

If most complaints cease at the first response, it follows that a few will remain dissatisfied to the point where they contact the practice again. Management at this stage is wholly dependent on the individual circumstances. However, it may be that repeated correspondence is not the most likely way to resolve complex issues. The written word does not cope well with 'what ifs' and 'yes buts', and perhaps the best way forward now is to meet with the complainant and discuss the outstanding details.

If a meeting is agreed to be the best way forward, it is important to be well prepared, not only in terms of necessary documentation and information, but also in terms of the attitude that you bring to the process. A well-organised chairman, a focused agenda, a commitment to openness and a genuine wish to recognise and resolve disputes are all ingredients of successful complaints management. Conciliation and mediation have been widely used in primary care, and the latest guidance suggests that they are to be encouraged. The complaints manager in the PCT is likely to have access to named, trained people who, with the consent of all parties, can assist greatly.

Dealing with complaints will inevitably involve having to cope with heightened emotions and angry people. It is very easy in these circumstances to lose sight of the substance of the complaint as you deal with the anger and frustration of the complainant. Tone and volume of voice are both very poor indicators of the validity of content. The NHS Zero Tolerance Policy[7] rightly demands that staff should not be abused or threatened at work, and in ideal circumstances complainants will always be polite and reasonable as they address concerns. In reality, it may be necessary to cope with some complaints as a two-stage process – emotions first and facts second.

Habitual complainants

Habitual or repetitive complainants can on very rare occasions cause great difficulty, as the demands made use up a great deal of time and effort that is disproportionate to the nature of the concerns expressed. Provision should be made in the practice complaints policy for describing criteria that define a habitual complainant and for identifying a procedure for coping.

The persistent or habitual complainer will probably:

- continue to pursue an issue when the local resolution process has been exhausted
- change the focus of a complaint when the investigation is nearing completion
- bombard various members of staff with telephone calls, fax messages and emails
- allege that documentary evidence has been falsified or deliberately lost
- deny that correspondence has been received
- complain to different parts of the NHS at the same time.

In these circumstances, assistance is necessary if the problem is to be managed properly. If you have never been on the receiving end of such a complainant, it is difficult to over-emphasise what an enormous drain on time and resources they can be. Evidence gained through careful documentation of every contact over a period of time is necessary to establish the 'habitual' nature of the problem. Once established, it is reasonable for verbal communication to cease and written communication to be limited to acknowledgement of receipt. The complaints manager from the PCT should be fully involved.

Independent review

In the vast majority of cases, local resolution will be sufficient to complete the process satisfactorily (97.4% of cases in 2002). Independent review remains an option in circumstances where local resolution has stalled. The Healthcare Commission has now assumed responsibility for the second stage of the process. *NHS Complaints Reform: making things right*[3] describes the options that the Healthcare Commission will have once they become involved. They can:

- make recommendations for further action from the NHS organisation complained about
- investigate the case in detail, either with the focus on resolving the individual complaint, or in the context of an inspection or inquiry about failures in the organisation
- refer cases that are particularly complex to the ombudsman.

It is clear from the above that once a complaint reaches the independent review stage, a large amount of effort and good will is necessary if a satisfactory outcome is to be obtained. A complaints policy that identifies the route through the process and gives guidance at each stage will be of great help in efforts to resolve complaints early on.

Complaints policy

The complaints policy needs to be tailored to the requirements of the individual practice, it needs to be understood and 'owned' by every member of staff, and it would be good practice to have it agreed as an appropriate tool for the resolution of difficulties by user groups and the local community. Policy documents have a habit of hiding on shelves and failing to become real working documents but this one should command high priority. Box 14.1 shows a 'model' policy that could be amended to fit the particular circumstances of your practice.

Box 14.1 Complaints policy

- A complaint is defined as *an expression of discontent that requires a formal response.*
- The practice will positively encourage comment and criticism and suggestions from practice users.
- Information for patients about how to register enquiries or complaints will be be visible and easily accessible in all parts of the practice.
- The practice will identify a senior member of staff who will assume managerial responsibility for the conduct of the complaints procedure. The name of that person will be easily available to practice users.
- All complaints received will be acknowledged in writing within 2 working days.

Continued

- Complaints will be investigated and a written response made within 20 working days. If this is unachievable, the reason for the delay will be explained and regular reports on progress will be provided. The response will address all the issues of concern.
- Practice staff will always treat complainants with courtesy and respect, the investigation undertaken will be objective, and the results of the investigation will be reported fully and openly.
- Changes made as a direct result of a complaint will be notified in writing to the complainant.
- Details of all complaints will be recorded and reviewed as an integral part of the practice clinical governance process.
- Any member of staff who is the subject of a complaint has the right to see both the complaint and the formal response.
- If disciplinary action is considered appropriate following a complaint investigation, the details remain a private matter between the staff concerned, and they will not form part of the formal response.
- Habitual or persistent complainants will be identified by specific criteria. Once they have been identified, communication will be limited to acknowledgement of written correspondence only.
- When an expression of dissatisfaction is received, the following flow chart may be helpful as you pilot your way through the process. Importantly it leads you to consider the problem from the wider 'risk management' perspective as well as the issues of concern to the patient.

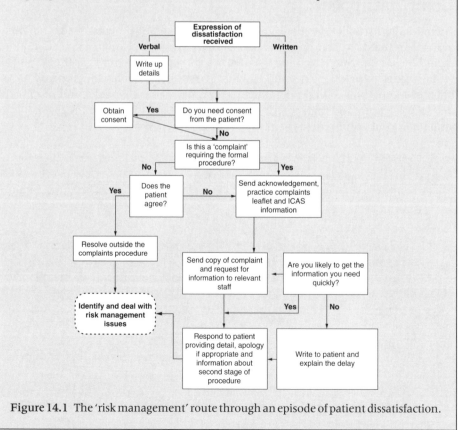

Figure 14.1 The 'risk management' route through an episode of patient dissatisfaction.

Complaints and compensation

Perhaps surprisingly, cash compensation is not high on the list of outcomes wanted by complainants. Nevertheless, on occasion the complaint letter specifically mentions that compensation is required. The 1996 procedure drew a clear distinction between complaints and litigation, pointing out that if litigation starts, the complaints procedure stops. In practice this distinction makes it very difficult to consider financial compensation in the context of complaint resolution, and it is very rarely considered appropriate. The Complaint Regulations (2004) underline that where you have clear evidence that the complainant intends to litigate, the complaints procedure is inappropriate.

The CMO's report on clinical negligence reform, entitled *Making Amends,*[8] was published in June 2003. Sir Liam Donaldson's report makes a number of recommendations that could, if introduced, allow compensation to be much more widely used as a way of dealing with complaints.

Three of the 19 recommendations are of relevance to NHS complaints.

- Recommendation 1: An NHS Redress Scheme should be introduced to provide investigations when things go wrong, remedial treatment, rehabilitation and care where needed, explanations and apologies, and *financial compensation in certain circumstances.*
- Recommendation 4: Subject to evaluation after a reasonable period, consideration should be given to extending the scheme to a higher monetary threshold and to *primary care settings.*
- Recommendation 8: The rule in the current NHS complaints procedure which requires a complaint to be halted pending resolution of a legal claim should be removed as part of the *reform of the complaints procedure.*

The report is still at the consultation stage, and it has a long way to go before the recommendations become part of the NHS procedure. However, it does perhaps indicate the direction of change.

Complaints and the PCT

Patients may choose to bypass the practice and complain directly to the PCT. PCTs have designated complaints managers, and have recently established PALS, either of which may be the first point of contact. PCTs do have a role in ensuring that the complaint is dealt with satisfactorily, and in circumstances where they are the first port of call they may wish to monitor the process.

The Board of the PCT is accountable for the performance of the organisation handling complaints, and where necessary should offer support to practices that are dealing with complaints. They have a responsibility for ensuring that adequate training and resources are available and also for ensuring that issues arising from complaints are properly integrated into clinical governance. The PCT Board will require regular reports on the type of complaints and the action taken.

Complaints and the practice list

A regular criticism from the ombudsman's office is that complainants are dealt with by simply being removed from the practice list. In these circumstances there would be no need to investigate, and of course it follows that no real learning would result. While a decision to remove a patient from the practice list remains one for the individual practitioner, it is highly unlikely that an inquiry would find in the practitioner's favour if the rationale for removal was simply the receipt of a complaint.

Patients should only be removed in circumstances where it is *reasonable* to do so – for example, if:

- the patient has moved away from the area
- staff have been the subject of violence or abuse
- the patient has involved the practice in criminal activity (e.g. the theft of drugs, prescription pads, etc.).

Patients may demonstrate a degree of unreasonable behaviour such that it becomes impossible to engage with them, and in these circumstances it may well be reasonable to remove them from the list. The habitual complainer may fall into this category. However, it would be good practice to canvas opinion from colleagues within the practice who may be able to identify alternative ways of dealing with the problem. 'Habitual-complainer' status is only achieved in exceptional circumstances, and is not a label to be applied lightly. If a decision is made to remove the patient, it follows that the patient should be given written reasons for that decision and advice about what to do next.

Complaints reduction

By far the most effective way of managing complaints is not to receive them in the first place. Reference was made earlier to the notion that complaints arise out of the gap that exists between expectation of service and the reality of experience. If the size of the gap can be reduced, it follows that the complaint numbers will fall.

The first thing to consider is the 'expectation' side of the equation. To what extent is the expectation held by your patients concerning what can or should be done for them when they engage with your service matched by the reality of what you and your practice colleagues can reasonably achieve?

Certainly the general public has high expectations. The NHS is at the top of the political agenda, and rarely does a day go by without a media story concerning advances in treatment, improvements in service or increased NHS funding. It is also true that for many the NHS is in fact the National Illness Service, and they engage with it only at times of acute need or crisis.

Changing or even identifying expectation is very complex, particularly if considered from a national perspective. Identifying local expectation and then engineering the service (the "reality" side of the equation) such that the two are closer together is perhaps more achievable, and it certainly seems to be one of the cornerstones of the NHS Plan. The newly created *patients' forums* have a remit to monitor and review the local services from a patient's perspective, and could play a central role in identifying local issues. At practice level it can be a very useful exercise to stand back for a moment and ask yourself the following questions.

1 Do patients who arrive in my surgery have an accurate impression of what goes on and what is likely to happen to them?

2 Is the practice information booklet or other type of information-providing system:
   - accurate?
   - relevant?
   - realistic?
   - seen by all of the patients?
3 Could we provide extra information to our patients over and above that which is provided already?
4 If our workload is such that we cannot do everything, have we prioritised our work and made the patients aware of this?
5 Is it likely that we make assumptions about the level of patients' medical knowledge and understanding that would not stand up to scrutiny?
6 Do we use jargon language that our patients do not understand?

The vast majority of complaint investigations reveal what you probably know already – that clinical staff are very good at 'treatments', but what some staff are less good at is explaining, listening, hearing, noticing and understanding when they are communicating with patients. The only way to align the patient's expectation with the reality of what your service can provide is to communicate with them effectively. If you succeed in this, complaint numbers will be low.

References

1 NHS Executive (1996) *Complaints, Listening, Acting . . . Improving*. NHS Executive, Leeds.
2 Wilson A (1994) *Being Heard*. Department of Health, London.
3 Department of Health (2003) *NHS Complaints Reform: making things right*. Department of Health, London.
4 Department of Health (2001) *Reforming the NHS Complaints Procedure: a listening document*. Department of Health, London.
5 Department of Health (2004) *The National Health Service (Complaints) Regulations. Draft consultation*. Department of Health, London.
6 Department of Health (2004) *The National Health Service (Complaints) Regulations*. Department of Health, London.
7 Department of Health (2000) *Zero Tolerance Survey of Reported Violent or Abusive Incidents*. Department of Health, London.
8 Department of Health (2003) *Making Amends. A consultation paper setting out proposals for reforming the approach to clinical negligence in the NHS*. Department of Health, London.

Chapter 15

Poorly performing doctors

Peter Mackenzie and Jamie Harrison

Key learning points

- Although the incidence of poor performance is not accurately known, it is likely to affect only a small proportion of doctors at any one time.
- Concerns about performance used to be either ignored, or assessed by unreliable local methods, which often led to draconian GMC investigation.
- PCTs now have a responsibility to supervise the management of alleged cases of poor performance.
- PCT mechanisms need to be open, fair and effective.
- The GMC has also recently reformed its processes.
- The NCAA is a new body with the potential to help both doctors and PCTs.

Why this issue has become important

Recent high-profile cases in the media concerning botched heart surgery in Bristol, retained children's organs at Alder Hey, and the murderous medical practice of Harold Shipman have led to growing national concern about the clinical performance of doctors.[1] In a recent annual report,[2] the CMO for England, Sir Liam Donaldson, highlighted the need to deal both fairly and quickly with poor performance, developing further the theme of clinical governance which he had previously introduced into the NHS.[3]

Writing in the *Student BMJ*,[4] he had previously explored why poor performance is not dealt with satisfactorily within the world of medicine, reflecting on three key themes:

- the high tolerance of deviant behaviour among doctors
- the fact that whistleblowing can be seen as disloyal
- the ambiguity of where to draw the line between acceptable and unacceptable practice.

Governments and society at large demand major changes in this area. The excuse that obtaining evidence of a colleague's poor performance is difficult is not tenable. Doing nothing is no longer an option.

The prevalence of poor performance

In 1999, the Government report *Supporting Doctors, Protecting Patients*[5] provided the following data on performance issues:

- 6% of the senior hospital workforce in any 5-year period may have problems
- there are 3 to 5 GPs per health authority area with some performance concerns, according to a Department of Health estimate
- 120 *alert letters* (warnings about doctors) had been issued since August 1997
- in a study of 300 responses from trusts, 46 doctors were suspended, of whom 29 hospital doctors had been suspended for over 6 months
- the Nuffield Trust has reported high levels of psychological disturbance in both hospital doctors and GPs, with levels ranging from 21% to 50%.

Yet there are difficulties with these figures, since they stem from a time when the only systematic response to poor performance was a GMC referral. It is likely that they underestimate the scale of the problem.

Why does poor performance occur?

Poor performance occurs for a variety of reasons, some related to the practitioner's state of health, some related to their medical knowledge, skills and general clinical competency, and some to do with the organisations and systems within which they work. It is therefore important to tease out factors such as physical or mental illness, substance misuse or addiction from more clearly 'clinical' causes of under-performance, such as becoming 'out of date' or losing technical skills. Organisational and system failures must also be considered.

Sir Donald Irvine has looked at causes of poor-quality medical care[6] (*see* Box 15.1). First, according to him, the culture of the NHS promotes the provider (clinician) rather than the patient. The Government emphasis on rapid access to healthcare puts quality development (IT, teamwork, good systems) under pressure. Accountability to self rather than to patients leads to paternalism, and too much reliance on waiting for 'the damage to be done' before intervening locally to stop poor performance, and a lack of co-ordination between the players involved in the supervision and regulation of practitioners, remains dangerous.

Box 15.1 Causes of poor-quality medical care (after Irvine[6])

- A provider-orientated culture
- Emphasis on speed of access at the expense of quality
- Self-accountability and paternalism
- Waiting for the damage to be done
- Lack of co-ordination for all involved in regulation

Irvine's solution, while he was president of the GMC, was to introduce explicit professional standards based on the document *Good Medical Practice* (GMP).[7] Securing compliance with GMP would be achieved through a process of revalidation, based on 5-yearly reviews of performance. Equally, it would be necessary to ensure that doctors participate in proper continuing further education, including building on their interpersonal skills. In addition, there would need to be structural change within the GMC itself.

How to identify and investigate allegations of poor performance

GMP now requires all doctors to take steps if they believe that the health, conduct or performance of a colleague may be putting patients at risk of harm. Equally, there is a plethora of routes by which an individual general practitioner can be investigated either following a single clinical incident or, more significantly, where there is a pattern of repeated poor performance. GPs can have their performance assessed by a PCT, the NCAA and the GMC. This section will examine each of these in turn.

PCT assessment procedures

Practical issues

An ideal PCT system would incorporate mechanisms for the early detection of performance problems, fair and reliable methods of assessment, swift, effective and fair decision-making processes, and some means of 'treating' the diagnosed problem.

Capability is still developing in this area, with PCTs beginning to learn how to manage their clinical governance requirements. Where concerns arise, the PCT can review performance indicators and allegations of poor performance (often leading to a simple dialogue with the practitioner or practice in most cases, followed by an agreed action plan), but where more serious or persistent concerns are found, a confidential case management approach is needed. This may necessitate the commissioning of a performance review, using a local performance assessment team (PAT), with findings fed back appropriately to the PCT. The RCGP has published a useful toolkit to guide practice,[8] which should be read in conjunction with that recently produced by the NCAA.[9]

Box 15.2 highlights ways in which concerns about a GP's performance might reach a PCT.

Box 15.2 A potential problem with a doctor

A single clinical encounter can give rise to a number of different possible investigations into an individual doctor, including any of the following:

- an NHS complaint
- an independent panel review
- health authority disciplinary inquiry
- ombudsman's inquiry

Continued

- GMC inquiry
- performance procedures
- conduct procedure
- health procedures
- inquest
- claim for negligence
- police inquiry
- clinical governance review
- analysis of PACT data by PCT
- Healthcare Commission review
- employer's investigation
- internal and public inquiries.

Performance assessment teams should be constituted for the task and their members should have (or develop) the necessary skills (*see* Box 15.3). Such teams should include both lay and clinical members, so that a visiting team might include two clinicians and one lay assessor. Teams are likely to be shared between PCTs, co-ordinated either by a strategic health authority (e.g. the South East London Strategic Health Authority) or by a postgraduate deanery (e.g. the Northern Deanery), or by a consortium of local PCTs, with one PCT leading the project. These teams will want to develop locally the capacity that the NCAA has achieved nationally (*see* below). Such teams will therefore need training and support, with the local postgraduate deaneries and NCAA being well placed to help. Equally, the LMC of the BMA has a history of giving valuable advice in this area.

Box 15.3 Competences of PAT members[10]

- Information-gathering skills
- Communication skills
- Teamworking skills
- Leadership skills
- Ability to adhere to assessment protocols
- Track record in own professional field

Recent guidance[11] to NHS trusts (which include PCTs) will make the Chief Executive responsible for appointing a case manager in cases where suspension or NCAA referral is contemplated. The case will need to be looked into quickly – exclusions from work will lapse after 4 weeks, imposing a tight timetable on this process.

Although this circular relates only to direct employees of NHS bodies, it can be expected that the rules for doctors on the list of a PCT will mirror this advice. PCTs can be expected to develop a body, probably under the Medical Director or

Clinical Governance Lead, to collect intelligence, manage cases and advise the Chief Executive. A workable model is shown in Box 15.4.

Box 15.4 Flow chart options for performance concerns

PCT Information Group
- Gathers data and processes allegations
- Appoints Case Managers
- Receives reports of cases
- Advises Chief Executive on possible actions

↓

Possible responses (not necessarily exclusive)
- No action
- Continued surveillance (should be explicit)
- Dialogue with the clinician or practice
- Appointment of a Case Manager
- Referral to a local PAT
- Referral to NCAA
- Referral to GMC
- Exclude from practice pending inquiry
- Occupational health assessment

↓

Possible 'treatments'
- No action
- Educational intervention
- Health intervention

Principles governing PCT performance procedures

A PCT is a public body that performs a public function. Although the investigation by a PCT of the performance of NHS GPs has not yet been confirmed by the courts to be a definite function of public law, we recommend that a PCT should incorporate the spirit and principles of public and European law fairness into any design of a performance investigation process.

The general principles of European law include the following:

- proportionality
- equality and respect for fundamental rights
- legitimate expectations
- legal certainty.

The principle of *proportionality* means that a public authority must not use a sledgehammer to crack a nut. *Equality* means that people in similar posts or positions should be treated similarly. Not only does this apply to nationality and age, but it also extends to doctors who may be in competition with the PCT. The principle of *legal certainty* states that those subject to a law should not be left with any uncertainty about their rights and obligations. Therefore PCTs must ensure that all GPs in their area are not penalised for being unaware of new legal changes that are brought in where the PCT has not given those GPs adequate notice of those changes.

Then there are rules of natural justice, which include the following.

* *Audi Alteram Partem (Hear the other side)*. Each side must have reasonable notice of the case that the GP has to meet, a chance to state their own case and to answer arguments against it, and the option to be represented.
* *Rule against bias*. If a PCT is investigating a doctor, it will often have a direct financial interest in the outcome of the case. It can be argued, therefore, that a hearing by the PCT is, prime facie, unfair. PCTs must ensure that any investigation conducted by them is scrupulously fair and lawful. The new guidance (*HSC 2003/012*)[11] is very helpful here.
* *Procedural Ultra Vires*. PCTs must comply with the rules and regulations that Parliament has laid down for them. *HSC 2003/012* applies to all employed staff from April 2004. It would seem prudent (and it also seems practical) for PCTs to manage contracted staff in the same way.

The RCGP[8] makes the point that mitigating circumstances should be explored, with attempts to resolve such issues. For example, is the doctor single-handed because no replacement partner can be found to ease the workload? Has there been a problem with the computer system or practice manager? Are there issues of ill health, stress or burnout and is the doctor both aware of, and addressing, such concerns? PCTs need to be sensitive to wider issues that may contribute to poor performance at work.

Making a diagnosis of why under-performance has occurred may need the expertise of the local PAT. Here the team visits the doctor or practice over 1 to 2 days, with pre-visit information collated as needed. Any visit must conform to the principles highlighted above, and will usually follow the processes outlined in Box 15.5.

Box 15.5 Processes of a performance visit

---

* Inspection of premises
* Inspection of records
* Interviews with doctor concerned
* Interviews with members of the primary healthcare team
* Interviews with external colleagues

(Consulting skills may also be assessed by direct observation, videotaping, or attendance at a simulated surgery using actors as simulated patients.)

If a PCT is wishing to investigate the performance of a local GP by conducting a performance visit, it must comply with the 'Code of Practice on Confidentiality' issued by the Department of Health on 2 September 2004.[12]

This Code of Practice sets out guidance and confidentiality of information held by contractors. The gist of this guidance is that if PCTs want to do an audit of a practitioner's work, consent will need to be obtained from patients whose records the PCT assessors wish to view. Normally the PCT would be expected to obtain the consent from those patients.

The report from the visit leads to the formulation of a plan for improvement, treating deficiencies in clinical performance through remedial or educative mechanisms rather than punishing an individual. Any restrictions on a doctor's practice should be proportionate, fair, and reviewed in a timely fashion. Support must be provided to the GP to include facilities and time to work on any concerns that have been identified. It may be helpful to the GP to have an appointed mentor who is independent of the performance review process. This mentor should work through a personal development plan with the GP.

The case should be managed carefully and in consultation with others, such as the local postgraduate deanery. There should be a potential endpoint, and performance should regularly be reviewed. Some doctors are sick. Since many performance issues are related to ill health, PCTs should have access to occupational health advice and support as part of the above processes. Should the above not prove satisfactory, or where a more formal assessment is required, referral to the NCAA for advice is the next possibility.

National Clinical Assessment Authority (NCAA)

The NCAA was established as a Special Health Authority in April 2001. The Department of Health's review of its 'arms length bodies' in 2004 recommended that the functions of the NCAA should continue and should be brought together with the National Patient Safety Agency (NPSA) although established as a separate, self-contained division within the Agency.[13] The aim of the authority is to provide a support service to NHS primary care, hospital and community trusts, the Prison Health Service and the Defence Medical Services when they are faced with concerns over the performance of an individual doctor. The NCAA also provides support to the employers of hospital and community dentists when there are performance concerns.

The NCAA provides advice, takes referrals and carries out targeted assessments where necessary. NCAA assessments involve trained medical and lay assessors. Once an objective assessment has been carried out, the NCAA will advise on the appropriate course of action. It does not take over the role of an employer, nor will it function as a regulator. The NCAA is established as an advisory body, and the NHS employer organisation remains responsible for resolving the problem once the NCAA has produced its assessment.

The reasons for referral to the NCAA are highlighted in Box 15.6.

The recent CMO's report included the following key points in relation to the NCAA.[2]

- The NHS has in the past had great difficulty in effectively addressing poor performance, partly because of inflexible, legalistic and daunting statutory procedures.

Box 15.6 Reasons for NCAA referral[12]

• Solely clinical issues	30%
• Clinical problem compounded by health or behavioural issue	80%
• Behavioural problem present	>50%
• Solely a behavioural problem	17%
• Underlying health problem	20%
• Health, clinical and behavioural problems all present	20%

• During the first 21 months the NCAA has taken 446 referrals, predominantly from older age groups, 4 in 5 referrals being male.
• The NCAA has been consulted in 36 cases where NHS trusts were proposing suspension, and in 30 cases the NCAA was able to offer alternative approaches.
• More PCTs need to use the NCAA in order to avoid inappropriate and prolonged suspensions.

Although suspensions are still relatively uncommon, with 30 doctors being suspended each year, Sir Liam Donaldson expects that in future suspension will last no longer than 1 month and that there will be an end to 'gardening leave'. This will prove to be a significant challenge to all concerned.

The components of NCAA assessments reflect those of local PCT performance assessment, with the addition of the expectation of an occupational and a behavioural assessment, and the possibility of a more exhaustive assessment of clinical practice (*see* Box 15.7).

Box 15.7 Components of NCAA assessments[9]

• Occupational health assessment
• Behavioural assessment
• Basic knowledge screen
• Review of information provided by the GP and the referring organisation prior to assessment
• Check of practice equipment
• Views of colleagues about the doctor's performance
• Patients' view of practice and satisfaction with consultations with the doctor
• Direct observation of practice (by one assessor sitting in with the GP while he or she consults)
• Medical record review
• Practice-based discussion – an opportunity to discuss with the doctor different aspects of his or her practice, both clinical and managerial

---

The outcome of NCAA assessments can be viewed in the following manner:

> As the purpose of the NCAA assessment is to provide useful recommendations, we want to involve the GP and the referring organisation at each stage. The steps to ensure this are:
>
> *Step 1.* Draft report of findings, conclusions and recommendations produced by NCAA – for comment by practitioner and referring organisation. Any comments from the referring organisation will be passed to the practitioner and vice versa.
>
> *Step 2.* Final report from the NCAA, with comments from the doctor and referring organisation appended.
>
> *Step 3.* Referring organisation and local GP education providers identify practical educational/managerial resources to implement the recommendations. This will likely involve the Deanery and the Workforce Development Confederation.
>
> *Step 4.* Meeting with practitioner and referring organisation, facilitated by the NCAA, to agree action plan including goals, review dates, responsibilities, arrangements for follow-up, monitoring and mentoring.
>
> *Step 5.* The referring organisation sends a copy of the action plan to the NCAA.[9]

The referring organisation will be responsible for following up progress after the NCAA assessment. However, if at the action planning meeting it is agreed that further NCAA assessment (e.g. selected parts of the full assessment) will be helpful, this can be arranged at, say, 6 or 12 months after the original assessment. As ever, the hope is for local resolution, with the doctor being encouraged to remain in practice with appropriate support.

The General Medical Council (GMC)[14]

There will be occasions when the severity of the allegations against a doctor demand referral to the GMC. The same applies when significant concerns arise from performance assessment processes (either local or via the NCAA). Equally, the GMC can become involved as a result of a direct complaint from the public.

The screening process

On 1 November 2004 the GMC streamlined its procedures for investigating complaints. This has been the most radical form of Council since it was established by the Medical Act of 1858. An investigation of concerns is now in two parts: the investigation phase and the adjudication phase. At the end of the investigation phase a doctor whose conduct is found to be inappropriate on the basis of a civil burden of proof (the balance of probabilities) may be given a warning. At the end of the adjudication phase, the current distinction between performance, conduct and health will be largely replaced by a single question: whether there are aspects of the doctor's conduct, performance or health that warrant interference with the doctor's registration. The sanctions of erasure, suspension, conditions and admonition (reprimand) will stay the same.

Because of significant delays in investigating complaints, the GMC has also introduced more Fitness to Practise panels manned by lay people and doctors who are appointed by the GMC but are not themselves GMC members.[15]

As an example, an analysis of GMC activity in March 2001 is shown in Box 15.8.[16]

Box 15.8 Analysis of GMC activity[16]	
Cases closed	424
On initial assessment	140 (33%)
Withdrawn/not pursued	108 (25%)
By screeners	137 (32%)
By Professional Performance Committee (PPC)	27 (6.4%)
By Professional Conduct Committee (PCC)	10 (2.4%)
Guilty	8
Not guilty	2

Once a complaint is received, it will be processed by the Registrar who is likely to invite one or two Case Examiners to consider the matter. Should the Case Examiners conclude that no action is indicated, the papers will be kept for a limited period. Until recently this period has been for six months for allegations of serious professional misconduct and three years for information suggesting a problem with a doctor's professional performance, after which time the papers are destroyed (unless new information has come to light in the interim).

The performance procedures

Unlike the conduct procedures, which are adversarial in nature and can be punitive in their effect, the performance and health procedures are like an inquiry. The aims are to put right deficiencies and to rehabilitate the doctor who is ill, subject to the overriding need to protect the public.

The idea of *seriously deficient performance* is a new one. The GMC has defined it as 'a departure from good professional practice, whether or not it is covered by specific GMC guidance, sufficiently serious to call into question a doctor's registration'.

The procedures were introduced in July 1997, and apply only to doctors' professional performance since that date.

The assessment

Where a doctor's performance is to be assessed, either with agreement or at the direction of the Assessment Referral Committee (to which there is the right of appeal), a further GMC member takes over from the screener to act as *case co-ordinator*. A panel or team of at least three individuals (two doctors and a lay person) will carry out the assessment. These are not GMC members. They are drawn from a list of people selected and trained by the GMC following public advertisement, and are led by a doctor from the same medical specialty as the doctor under investigation. The GMC provides the team with the doctor's comments and any other evidence that the doctor has submitted, together with other relevant information, including the original complaint.

The team visits the doctor at his or her place of work, to review patient records and discuss particular cases, interviewing both the complainant and others, to formulate an overall picture of the doctor's performance. This process is as sensitive and confidential as possible, and as far as is humanly possible it is a private matter between the doctor and the GMC.

Assessment methods

Depending on the nature of the complaint, a decision may be taken to assess the doctor's skills using 'standardised' patients in role-play situations. Alternatively, with the consent of patients, the doctor may be directly observed in actual consultations. There may be specific tests of his or her medical knowledge or skills. Such tests may include the use of multiple-choice questions (MCQs), extended matching questions (EMQs) or objective clinical scenarios (OSCEs), such as how to break bad news to an actor who is simulating a patient. The assessors will also undertake third-party interviews with a variety of people (only some of whom are doctors) who work regularly with the doctor who is being investigated.

The doctor is expected to co-operate fully with the assessment. Failure to do this normally leads to a referral to a Fitness to Practise Panel (FPP), whose powers are more extensive. These include the powers to suspend the practitioner until he agrees to undergo a performance assessment.

At any stage of the performance procedures the doctor concerned may choose to seek voluntary removal from the GMC Register. The GMC will allow this, with automatic discontinuation of the assessment. Such a decision should not be taken lightly, and the doctor is well advised to seek advice from friends, experienced colleagues and his or her defence organisation. The GMC will not, incidentally, normally grant an application for voluntary erasure if the concerns raised are a matter of professional conduct.

What happens next?

The assessment panel reports to the case co-ordinator on what has been found, making recommendations on what needs to be done to put right any identified deficiencies. The doctor will also receive the report and can comment on it to the GMC. If the panel has not reported serious concern about performance, there will probably be no further action.

If the panel has identified serious deficiencies, recommendations will be made about what the doctor should do to put things right, inviting agreement to a *statement of requirements* intended to address specific problems. These might include, for example, retraining, counselling or limiting clinical practice in certain ways. At this stage the procedure remains voluntary – the GMC will want to work with the doctor's co-operation so that the remedial action has the maximum chance of being successful.

Should either the doctor concerned fail to agree with the requirements put forward by the case co-ordinator, or the co-ordinator believes that the deficiencies in performance are serious enough to warrant it, the case will be referred to a FPP, which will decide whether to suspend the doctor's registration or impose conditions upon it.

Remedial action

If the doctor agrees to comply with the requirements, it becomes their responsibility to put right the deficiencies that the panel has identified. The GMC can put the doctor in touch with sources of advice such as a postgraduate dean or a director of postgraduate GP education.

The doctor's case will not be closed until the GMC is satisfied that his or her standard of professional performance has reached the required level. This may need more than one round of remedial action. Each time the GMC will want to reassess performance to see what progress has been made. If at any time it decides that performance is not improving, or that there is a failure to co-operate, the case will be referred to the FPP.

Fitness to Practise Panel

A FPP hearing allows legal rules of procedure. The doctor may be legally represented and witnesses may be called to give evidence and be cross examined.

If at the end of the hearing the FPP decides that the doctor's fitness to practise is impaired then they do one of the following:

- put conditions on the doctor's registration
- suspend the doctor's name from the Medical Register so he cannot practise during the period of suspension
- erase the doctor's name from the Medical Register
- a warning may on occasions be appropriate where concerns have indicated a significant departure from the principles set out in the GMC's guidance *Good Medical Practice*, or if there is a significant cause for concern following assessment but a restriction on the doctor's registration is not necessary.

A doctor is entitled to appeal to the High Court or Court of Session in Scotland, about any decision by the FPP. The Panel decision will not take effect until either the appeal period expires or the appeal is determined. However the Panel can impose an immediate order of suspension or conditions if it believes this is needed to protect the public or is in the best interest of the doctor.

Proposed changes at the GMC

Following consultation with the Government in May 2002, it was decided that the mechanism for investigating and dealing with complaints will change. There will be two stages.

Stage 1: Investigation

The old 'screening' stage will be replaced by a single stage under the control of the Investigation Committee. The test to apply is simply '*Is there a realistic prospect of establishing that fitness to practise is impaired to a degree justifying action on registration?*'

This is a stricter test than the one currently applied by the screeners, namely 'Could the complaint, if proved, raise an issue of seriously deficient performance?'.

If the case passes this test, it will move to the second stage.

Stage 2: Adjudication

This is separate from the investigation stage, and no GMC member will be involved in the case. Committees are to be abolished and the cases heard by new Fitness to Practise Panels. Although the Panels will hear a variety of case types, there is a single focus on whether fitness to practise is impaired. Appeal from this Panel is to be to the High Court and not the Privy Council.

The Panels can issue warnings, which are for either a 'significant departure from *Good Medical Practice* or, where there is *real cause for concern* following assessment.' Although registration is not to be affected by warnings, they will feed into appraisals and/or revalidation. These changes were implemented during 2004.

Conclusion

Poor performance by doctors is an issue of clinical risk. Their patients are at risk of suboptimal outcomes or avoidable adverse outcomes. It is also an issue for the doctors themselves, as failure to identify difficulties at an early stage is a missed opportunity for the doctor's own personal development.

It is clear that poorly performing doctors can no longer be ignored or thought to be someone else's business. Doctors in particular have a responsibility to face up to performance issues relating both to their own personal clinical practice and to that of their colleagues. The newly emerging PCTs and SHAs also have a responsibility to monitor and engage with issues of performance. Ideally, poor performance should be detected at an early stage, with remedial programmes instigated. This is the way ahead.

Yet poor performance remains a source of anxiety in primary care. Greater awareness of the issue, and an acceptance of responsibility for monitoring its prevalence, are leading to an increased demand for robust and effective mechanisms to tackle perceived concerns. This is leading to the development of local performance assessment teams, building on the experience of local postgraduate deaneries, the newly formed NCAA and the GMC.

Equally, local strategies for remediation are required. These include, for example, the development of a network of advanced training practices in the Northern Deanery, where poorly performing doctors can receive support, advice and a protected environment in which to recover and find teaching and training. Given the initial cost of training doctors, and the current issues of recruitment and retention of GPs, it is only wise to maximise the doctor workforce within primary care.[17]

Acknowledgements

The authors would like to acknowledge the contribution of Alan Kershaw (Former Director of Standards and Education at the GMC) in the preparation of material relating to GMC procedures.

Postscript

In January 2005 after this chapter had been written, the Government announced a review of the current arrangements for protecting patients in response to the Shipman Inquiry.

The review to be led by the CMO, Sir Liam Donaldson, will identify measures to:

- strengthen procedures for assuring the safety of patients in situations where a doctor's performance or conduct poses a risk to patient safety or the effective functioning of services
- ensure the operation of an effective system of revalidation
- modify the role, structure and functions of the GMC.

An advisory group will support the CMO throughout the review and is drawn from organisations representing consumers, healthcare quality and professional interests.

References

1 Harrison J, Innes R and van Zwanenberg T (2003) *Rebuilding Trust in Healthcare.* Radcliffe Medical Press, Oxford.
2 Chief Medical Officer (2002) *The Annual Report of the Chief Medical Officer.* Department of Health, London.
3 Donaldson L (2004) Clinical governance: a quality concept. In: T van Zwanenberg and J Harrison (eds) *Clinical Governance in Primary Care* (2e). Radcliffe Medical Press, Oxford.
4 Donaldson L (1996) Facing up to the problem of the poorly performing doctor; www.studentbmj.com/back_issues/0896/08ed2.htm
5 Department of Health (1999) *Supporting Doctors, Protecting Patients.* Department of Health, London.
6 Irvine D (2001) *Patients and doctors: all change?* Presentation to the University of Northumbria at Newcastle, 22 November 2001.
7 General Medical Council (1998) *Good Medical Practice.* General Medical Council, London.
8 Royal College of General Practitioners (2001) *Toolkit for Managing GPs Whose Performance Gives Concern.* www.rcgp.org.uk/quality_unit.toolkit
9 National Clinical Assessment Authority (2004) *NCAA Toolkit;* www.ncaa.nhs.uk/toolkit
10 South East London Strategic Health Authority (2003) *Job description for local assessors.* Personal communication from Dr Sadru Kheraj, 21 January 2004.
11 Department of Health (2003) *HSC 2003/012. Maintaining high professional standards in the modern NHS: a framework for the initial handling of concerns about doctors and dentists in the NHS;* www.dh.gov.uk/PublicationsandStatistics/LettersandCirculars
12 Department of Health (2004) *Confidentiality and Disclosure of Information: General Medical Services, Personal Medical Services and Alternative Provider Medical Services Code of Practice.* Department of Health, London; www.dh.gov.uk/PublicationsAndStatistics/ Publications/PublicationsPolicyAndGuidance/PublicationsPolicyAndGuidanceArticle/ fs/en?CONTENT_ID=4088718&chk=6qzD1b
13 Department of Health (2004) *Reconfiguring the Department of Health's Arms Length Bodies.* Department of Health, London.
14 Medical Protection Society (2000) *Fit to Practise? How the GMC handles complaints about doctors;* www.medicalprotection.org/assets/pdf/booklets/fit_to_practise.pdf

15 Panting G (2004) GMC revises its fitness to practise procedures. *Guidelines in Practice*. 7: 41–5.
16 Drife J (2002) *The GMC: past, present and future.* Presentation to the Medical Protection Society, London, 31 October 2002.
17 Harrison J and van Zwanenberg T (2002) *GP Tomorrow* (2e). Radcliffe Medical Press, Oxford.

Chapter 16

Safeguarding children in primary care

Jane Cowan

Whenever a child is deliberately injured or killed, there is inevitably great concern in case some important tell-tale sign has been missed. Those who sit in judgement often do so with the great benefit of hindsight. So I readily acknowledge that staff who undertake the work of protecting children and supporting families on behalf of us all deserve both our understanding and our support. It is a job which carries risks, because in every judgement they make, those staff have to balance the rights of a parent with that of the protection of the child.[1]

Key learning points

- Safeguarding children is paramount.
- All health professionals in primary care should be aware of what to do if they think that a child is at risk.
- High standards of documentation are required to ensure that relevant information is available for those looking after the interests of the child.
- Effective, appropriate and timely communication between primary healthcare professionals and other agencies is essential.
- Children in families where there is domestic violence may be at increased risk.
- GPs should be aware of their own training needs in child protection matters.
- Practices can use the new GMS contract to focus on training needs and risk management initiatives in child protection.

In undertaking his inquiry into the death of Victoria Climbié, Lord Laming reviewed the roles and responsibilities of the various workers employed by the health service, the police and social services. Although the emphasis on the contribution made by health service employees centred predominantly on systems within secondary care, Lord Laming nevertheless looked in some depth at the involvement of GPs and health visitors.

Lord Laming reinforced the view that GPs and health visitors have an 'equally vital role to play in protecting children',[1] and this chapter aims to explore and confirm that view.

The chapter mainly refers to PCTs and the general practices within them. However, the principles are applicable to local health boards and other primary care organisations in Wales, Northern Ireland and Scotland. The majority of the documents referred to originate from the Department of Health in England, but most are produced in either the same or similar format across the other three countries in the UK. Much of the advice reflects practice in all four countries and identifies the legislative differences where appropriate.

Child protection responsibilities of primary care trusts (PCTs)

In January 2002, a letter from the Department of Health was sent to all primary care trusts outlining the changes that would be occurring with the shift of responsibility from the Health Authorities to the PCTs.[2]

An annex attached to the letter set out 'the implications for the constituent parts of the NHS and the support that is to be made available for PCTs in developing competency in child protection'.[2] Although somewhat cumbersome, this essentially established what the new PCOs were expected to do in order to comply with Department of Health requirements, thereby clarifying and improving child protection arrangements.

Key individuals within the primary care organisation (PCO)

To meet the needs of the changing responsibilities for child protection, the PCOs have to make arrangements to ensure that the key individuals within the organisation are identified and their roles and responsibilities are clearly defined.
   These include:

- a named public health professional
- designated professionals (usually a senior paediatrician and a senior nurse)
- named professionals (a doctor and a nurse).

The roles of the named professionals in primary care are important for liaison and teaching purposes. The named doctor (usually a GP) takes a professional lead and should have expertise in children's health and development, and an understanding of the care problems and issues in relation to safeguarding children and the need to promote their welfare.

   The named professionals will also be responsible for undertaking any internal case reviews for the trust (PCO) unless there is a clear conflict of interest – for example, they may have been involved themselves in the particular case. The named professionals will work closely with the designated professionals and as such should be able to provide valuable insight into specific problems encountered in primary care.

Training requirements set by the PCT

Following the Department of Health guidance issued in January 2002,[2] PCTs were to 'ensure that all health professionals, including GPs, practice nurses, practice managers, receptionists and any other staff whom they employ are given opportunities to attend child protection training as required'.

This creates a demand for a considerable training resource within any PCO, as there will be hundreds of members of staff who will need access to training with all that it entails. This is dealt with in more detail later in this chapter in the section on the specific responsibilities of the GP practice.

What to Do if You're Worried a Child is Being Abused[3]

In May 2003, a multi-agency document with a summary and flow chart with the above title was made available directly from the Department of Health and from within trusts.

This guidance should therefore be widely available within all GP practices and read at some time by all staff. One could argue that, as part of any induction programme for new staff joining a practice, whether or not they are health professionals, a requirement should be placed upon them to read some basic information about safeguarding children. This would be in anticipation of any further formal access to the practice child protection training programme.

The guidance is relatively simple and straightforward, making the position clear for all those who may encounter a situation where they consider a child or children to be at risk of harm. It is not acceptable for a health professional to fail to act upon concerns about a child. At the very least, good-quality information should be taken and recorded properly, as it may be a vital part of the jigsaw in the future when a child's welfare is being considered.

The information in Box 16.1 is taken directly from the summary document.

Box 16.1 Extract from summary document on safeguarding children

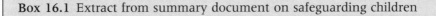

Everyone working with children and families should:

- be familiar with and follow your organisation's procedures and protocols for promoting and safeguarding the welfare of children in your area, and know who to contact in your organisation to express concerns about a child's welfare
- remember that allegations of child abuse or neglect may lead to a criminal investigation, so don't do anything that may jeopardise a police investigation, such as asking a child leading questions or attempting to investigate the allegations of abuse
- refer any concerns about child abuse or neglect to social services or the police. If you are responsible for making referrals, know who to contact in police, health, education and social services to express concerns about a child's welfare

Continued

- when referring a child to social services, consider and include any information you have on the child's developmental needs and their parents'/carers' ability to respond to these needs within the context of their wider family and environment. Similarly, when contributing to an assessment or providing services, you should consider what contribution you are able to make in each of these three areas. Specialist assessments in particular are likely to provide information in a specific dimension, such as health, education or family functioning
- communicate with the child in a way that is appropriate to their age, understanding and preference. This is especially important for disabled children and for children whose preferred language is not English. Where concerns arise as a result of information given by a child, it is important to reassure the child but not to promise confidentiality
- see the child as part of considering what action to take in relation to concerns about the child's welfare
- record full information about the child, at first point of contact, including name(s), address(es), gender, date of birth, name(s) of person(s) with parental responsibility (for consent purposes) and primary carer(s) if different to these persons. Keep this information up to date. In schools, this information will be part of the pupil's record
- record all concerns, discussions about the child, decisions made, and the reason for those decisions. The child's records should include an up-to-date chronology, and details of the lead worker in the relevant agency (for example, a social worker, GP, health visitor or teacher).

Source: 'What to Do if You're Worried a Child is Being Abused, published by the Department of Health in May 2003[3]

If the lead GP in any practice were to review the above recommendations within his or her own practice, it is likely that there would be some discrepancies and inconsistencies in process among individuals. There is often great anxiety about what should be written down and where, who should be involved and the role of the other agencies. In the light of the extensive guidance that is available within the health service with regard to child protection, together with the local guidance that will be provided under the auspices of the Area Child Protection Committees, there is no excuse for failing to review practice and adopt a common approach in primary care.

Guidance from the Royal College of General Practitioners

In October 2002, the RCGP produced a position statement on child abuse.[4] This document, which is available on the RCGP website, is recommended reading for named professionals in primary care and for any GPs who are taking the lead within their practice and who are involved in developing policy and practice to safeguard children.

The document recognises the difficult professional position in which many GPs find themselves, and the anxieties that exist in terms of maintaining skills, understanding the process and making appropriate referrals.

Despite these problems, GPs have a responsibility to understand their local networks for the protection of children, and are required to contribute to the process as necessary.

Understanding your local arrangements for safeguarding children

As discussed earlier, the PCO must ensure that child protection is of paramount importance in the organisation. To achieve this, effective active communication and networking are needed between practices within the PCO and between other health care providers and agencies.

The designated professionals for the organisation should facilitate education and training, represent concerns on the Area Child Protection Committee (ACPC), and liaise on your behalf with social services, the police and education. In situations where the GP or another member of the primary care team is having difficulty accessing services for children in need or at risk, advice should be sought from the child protection team.

Copies of information provided by the ACPC in the form of local policy and guidance must be readily accessible in the practice and widely available to all staff.

Working with social services

The role of social services staff is crucial to the protection of children. As an agency, they too suffer the staff shortages and recruitment problems that have a direct impact on the services which they are able to provide.

The skills required to work with children in need and children at risk are considerable. Difficulties often arise between agencies due to:

- staffing problems
- poor communication
- poor documentation.

Parents also often have a very unhealthy suspicion of social services, fearing that involvement may lead to the removal of their children if any concerns about neglect or parenting skills are raised.

Improving the profile of the social services team is of benefit to all in the community, and in the realms of child protection most social services in local authority areas produce excellent parent information packs explaining simply and effectively the processes that occur when children and their families engage (willingly or reluctantly) with their services.

We recommend that all staff be made aware of this in order to dispel any misapprehensions about the service. The availability of relevant social services literature in the practice may be of value for staff, patients and their families.

Clinical records

It is evident from case studies, anecdotal reports and national inquiry documents over the years that record keeping in child protection cases still falls below a reasonable standard.

In keeping poor records we continue to fail children. A lack of well-recorded clinical information and minimal detail of relevant facts (e.g. about family circumstances) can adversely affect the assessment of children for child protection purposes when multi-agency involvement occurs. The child protection process has to be fair to the parents as well as to the children. In omitting to record enough relevant details throughout a child's clinical history of contact with the practice, the GP and other staff cannot reasonably provide well-evidenced views, and have to rely instead only on their memory of interactions and conversations with either the family or other staff and professionals from outside the practice.

In reviewing the contact that Victoria Climbié had with general practice, Lord Laming noted that there were three issues that required particular attention.[1] These were:

- the manner in which new child patients are registered with GPs
- the information that should be gathered during the registration process and the manner in which information should be shared
- training in child protection and knowledge of local policies and procedures.[1]

To date, audit of record keeping in cases of concern in the primary care setting appears to be minimal. In developing local policy, audits of this nature will be relevant. Particular emphasis should be placed on where data are stored in practices (for both paper and electronic records).

The following areas should be considered in relation to record keeping:

1 initial registration of new child/family
2 identifying who has parental responsibility
3 levels of access to IT records
4 storage of documents
5 identifying the vulnerable child/family at each consultation
6 documenting injuries
7 coding systems
8 robust records transfer policies
9 GMS contract requirements for records.

Initial registration of new child/family

This process differs from one practice to another. The numbers of young people and children moving into and out of practices at any one time have in the past precluded any form of specific registration examination in many organisations. Therefore potential opportunities have been lost for a baseline assessment of a child and his or her needs.

It is accepted that for the majority of children such an assessment may be deemed unnecessary, but for some this may be a crucial time. In those families where children are abused there is often a frequent pattern of moving between

GP practices, poor school attendance, and failure to comply with healthcare surveillance programmes. A review of children moving into a new area or joining another practice may provide an opportunity for the practice nurse or health visitor to establish the trends within the family and in particular register the school attended. If concerns are raised then contact can be made with the appropriate school health service or education authority.

Identifying who has parental responsibility

It is not normal practice in most GP practices to establish for each registered child who has parental responsibility (*see* chapter 12 for definitions). However, experience suggests that in primary care many healthcare interventions are undertaken without specific knowledge of whether the mother's partner has parental responsibility for the children with whom he is living. Assumptions can all too easily be made, and this may interfere with proper process.

Likewise, if a child is in the care of a local authority under the terms of, for example, an Emergency Protection Order or an Interim Care Order, it is incumbent on the professionals to establish who is entitled to give consent.

Levels of access to IT records

Many practices have differerent levels of access to the IT system based on clinical responsibility and need. It is possible that a health professional with concerns about a particular child or family may be unable to access clinical data held on the IT system in order to record or ascertain whether there is relevant information. Similarly, if a healthcare professional is in possession of information that has been obtained outside the practice environment or has received a phone call pertinent to a child protection matter, there may be difficultly in sharing this information effectively within the practice.

Nursing staff working in the community often find it difficult to share clinical or socially relevant information as they maintain their own clinical records, which are rarely seen by or discussed with the GP, and they are often not entitled or invited to contribute to the main health record. These gaps in communication are not in the best interest of the child.

There are frequently unrealistic concerns among doctors that the non-medical members of staff may not be able to deal with confidential clinical material in the manner expected. This attitude can undermine professional working relationships, and it demonstrates a lack of understanding of the codes of practice that shape and determine the work of nursing staff and therapists.

We recommend that practices and PCTs address this as a training issue. The development of multi-professional trust in relation to confidentiality is essential for the effective sharing of information.

Storage of documents (including case-conference minutes)

A variety of systems exist for storage of records in primary care. Even within one practice consisting of several partners, differences of opinion may lead to inconsistencies with regard to how child protection information should be stored.

If a child becomes part of the child protection process, large quantities of paper start to accumulate as a result of assessment documents, reports prepared for conferences, case-conference minutes, etc. These can become bulky and unwieldy, and are seldom referred to in the routine consultation process. The vulnerability of the child (and the professional) will increase if paperwork is filed separately from the main record without proper reference to it. This can happen for several reasons, but it should be addressed by each practice based on local policy and guidance.

Case-conference minutes are produced by social services and sent to all those who attended the conference, and those who were invited but were unable to attend. In most cases the parents receive a copy of the minutes. The information contained within them is distilled from the reports from health, education and social services and the police, and forms a key part of the records of any professional with responsibility for the care of the child or children referred to. For those parents who attend with their children for any consultation, it is expected that the doctor will be aware of the involvement of social services and other agencies. The parent is likely to assume that the GP knows that their child is on the child protection register, if that is the case.

If the case conference minutes and other relevant documentation are to be scanned into the IT system and the originals destroyed, it is essential that if the child moves practice, all of the scanned documents are forwarded, or retrieved and forwarded in paper format. Likewise, any other pieces of information that are stored within the practice systems must be disclosed fully when children move on.

Ordinarily, if the system is working well, the designated professionals for child protection will ensure that files are moved into new areas when children leave. Children under the child protection umbrella who leave an area without social services or health services being informed often only have their problems pieced together when they register elsewhere and records are requested. If the complete file is not forwarded, the child may become more vulnerable.

Some practices file case-conference minutes and other relevant details in a paper file, using the electronic file for routine work. A system should be established to ensure that the user of the electronic file is aware that relevant information exists elsewhere, particularly if locum doctors or others new to the practice may be unaware of the history of families where children are at risk or have already been harmed.

Identifying the vulnerable child/family at each consultation

A significant number of children who are at risk do not of course come to the attention of those engaged in specific child protection roles. These vulnerable children are dependent on the vigilance of others in considering their welfare.

Raising awareness of the problems and lowering thresholds for suspicion of harm are two ways in which primary care services can contribute to the safeguarding of children. It is often the case that the GP who sees the child with minor symptoms may not be exposed to any behaviour by the parents that raises suspicions. Likewise, the GP is often unaware of any concerns that may exist within the education service or among other healthcare professionals, due to communication problems between agencies or individuals.

The way to identify these children is by improved communication within the primary care team, discussing common concerns with appropriate staff and making appropriate records, thus allowing other colleagues to be informed of the potential problems. The proper sharing of information and concerns in order to safeguard children is essential if we are to improve the lives of children who are abused.

Documenting injuries

Meticulous recording of clinical signs and symptoms is essential in child protection work. The successful prosecution of a perpetrator may be dependent on this.

Occasionally children will present to the surgery with minor ailments when other minor injuries, scratches, bruises, etc. are noted by or commented upon by either the GP or the parent. In the majority of cases, particularly in the active preschool child, these injuries are sustained purely accidentally. However, in some children this is sadly not the case.

The healthcare professional in the practice must be able to record fully any injuries, marks or unusual signs if they consider that these are worth noting. It is inappropriate to suggest that each child needs to have every bruise recorded, but there are families who, by virtue of their circumstances, may have children who are in need. Even if injuries have good explanations and appear to be beyond suspicion, the fact that a child is repeatedly able to harm him- or herself may be suggestive of neglect.

If injuries are to be recorded, this is best done in a way that is easily reproducible. In some practices, staff use body charts to record injuries, scars, etc. and then scan these into the system. If there are other robust mechanisms for recording this information, it is essential that all members of staff save material in the same way. It is then easily available if any staff members are asked to produce reports for the purposes of case conferences or proceedings.

Coding systems

Although it is possible to use clinical coding to identify children who are on the child protection register, this is not always the case for children who are thought to be vulnerable but who are not part of the formal process.

In some PCOs, work has been ongoing to determine an effective way of coding for children who appear to be vulnerable and need monitoring. Examples include those families where there is a history of domestic violence or of severe drug and alcohol problems in the parents. This is not to suggest that in those families parenting is ineffective, but rather that it is important to maintain a lower threshold for intervention if the children appear to be suffering as a result of neglect due to other overriding problems within the household. In these cases some practices are using a coding system indicating 'shared care' (i.e. that there is health visitor or other healthcare professional involvement).

There may be a problem in ensuring consistency within the practice or the PCO. What may appear to be a vulnerable child in the eyes of one practitioner may not merit coding as such by another. Practice policy should be developed following local guidance. All relevant members of the primary healthcare team should be involved in developing and reviewing policy to improve consistency.

GPs will often raise concerns about breaching confidentiality or casting aspersions on the family by using such methods. Under current law, there is no reason why a healthcare professional cannot document anxieties about a child or family to draw this to the attention of others involved on a 'need-to-know' basis. Indeed the parents *should* be aware of concerns that healthcare teams may have about a particular child or children, and we recommend that the GP or health visitor informs the family that they are 'keeping an eye' on the situation'.

Review of cases where there is concern will allow the coding to be removed once the professionals are reassured that the situation has changed for the benefit of the child.

It is useful to record who the key workers are or which other agencies are involved so that appropriate communication is maintained. This should be done wherever possible with the consent of those with parental responsibility. It should also be done in a way that allows it to appear on an easily accessible part of the electronic record.

Robust records transfer policies

The transfer of records out of practices has been alluded to earlier with regard to case-conference minutes. Practices should develop a policy to ensure the effective transfer of all children's records.

Advice should be available from the named professionals. In cases where children are on the child protection register there will be a local policy determining the way in which records are transferred.

GMS contract requirements for records[5]

Reviewing the new contract under annexes A, B and C, there are several areas setting out standards for records that are pertinent to the agenda for safeguarding children[5] (*see* Tables 16.1, 16.2 and 16.3).

Table 16.1 Annex A of the new GMS contract

Records 1	Each patient contact with a clinician is recorded in the patient's record, including consultations, visits and telephone advice
Records 2	Entries in the clinical records are legible
Records 3	The practice has a system for transferring and acting on information about patients seen by other doctors out of hours
Records 14	The records, hospital letters and investigation reports are filed in date order or available electronically in date order
Records 15	The practice has up-to-date clinical summaries for at least 60% of patients
Records 19	At least 80% per cent of newly registered patients have had their notes summarised within 8 weeks of receipt by the practice

Table 16.2 Annex B of the new GMS contract

11	The practice has a system to allow patients access to their records on request in accordance with current legislation
12	There is a designated individual (data controller) responsible for confidentiality
13	If the records are computerised, there are mechanisms to ensure that the data are transferred when patients leave the practice

Table 16.3 Annex C of the new GMS contract

Section 1	Clinical audit
	Organisational audit
Section 8	IM & T

Disclosure of clinical information

Guidance from the GMC, the MPOs and the Department of Health is consistent with regard to disclosure of clinical information in child protection matters. The guidance reflects the current legislation and is based upon the following:

- the Children Act 1989
- the Human Rights Act 1998
- the Data Protection Act 1988
- common law duty of confidence
- the United Nations Convention on the Rights of the Child (ratified by the UK government in 1991).

In most cases where disclosure of clinical information is required/requested, the consent of the parent is usually obtained and the process should not lead to problems. However, occasions do arise where specific consent has not been obtained, or may have been refused, by those with parental responsibility and it is the healthcare professional's opinion that disclosure is in the best interests of the child. Under those circumstances, specific advice should be sought if the matter is not entirely clear.

Advice on disclosure may be available from the following individuals or organisations:

1 locally:
   • named GP for child protection
   • designated doctor or nurse for child protection
   • Caldicott Guardian for local PCT or LHB
   • PCT or LHB legal advisers
2 nationally:
   • MPOs
   • GMC
   • BMA
   • NMC.

Practices should have some basic ground rules on disclosure of information that are understood by all relevant staff. The disclosure may not be limited to clinical records, but may extend to records of telephone conversations and general observations about a particular child and his or her family circumstances. If such information is disclosed with or without valid consent, it should be recorded appropriately, including the name of the person or organisation to whom the disclosure was made.

Again, useful advice can be found within the summary of the document referred to previously if you are concerned about a child being abused.[3,6] Both the summary and the full document are available on the Department of Health website.

Examples from the document are given in Box 16.2. The booklet has an appendix of several pages that deals with disclosure issues and is very helpful when formulating practice policy or considering individual cases.

Box 16.2 Examples taken from the document *What to Do if You're Worried a Child is Being Abused*, published by the Department of Health in May 2003[6]

Whose consent is required? The duty of confidence is owed to the person who has provided information on the understanding it is to be kept confidential and, in the case of medical or other records, the person to whom the information relates.

Has consent been given? You do not need express consent if you have reasonable grounds to believe that the person to whom the duty is owed understands and accepts that the information will be disclosed. For example, a person who refers an allegation of abuse to a social worker would expect that information to be shared on a 'need-to-know' basis with those responsible for following up the allegation. Anyone who receives information, knowing it is confidential, is also subject to a duty of confidence. Whenever you give or receive information in confidence you should ensure there is a clear understanding as to how it may be used or shared.

Should I seek consent? If you are in doubt as to whether a disclosure is authorised, it is best to obtain express consent. But you should not do so if you think this would be contrary to a child's welfare. For example, if the information is needed urgently, the delay in obtaining consent may not be justified. Seeking consent may prejudice a police investigation or may increase the risk of harm to the child.

What if consent is refused? You will need to decide whether the circumstances justify the disclosure, taking into account what is being disclosed, for what purposes and to whom.

Key points in information disclosure can be summarised as follows.

- The welfare of the child is paramount.
- Be aware of the law that determines confidentiality and disclosure.
- Consent from relevant parties is preferable prior to disclosure.
- Understand the concept of the 'Need-to-know' basis.
- Consider the rights and needs of the young person.
- Seek advice early on.

Clinical signs and symptoms of child abuse

It is beyond the scope of this book to embark upon clinical matters. There are many simple texts available that are of help to the primary care practitioner, and several teaching packs (including CD-ROMs) with high-quality clinical information.

The local child protection team should be able to help with resources, and often keeps teaching packs to be used in addition to any other local material. Video tapes produced by the NSPCC are often very helpful in refreshing clinical skills in this area.

Domestic violence and safeguarding children

The Home Office defines domestic violence as 'Any violence between current and former partner in an intimate relationship, wherever or whenever the violence occurs. The violence may include physical, sexual, emotional and financial abuse'.[7]

The incidence of domestic violence in the UK is increasing, and its impact on children should not be underestimated. Recent initiatives from the Government are aimed at reducing harm to victims, and include the introduction of the Domestic Violence, Crime and Victims Bill in the House of Lords in December 2003. The strategy on domestic violence includes key elements based on prevention, protection, and justice and support. Children and young people naturally feature in this.

The Domestic Violence Data Source (DVDS) states that 'Research has indicated that roughly half of those experiencing domestic violence have children under 16 living in the household'.[8]

It is therefore incumbent on those working in primary care to understand the nature of domestic violence (again, no respecter of means or profession) and the potential impact that it has on children known to and registered at the practice. Given that research also suggests that one in four women will be a victim of domestic violence in their lifetime, the GP must remain alert to this possibility and the effects that it may have on the patient and her children.

Domestic violence is not confined to women. In a consultation paper produced by the Government in 2003,[9] data suggested that one in six men are likely to be victims of domestic violence in their lifetime, and 30 men per year are killed by a partner or former partner. Where this is suspected, the children in that relationship are as vulnerable when the woman is the perpetrator.

The DVDS includes the following examples of how the effects manifest in children:

• physical and emotional injury, neglect or other harm
• low self-esteem
• problems relating to others
• feelings of isolation, hostility or guilt
• inappropriate understanding of the acceptability of violence
• taking on responsibility for parenting other siblings
• academic under-achievement, exclusion from school.

Raising awareness within the practice, and possible means of identifying and monitoring domestic violence are suggested later in the chapter.

Children in families where violence exists are particularly vulnerable with respect to both emotional and physical abuse.

Child sexual abuse

Cases of possible sexual abuse can sometimes be difficult to diagnose, and may only surface following investigations or treatment for a condition that presented almost routinely to the GP. Examples would include the child with persistent vulvovaginitis, or intermittent bloodstaining of the undergarments in the pre-pubertal girl.

GPs should retain an open mind at all times, being sensitive to the demeanour of the child, the parent/carer, the family circumstances, etc. Appropriate communication of concerns to colleagues who may be involved with the family (e.g. health visitors or school nurses) may raise the index of suspicion.

Perpetrators may be close or extended family members, friends or neighbours and, as with all child protection issues, child sexual abuse is no respecter of class. In those children in whom sexual abuse may be suspected, or when a parent or carer suggests to the GP that sexual abuse may have taken place, the GP must be aware of local practice. Particular attention must be paid to the history as given to the GP or the carer, and at all times great sensitivity is needed when dealing with the child or young person.

This area of clinical practice is fraught with difficulty, but careful elucidation of clinical signs can ultimately lead to successful prosecutions of perpetrators. *The role of the GP is therefore not to undertake clinical examination specifically for the purpose of determining whether sexual abuse has taken place, but to establish what additional help and advice are needed and whether the child is in immediate danger.*

It is a widely held belief that unnecessary and overzealous examination of a child by more than one healthcare professional for the purpose of confirming whether child sexual abuse has taken place is in itself an abuse of the child or young person. Caution is necessary under these circumstances.

- In suspected child abuse, *having established that the child is safe*, seek advice immediately from the child protection team using local referral pathways to ensure that any clinical examination undertaken is in the best interests of the child.
- Document fully and carefully any information provided by the child, parent or carer.
- Explain what steps you are taking and what happens next.
- Reassure the child/carer/parent that they were right to bring their concerns to your attention.
- Do not belittle or attempt to refute any allegations that the child may make – leave that to those more experienced in the field.

Guidance provided in 2002 by the Royal College of Paediatricians and the Association of Police Surgeons[10] has clarified the need to adopt a consistent approach to the management of the child when sexual abuse is suspected.

Children in whom illness is fabricated or induced

Although fabricated or induced illness is unusual, guidance from the Department of Health suggests that an average PCT is likely to see one case per year. As such, the Department of Health[11] requires PCTs to ensure that appropriate training is provided for 'professional staff at all levels and in all disciplines'.

The guidance published in August 2002[11] makes the following suggestions.

- GPs and all members of the primary healthcare team are well placed to recognise the early signs and symptoms of fabricated or induced illness in a child.
- Professionals in primary healthcare teams may have unique knowledge of uncorroborated, odd or unusual presentations.
- Professionals may be aware of children who frequently attend the clinic where there is a discrepancy between the reported signs and symptoms and those observed.
- These cases present dilemmas for staff with regard to conflict of interest and confidentiality.
- Guidance and advice are needed, and the procedures in the Department of Health document should be followed.
- There are often many opportunities for nurses, midwives and health visitors to notice unusual behaviours and, as such, training and heightened awareness are crucial.

Given the above, training updates in this area are required in many practices. These can be arranged in conjunction with the general child protection training programme.

GPs should be encouraged to discuss any specific case concerns they have with their designated doctors in child protection in accordance with local policy. Clinically these can be complex cases. As a result, relationships with the family can become strained for the GP, who is often asked to undertake more and more referrals and investigations without any obvious benefit for the child.

When should children be referred in cases of suspected abuse?

Many GPs express a lack of confidence in cases where they have suspicions that the needs of a child are not being met, but have insufficient evidence to warrant a referral. It is known that thresholds for acceptance of referrals vary between social services departments, particularly when they are hard pressed.

Within each PCO area there should be sufficient access to advice for the GP and members of the primary healthcare team from within health and social services to help with the decision making. The Department of Health flow charts produced in May 2003 assist with this.[3]

Some PCTs develop their own flow charts that reflect local practice. One good example of this is the double-sided laminated chart which is produced by East Cheshire PCT child protection team and issued to all practices following a period of intensive training. This enables clearly visible advice to be at hand in all of the consulting rooms. The chart distinguishes between the child in need and the child at risk, identifies when consent is required, and gives the local contact numbers for named and designated professionals, social services offices and the emergency duty team.

The GMC published updated advice on confidentiality in April 2004,[12] and this is available on their website.

> If you believe a patient to be a victim of neglect or physical, sexual or emotional abuse, and you consider that the patient cannot give or withhold consent to disclosure, you must give information promptly to an appropriate responsible person or statutory agency, where you believe that the disclosure is in the patient's best interests. If, for any reason, you believe that disclosure of information is not in the best interests of an abused or neglected patient, you should discuss the issues with an experienced colleague. If you decide not to disclose information, you must be prepared to justify your decision.

Attending case conferences

This is commented upon in the RCGP position statement.[14] Attendance at case conferences remains a problem for many GPs due to time commitments, locum cover and the often short notice period.

Many initial case conferences are convened when the GP has very little involvement in the care of the child and may not have prepared any information or reports for consideration. Few GPs are familiar with the *Framework for the*

Assessment of Children in Need and their Families,[13] and they are likely to be unfamiliar with the processes leading up to the decision to call an initial case conference. For example, a child who is not known to the GP, but is registered with the practice, may have had some input from the health visitor or school nurse, but no specific health problems. The GP may consider that they have a limited role in attending a multi-disciplinary conference, and would prefer to send a report.

This is reasonable in some cases. We recommend that the GP produces some information in time for the conference and communicates effectively with other members of the primary care team prior to the conference hearing (it is likely that another member of the primary care team will attend the conference).

Unfortunately, a number of opportunities for sharing information are lost, and unless the designated or named professionals are able to play an active role, there are occasions when the lack of any medically qualified individuals at a case conference may compromise the child or children in question.

Figure 16.1 is a flow diagram illustrating the processes that lead to a case conference.

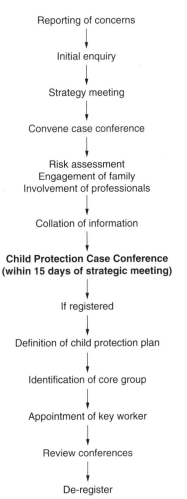

Reporting of concerns

↓

Initial enquiry

↓

Strategy meeting

↓

Convene case conference

↓

Risk assessment
Engagement of family
Involvement of professionals

↓

Collation of information

↓

**Child Protection Case Conference
(wihin 15 days of strategic meeting)**

↓

If registered

↓

Definition of child protection plan

↓

Identification of core group

↓

Appointment of key worker

↓

Review conferences

↓

De-register

Figure 16.1 Flow diagram illustrating the processes that lead to a child protection case conference.[4]

The child protection register

Following an initial case conference, if a decision is made that the child is at continuing risk of significant harm, they will then be registered on the child protection register.

The register is maintained by social services and records all the children in a local authority area who are considered to be suffering from or at risk of suffering significant harm.

The majority of children on child protection registers are able to remain in their families with support from a selection of child protection agency workers.

Any healthcare professional or member of the police should be able to access the register if they have concerns about a particular child or children at any time (on a 24-hour basis) to ascertain whether the child is on the register or not, as this may influence clinical and care decisions.

The NSPCC collates information and publishes statistics about children in need, and it has a range of data available for those involved in this work.[14]

Data collected from the various Health Departments in England, Wales, Scotland and Northern Ireland, and available on the NSPCC website,[14] show that for the year ending 31 March 2002 there were 31 220 children's names on child protection registers in the UK. Most of these were in England – reflecting the majority of the population in the UK.

The register also demonstrates the age range of children who are registered at any one time. Younger children (aged under 4 years) appear to be most vulnerable.

The numbers on the register change constantly as children are moved on and off it depending on circumstances, new cases coming to the attention of the professionals, young people reaching independence, etc.

Criteria for placing a child on the child protection register in England include the following:

- neglect
- physical abuse
- sexual abuse
- emotional abuse.

The definitions of each of the categories are always available in local guidance and child protection handbooks produced by ACPCs.

The primary care team and 'looked-after' children (children in the care of the local authority)

By virtue of the number of children who are looked after in the UK at any one time, each practice would expect to see a few per year. In a resource containing data provided by the Department of Health in 2002,[14] the following was stated: 'in a PCT serving 100 000 total population, approximately 160 children would be expected to experience being looked after in one year, of whom approximately 50 would be new entrants', new entrants being those children who had not previously experienced the care system.

Taking a 'snapshot view' from data provided for 31 March 2001,[14] twice as many children (59 000) in England were being looked after as were on the child protection register (27 000), although some of those registered were likely to have been looked after at the time of the survey.

All these children will have health needs, and all will be required to be assessed as part of the process of being looked after. This has implications for the primary healthcare team. The principles behind the work that is required to a great extent mirror those for the more general child protection discussion in this chapter.

The Department of Health[15] sets out the contributions expected from the primary healthcare team. Health information is an important feature of this, and some examples are set out below as they are relevant to the overall processes in primary care and what primary care teams should do.

- Provide, when needed, summaries of the health history of a child or young person who is looked after, including their family history where relevant and appropriate, and ensure that this information is passed promptly to healthcare professionals undertaking health assessments, subject to appropriate consents.
- Maintain a record of the health assessment and contribute to any necessary action within the health plan.
- Ensure that the clinical records make the 'looked-after' status of the child or young person clear, so that their particular needs can be acknowledged.
- Regularly review the clinical records of 'looked-after' children and young people who are registered with the primary care team.[15]

The new GMS contract and child protection

Apart from the references made earlier in the chapter to medical records and the contract, there are several specific clauses to be addressed in the new contract that are relevant to child protection.[5] These are set out in Tables 16.4, 16.5 and 16.6.

Table 16.4 Annex A of the new GMS contract

Education 4	All new staff receive induction training
Management 1	Individual healthcare professionals have access to information on local procedures relating to child protection

Table 16.5 Annex B of the new GMS contract

6	The practice has a policy for consent to the treatment of children that conforms to the current Children's Act or equivalent legislation
20	Individual healthcare professionals should be able to demonstrate that they comply with the national child protection guidance, and should provide at least one critical event analysis regarding concerns about a child's welfare if appropriate

Table 16.6 Annex C of the new GMS contract

Section 1	Clinical audit and organisational audit
Section 2	Risk assessment Significant event audit/reporting Confidentiality
Section 4	Patient protection Social services Working partnerships Networking with colleagues from other practices

Many of the above contractual requirements have been touched upon in this chapter and can hopefully be dealt with by review of current systems and processes in the practice for safeguarding children. It may be possible within the PCO to utilise the named professionals to help develop policies and procedures for all practices that will deliver the contract specifications and thereby enhance the provision for children in need.

Assessing knowledge and training

The following recommendation was made by Lord Laming:[1]

> All GPs must devise and maintain procedures to ensure that they, and all members of their practice staff, are aware of whom to contact in the local health agencies, social services and the police in the event of child protection concerns in relation to any of their patients. (Paragraph 12.29)

To maintain safe practice, training is essential. Baseline assessments of training needs in primary care often reveal significant deficiencies. The level of awareness has undoubtedly risen following the publication of the Climbié Report,[1] and no doubt the number of practices with policies will increase as well.

Nursing staff working in the community usually access more child protection training and support (and are more likely to attend multi-disciplinary training events) than GPs. Nursing staff also receive clinical supervision in this area.

Each practice must establish the training needs that exist, taking into account the recommendations from the Laming Report,[1] the new GMS contract[5] and general professional requirements. Working with the local child protection team should lead to some solutions and will assist the development of updated local practice policies.

Practice policies and key documents

There are many reference documents available in all four countries of the UK that outline policy and practice for safeguarding children. Realistically, however, these are not going to be used on a regular basis within most practices.

It may be helpful to seek the advice of the local named GP with responsibilities for child protection and the PCO to ascertain what is considered essential.

The local ACPC may have a list of recommended documents for primary care. At the very least a copy of its own guidance is essential.

We recommend that practices use the new contract as an impetus for improving child protection processes in primary care – with potentially valuable outcomes.

References

1 Laming, Lord (2003) *The Victoria Climbié Inquiry.* The Stationery Office, London; www.victoria-climbie-inquiry.org.uk

2 Department of Health (2002) *Letter from Jacqui Smith, Minister of State for Health, to Chief Executives of Primary Care Trusts.* Department of Health, London.

3 Department of Health, Home Office and Department for Education and Skills (2003) *What to Do if You're Worried a Child is Being Abused.* Department of Health Publications, London.

4 Royal College of General Practitioners (2002) *A Position Paper from the Royal College of General Practitioners with Endorsement from the Royal College of Paediatrics and Child Health, the National Society for the Prevention of Cruelty to Children, the British Association of Medical Managers and the NHS Confederation.* www.rcgp.org.uk/rcgp/corporate/position/childprotection.pdf

5 Department of Health (2004) *Standard General Medical Services Contract.* Department of Health, London; www.dh.gov.uk/assetRoot/04/09/22/38/04092238.pdf

6 Department of Health, Home Office and Department for Education and Skills (2003) *What to Do if You're Worried a Child is Being Abused. Summary.* Department of Health Publications, London.

7 www.womenandequalityunit.gov.uk/domestic violence/

8 www.domesticviolencedata.org/1_services/child_ser.asp

9 www.homeoffice.gov.uk/docs2/violence.html and www.homeoffice.gov.uk/docs2/domesticviolence.pdf

10 Royal College of Paediatrics and Child Health and Association of Police Surgeons (2002) *Guidance on Paediatric Forensic Examinations in Relation to Possible Child Sexual Abuse.* Royal College of Paediatrics and Child Health, London.

11 Department of Health, Department for Education and Employment and National Assembly for Wales (2002) *Safeguarding Children in Whom Illness is Fabricated or Induced. Supplementary guidance to 'Working Together to Safeguard Children'.* Department of Health, London; www.dh.gov.uk/PublicationsAndStatistics/Publications/PublicationsPolicyAndGuidance/PublicationsPolicyAndGuidanceArticle/fs/en?CONTENT_ID=4006042&chk=dG%2Bgny

12 General Medical Council (2004) *Confidentiality: protecting and providing information.* General Medical Council, London; www.gmc-uk.org/standards/secret.htm

13 Department of Health, Department for Education and Employment and Home Office (1999) *Framework for the Assessment of Children in Need and Their Families.* The Stationery Office, London.

14 *NSPCC Inform: the online child protection resource*; www.nspcc.org.uk/inform/Statistics/CPStats/CP_Family.asp#youngpeople

15 Department of Health (2002) *Promoting the Health of Looked After Children.* Department of Health Publications, London.

Chapter 17

The impact of guidelines on practice

Brian Hurwitz

Key learning points

- The Bolam standard still applies.
- There appears to be no managerial or legal expectation in the UK that doctors should automatically follow guidelines.
- Guidelines currently play a subservient role to that of the expert witness in court proceedings.
- Guidelines vary in quality. Blindly following poor, inappropriate or out-of-date guidelines can harm patients and confer medico-legal risk.
- Guidelines are likely to assume a greater prominence in future.
- In particular, NICE guidelines are likely to have special legal significance.

The legal status of clinical practice guidelines

Guidelines have no defined legal position. However, any doctor not fulfilling the standards and quality of care in the appropriate treatment that are set out in these Clinical Guidelines will have this taken into account if, for any reason, consideration of their performance in this clinical area is undertaken.[1]

Guidelines are no substitute for expert evidence about acceptable practice. Compliance with well-recognised guidelines is likely to exculpate (exonerate). Deviation from well-recognised guidelines may be Bolam-defensible.[2]

Introduction

The authority and standing of clinical practice guidelines were first recognised to be an important professional and legal issue by Plato in the fourth century BC. Plato was interested in the difference between human skills grounded in practical expertise and those based solely upon following instructions or obeying rules. The pervasive influence of guidelines on the practice of modern medicine, and the varied approaches to guideline development that coexist today (with consequent

---

This chapter previously appeared in Whitty P and Eccles M (eds) (2004) *Clinical Practice Guidelines in Mental Health: a guide to their use in improving care*, published by Radcliffe Publishing.

effects on clinical guideline quality) mean that the legal status of guidelines continues to be debated.

Plato invented the following thought experiment to explore the matter. Doctors were to be stripped of their clinical freedom – 'no longer allowed unchecked authority' – and to form themselves into councils to determine majority views about how best to practise medicine in all situations. The deliberations and majority decisions of such panels, composed of clinical and non-clinical members, were to be codified and published in order 'to dictate the ways in which the treatment of the sick was to be practised'.[3] Plato considered the hallmarks of expertise to be flexible responsiveness and improvisatory ability – aspects of medical practice that are still recognised today, and which Plato believed would be endangered by the use of guidelines.[3] However effective healthcare by guideline turned out to be (and Plato was prepared to concede its potential), such care would constitute a debased form of practice, because guidelines, he concluded, presupposed standardised treatments for average patients rather than customised treatments for particular patients, and because the knowledge and analysis that go into the creation of guidelines are not rooted in the mental processes of clinicians, but in the minds of guideline developers who are distant from the consultation. Very similar concerns continue to trouble present-day clinicians.

> There is a fear that in the absence of evidence clearly applicable to the case in hand, a clinician might be forced by guidelines to make use of evidence which is only doubtfully relevant, generated perhaps in a different grouping of patients in another country and some other time and using a similar but not identical treatment. This is . . . to use evidence in the manner of the fabled drunkard who searched under the street lamp for his door key because that is where the light was, even though he had dropped the key somewhere else.[4]

> The extent to which guidelines depend on opinion is disturbing for anyone who believes they should be evidence-based. Guidelines are evidence filtered through opinion. The opinion is crucial – but whose opinion should it be? The NICE committee is made up of a variety of experts in different disciplines who take specific advice from a small number of specialists in the relevant field. These specialists may or may not hold an opinion widely shared by their (equally expert) colleagues.[5]

In Plato's view, once a profession committed itself to providing healthcare through guidelines (a position now demanded by the UK Government[6,7]), he could see no alternative but to ensure compliance with them, even if this entailed resorting to legal action. Such guidelines, he believed, would have to be understood almost as clinical laws, for once expertise no longer resides within the patient's clinician but is represented in guidelines instead, corruption of or deviation from such guidelines would result in medical treatments being grounded in personal whim or quackery.

Plato's reference to the legal arena was remarkable in its prescience. Only comparatively recently have guidelines begun to feature in modern-day health care regulations and in case law.[8-12] Today, the GMC advises clinical teams 'normally to use recommended clinical guidelines.'[13]

Guidelines and legislation

Legislation in Europe and the USA has harnessed guidelines to a variety of healthcare regulatory tasks.[14,15] An example in the UK is the Human Fertilisation and Embryology Act 1990 which established a regulatory Authority (Human Fertilisation and Embryology Authority, HFEA) empowered to develop guidelines.[16] HFEA initially decided to restrict to three the number of fertilised eggs that can legally be placed in a woman's uterus during treatment by *in-vitro* fertilisation (IVF), and later reduced this number to two. The mandatory nature of HFEA's guidance on this matter in the event of transgression is made plain by enforceable penalties, including revocation of the licence to practise IVF. HFEA's 'guidance' on this is backed by Parliamentary authority and carries the force of a prescriptive legal rule.

In France, mandatory practice guidelines introduced under a 1993 statute, Loi Teulade 93–8, cover investigations, prescribing and certain medical procedures. Initially developed by the social security administration responsible for reimbursing private practitioners and the doctors' unions, guideline development has now been taken over by an independent organisation, the Agence Nationale pour le Dévelopement de l'Evaluation Médicale. Once published, the guidelines constitute an enforceable agreement between doctors and the social security administration.[17,18]

Standards of medical care

The legally required standard of medical treatment that a doctor generally owes to a patient derives in the UK from the case of Bolam v Friern Hospital Management Committee (1957).[19] In the words of the judge of this case, 'the test is the standard of the ordinary skilled man exercising and professing to have that special skill.'[19] The judge in the Bolam case recognised that there could be two or more schools of thought regarding proper medical treatment. Therefore doctors can usually rebut a charge of negligence if they have acted in conformity with a body of other responsible doctors.[19]

Box 17.1 Negligence

Medical negligence is a composite finding comprising three essential elements. The complainant, formerly the plaintiff, the person bringing the action, must show that:

1 the defendant doctor owed the complainant a duty of care and
2 the doctor breached this duty of care by failing to provide the required standard of medical care, and
3 this failure actually caused the plaintiff harm – a harm that was both foreseeable and reasonably avoidable.

Clinical guidelines could influence the manner in which the courts establish the second element of this composite.

Expert testimony helps the courts to ascertain what is accepted and proper practice in specific cases, ensuring that professionally generated standards derived from real clinical situations are generally applied by the courts, rather than standards enunciated in the rhetoric of clinical guidelines. In Cranley v Medical Board of Western Australia (1990),[20] an Australian GP stood accused of misconduct because he had prescribed injectable diazepam to heroin addicts, contrary to the Australian National Methadone Guidelines. He was initially found guilty of 'infamous and improper conduct', but after hearing of a minority medical opinion supporting the treatment of opiate addicts within the harm reduction framework followed by Dr Cranley, the Supreme Court of Western Australia upheld his appeal.[20]

As a norm, the Bolam test is supposed to represent an aggregate of individual clinical judgements informed by scientific evidence and professional experience. Its advantages are held to be that it takes account of evolving standards of care and is a professionally led (although legally imposed) standard. It allows for differences of opinion, and is sufficiently broadly expressed to encompass medical practice that is predominantly scientific, or as much a craft as a science.

However, unlike the tests of negligence adopted in other common-law jurisdictions, such as Canada (where the test is based on 'that degree of care and skill which could *reasonably be expected* of a normal prudent practitioner of the same experience and standing'),[21] the Bolam test appears to be more a 'state-of-the-art' descriptive test of what *is* done in practice, rather than a normative test of what *ought* to be done. Under Bolam, widespread adoption of guidelines could result in guideline-informed care becoming viewed as the customary norm, with departure from guidelines then being seen as prima facie evidence of a case to answer.[22,23]

A leading UK barrister has concluded that the combined effects of guidelines and evidence-based medicine are that 'many areas of medicine and surgery, which attract the attention of civil litigators, are or will be governed by clinical guidelines. Increasingly, it will be possible to plead just one particular of negligence: "Failing to follow guideline X".'[2] Given the poor quality of many clinical guidelines currently in circulation, this consequence should be guarded against (*see* Box 17.2).[24] Some guideline quality markers may be a crude indication of overall guideline quality, but the potential for poor-quality guidelines to influence the legal standard by which a doctor is judged is compounded by the failure of the courts generally to call expert witnesses to scrutinise the robustness and quality of guidelines.[25,26]

Box 17.2 Quality indicators of clinical guidelines published in peer-review journals over a 10-year period

---

Of 431 clinical guidelines published in English, listed in Medline, and produced by specialty societies between January 1988 and July 1998, 88% were found to give no information on the searches used to retrieve relevant published studies, 67% failed to report any description of the type of stakeholders involved in guideline development or use, and 82% provided no explicit grading of the strength of recommendations.[24]

The Bolam test in the UK operates on a case-by-case basis. Lord Woolf, the Lord Chief Justice of England, speaking extra-judicially to the Royal College of Physicians of London about legal standards of care, explained that:

> The general approach of the courts is to apply the standards that the medical profession adopts. Thus we judge whether there has been negligence in the treatment of a patient by asking whether or not the medical treatment, which is the subject of complaint, accords with standards which *any* recognised section of the medical profession regards as acceptable. . . . By adopting this standard the courts have managed to hold the balance fairly between the interests of the patient and the interest of the profession. By striking the right balance, the courts reduce the risk of proper medical practice being undermined by fear of litigation, and recognise the need for compensation to be paid where treatment is of an unacceptable standard.[27]

Hitherto, the main justification for judicial reliance upon customary care standards has been the belief that technical medical matters are beyond the detailed knowledge of judges and lay people and are best left to 'experts'. Since guidelines offer doctors and patients explicit examples of standards of care articulated in considerable detail for use in specific clinical circumstances, they could be thought to remove the need for expert testimony in court, as the courts would have direct access to relevant standards from guidelines.[22,24]

However, guidelines may not in fact reflect customary standards of care at all. Indeed, some appear designed to hasten the incorporation of research findings into routine practice.[28] This inevitably challenges the law's use of a customary care standard that does little to narrow gaps between everyday clinical practices and evidence-based practice. In an evidence-linked era, Bolam may be thought to demand too little to encourage higher standards of care. Condemned as 'a blot on English medical law', the Bolam test has been disparaged as the result of undue judicial deference to medical opinion. However, despite no longer being as influential as it once was, Bolam has not yet been superseded in the UK by a legal standard entirely determined without reference to a responsible body of medical practitioners (*see* Box 17.3).[29,30]

Box 17.3 Guidelines are no substitute for expert evidence

Guidelines could be introduced to a court by an expert witness as evidence of accepted and customary standards of care, but they cannot be introduced as a substitute for expert testimony. Courts are unlikely to adopt standards of care advocated in clinical guidelines as legal 'gold standards', because the mere fact that a guideline exists does not of itself establish that compliance with it is reasonable in the circumstances, or that non-compliance is negligent.

> Guidelines are no substitute for expert evidence about acceptable practice. Compliance with well recognised guidelines is likely to exculpate (exonerate). Deviation from well-recognised guidelines may be Bolam-defensible.[2]

Author or sponsor liability

The possibility that bias might creep into guideline development has been a concern in France, where complaints have been laid before the Fraud Squad alleging improper conduct by participants in the French guidelines programme.[17] It is also a concern of the American Medical Association (AMA), which believes that 'bad faith claims could be lodged against developers who stand to benefit from the content of a guideline and who design results to comport with desired cost containment goals.'[31]

In the USA, the AMA has outlined the scenarios which could found a claim against guideline developers or sponsors in the event of faulty guidelines being associated with patient harm. These include negligence in 'analysing or interpreting data, or translating data into a guideline, ignoring well-known and scientifically valid data, and utilising data that were known, or should have been known, to be insufficient or faulty.'[30] However, to date no cases have arisen in either US or UK jurisdictions in which the courts have been required to decide whether guideline authors were liable for incorrect or misleading statements (*see* Box 17.4).[2,30–34]

Box 17.4 American Medical Association advice to US guideline developers

The AMA believes developers of guidelines should:

assume that their research methodology and resulting conclusions will subsequently be subject to legal review and to proceed with the assumption that they may be challenged in court. In keeping with this approach, the guidelines' underlying methodology, supporting research, recommendations, and conclusions should be fully documented and preserved for inspection by others at a later time.'[30]

In non-medical spheres, UK courts have decided similar questions where people have suffered economic loss by relying upon written statements of advice.[35] However, the general position in the UK is that there can be no duty of care between the author of a document or book and its myriad potential readers, unless the authors could foresee that their written advice would be directly communicated to a reader, who would have little choice but to rely upon it without independent enquiry. Such advice would require to possess quite extraordinary authority for doctors to be expected to follow clinical guidelines without further inquiry.[36]

Box 17.5 Author/sponsor liability

While an action could be taken against a clinician for not keeping up to date, a College is probably not actionable, as it would be difficult to show it owes a duty or obligation directly to the patient.[37]

The status of advice offered by guidelines should be made as clear as possible to clinicians. For example, the prefatory statement in the NICE guidelines on *Core Interventions in the Treatment and Management of Schizophrenia in Primary and Secondary Care* states that:

> This guidance represents the view of the Institute, which was arrived at after careful consideration of the evidence available. Health professionals are expected to take it fully into account when exercising their clinical judgment. The guidance does not, however, override the individual responsibility of health professionals to make decisions appropriate to the circumstances of the individual patient, in consultation with the patient and/or guardian or carer.[38]

Although reading like a disclaimer, the authors emphasise that users of the guideline are expected to behave as learned intermediaries, exercising customary clinical discretion and consulting other sources of relevant information.

Discretion

Some health service lawyers have commented that as guidelines receive increasing acceptance in the clinical community, acting in accordance with a clinical guideline could be viewed as acceptable medical practice *per se*. However, guidelines can create a false sense of consensus, can mask or underplay controversy, and may rapidly become out of date as a result of new findings. Most guidelines face more or less well-grounded degrees of dissent most of the time. For example, in 2003 the *Drug and Therapeutics Bulletin* systematically reviewed the role of intravenous magnesium administration in the treatment of severe asthma, and concluded that:

> The current British Guideline on the Management of Asthma, published jointly by the British Thoracic Society and the Scottish Intercollegiate Guidelines Network, suggests that a single iv dose of magnesium sulphate should be used for the treatment of patients with acute severe asthma.[39] However, the available data are weak and conflicting and do not justify this unlicensed use of the drug.[40]

In general, doctors are expected to use appropriate clinical discretion when deciding upon medical treatment, and the courts continue to place the testimony of expert witnesses about what constitutes reasonable practice above the recommendations of prestigious works of reference (*see* Box 17.3). Even where a guideline has been laid down as a legal standard, courts require sensible discretion to be used in its appropriate application.[41]

In administrative law, the essence of discretion is 'a readiness to deal with each case on its merits.'[42] The NHS Executive acknowledges that when endorsed by prestigious professional bodies or even commended by the NHS Executive:

> clinical guidelines can still only assist the practitioner; they cannot be used to mandate, authorise or outlaw treatment options. Regardless of the strength of the evidence, it will remain the responsibility of the practising clinicians to interpret their application . . . . It would be wholly inappropriate for clinical guidelines to be used as a means

of coercion of the individual clinician, by managers and senior professionals.'[43]

Rigid, uncritical adherence to guidelines is not the formal, administrative or managerial expectation in the NHS. Translation of precepts into action involves interpretation,[44] as emphasised in guidelines on the treatment of hypertension produced by the World Health Organization:

> Guidelines should provide extensive, critical and well-balanced information on benefits and limitations of the various diagnostic and therapeutic interventions so that the physician may exert the most careful judgement in individual cases.[45]

However, concern remains that guidelines could erode clinical abilities, diminish clinical judgement, and reduce medical practice to 'cookbook medicine' and the thoughtless activities of physician automata.[46] In the USA, tensions surfacing between treatment protocols and doctors' clinical judgement have led the courts to rule that clinicians may not claim as a defence to negligence that their clinical judgement has been corrupted by guidelines.[47]

Although some judgements required of doctors in discrete areas of medicine can be more or less explicitly specified, this should not be thought to reduce clinical judgements to nothing other than 'decisional algebra', which can be objectified in expert systems, algorithms, protocols or guidelines. Clinical practice frequently involves judgements about complex individual circumstances in the context of different degrees of uncertainty. Medical decision making depends on opinionated assessments that are grounded in knowledge of appropriate scientific findings, which are informed by clinical experience and take account of patients' wishes. Such decisions are not simple transductions of input information resulting in output decisions. Clinical judgements frequently go beyond explicit input information, adding considerations of feeling, attitude and value to the output.[48] As one distinguished professor of cardiology has expressed it, 'treatment can depend on something as subtle and unquantifiable as the glint in a patient's eye.'[49] Applying guidelines to individual care is always likely to require judgement, even when recommendations are properly evidence-linked.[50] Sir Michael Rawlins, the Chairman of NICE, accepts that 'No guideline can cover 100 per cent, because people vary. It's up to the doctor or other health professional to decide when the guideline is no longer applicable and what to do in its place.'[51]

The implications of Sir Michael's view – that up to a fifth of clinical decisions taken in situations prima facie covered by guidelines may yet quite properly deviate from them – does not detract from the advice issued by Vivienne Nathanson, head of the Science, Ethics and Policy Unit of the BMA (and endorsed by Sir Michael Rawlins[51]) that doctors should record treatment decisions in patients' notes in ways that 'show that they have considered the guidelines.'[52]

National Institute for Clinical Excellence (NICE) and guidelines

How, if at all, does the arrival of NICE alter the legal status of guidelines? NICE was set up to give guidance to the NHS as a whole, to the Government, and ultimately to patients, in several areas of healthcare, including the creation of clinical guidelines.[53] According to the Department of Health memorandum setting out the ground rules under which NICE operates, the Institute is required to follow a transparent and well-structured process, giving appropriate interested parties the opportunity to submit evidence, and to comment on draft conclusions. The memorandum conceptualises the Department of Health's view of the legal status of NICE guidance in the following terms:

> All guidance must be fully reasoned and written in terms which make clear that it is guidance. Guidance for clinicians does not override their professional responsibility to make the appropriate decision in the circumstances of the individual patient, in consultation with the patient or guardian/carer and in the light of any locally agreed policies. Similarly, guidance to NHS trusts and commissioners must make clear that it does not take away their discretion under administrative law to take account of individual circumstances.[53]

NICE has been charged with ensuring that the implications of its recommendations are transmitted to NSFs and related quality-of-care initiatives, such as the following NHS information and advice channels: PRODIGY guidelines, the National electronic Library for Health, protocols used by NHS Direct and NHS Walk-in Centres, and any material for patients produced by NHS Direct Online.[53]

NICE is therefore structurally and strategically positioned to be at the hub of a series of influential mechanisms designed to facilitate implementation of guidance. How realistic, therefore, is the Department of Health's simultaneously held view that NICE-approved guidance should not be thought to undercut or override clinicians' professional responsibility to make appropriate decisions in the circumstances of the individual patient?

A 1999 legal case, which arose from a desire to limit a drug's use within the NHS, has clearly indicated that the language in which advice is couched can significantly influence how guidance is likely to be interpreted. Its language can also bear on the lawfulness of its guidance. In R v Secretary of State for Health ex parte Pfizer Ltd (May 1999)[54] the lawfulness of a Health Service Circular (1998/158)[55] dated 16 September 1998 was challenged in the High Court. Although the circular in question contained the heading '*Material which is for guidance only and aims to share good practice*', the judge ruled that the circular in question was advice in presentation only, and that in substance and effect it was a direction which unlawfully curtailed the clinical discretion of UK GPs – a discretion, moreover, which has statutory underpinning:[56] 'the problem with the circular is that the advice was given in a manner which meant that GPs would inevitably regard it as overriding their professional judgement . . . .'.[54]

The case highlights the potential power of a clinical guideline agency such as NICE. On the one hand, the model hitherto construed to characterise physician–guideline relationships posits doctors as free agents, capable of appropriately taking advantage of authoritative guidance without entering into a relationship of professional *reliance* upon guideline guidance. On the other hand, as the analysis of Health Service Circular 1998/158 indicates, executive implementation of authoritative guidance carries with it a danger that guidance can all too easily be packaged as (and therefore mistaken for) instructions. If this happens, it will significantly undermine the ability of clinicians to act as their own 'master editors' of advisory information, able to modify and blend guideline advice with their own experience in the context of the advice of local treatment policies. It may be that this model of practice is now a diminishing ideal, one perhaps only applicable to specialists in their own field of expertise, who have the appropriate depth of experience and knowledge to avoid over-reliance on clinical guidelines.[5,49]

Conclusions

Despite stirrings afoot to replace the customary Bolam standard of medical care with a normative standard that would be more susceptible to determination without reference to a professional body of medical opinion, there appears to be no managerial or legal expectation in the UK that doctors should automatically follow guidelines. Clinical guidelines are not generally credited by the courts with a special 'self-evident' status, and guidelines currently play a subservient role to that of the expert witness in court proceedings.[34] The only published study of actual guideline use in litigation revealed that, in the USA, guidelines play 'a relevant or pivotal role in the proof of negligence' in less than 7% of US malpractice actions.[57]

Nevertheless, clinical guidelines look set to become more influential with regard to both the way doctors practise and the manner in which they are to be held accountable. The GMC has announced a general expectation that doctors 'will normally follow guidelines',[13] and the courts tend to look to the GMC concerning matters of ethical guidance.[58] The creation of NICE, with its *dual role* of developing authoritative guidelines and disseminating them through official NHS channels, means that its guidelines are likely to be credited with a distinctive title to be believed from a legal point of view.[59,60]

In future, adherence to NICE guidelines which are allegedly associated with patient harm is therefore likely to exonerate the defendant doctor, unless it can be shown that the guidelines followed are faulty or inappropriately or unthinkingly applied in a particular case. Deviation from NICE guidelines is likely to inculpate a defendant unless he or she can show that NICE guidelines not followed are faulty, or face sufficient counter-evidence to justify a body of responsible doctors deviating from them.

Clinical discretion remains at the core of what it means to be a doctor exercising professional judgement. However, discretion in the circumstances of modern healthcare is characterised by many potentially competing pressures – from patient choice, clinical guidelines, targets, costs and incentives. The kind of discretion to be exercised in the use of guidelines should probably be understood to be different from that exercised when using other decision-making aids, such as textbooks, lecture notes or expert systems. Guidelines are 'standardised specifications of care'[52] which are inherently designed to constrain clinical discretion in ways never envisaged by the authors of textbooks.

However, against the increased constraint on clinical discretion that guidelines undoubtedly exercise, and unlike the consensus guidelines envisaged by Plato, modern-day evidence-linked clinical guidelines seek to make transparent the strengths, weaknesses and relevance of research evidence to clinical care. Such guidelines generally take years to prepare, and for most of their lifespan they coexist with evidence that is frequently thought to challenge aspects of their guidance. In addition, many guidelines of poorer quality remain in circulation. Guidelines cited in court proceedings should therefore be scrutinised by experts for their quality, validity and currency, and for their relevance and applicability to the case in question.

References

1 Department of Health (1999) *Drug Misuse and Dependence: guidelines on clinical management*. Department of Health, London.
2 Foster C (2002) Civil procedure, trial issues and clinical guidelines. In: J Tingle and C Foster (eds) *Clinical Guidelines: law, policy and practice*. Cavendish Publishing, London.
3 Annas J and Waterfield R (eds) (1995) *Plato: The Statesman*. Cambridge University Press, Cambridge.
4 Grimley Evans J (1995) Evidence-based and evidence-biased medicine. *Age Ageing.* **24**: 461–3.
5 Hampton JR (2003) Guidelines – for the obedience of fools and the guidance of wise men? *Clin Med.* **3**: 279–84.
6 Secretary of State for Health (1997) *The New NHS: modern, dependable*. The Stationery Office, London.
7 Department of Health (2001) *A Commitment to Quality: quest for excellence*. The Stationery Office, London.
8 *Loveday v Renton and Wellcome Foundation Ltd (QBD)* [1990] 1 *Med LR* 117–204.
9 *Re W (A minor)* [1992] 3 *WLR* 758–82.
10 *Ratty v Haringey HA* [1994] 5 *Med LR* 413.
11 *Airedale NHS Trust v Bland* (Guardian *ad litem*) [1993] 1 *All ER* 821–96.
12 *Early v Newham Health Authority* [1994] 5 *Med LR* 215–17.
13 General Medical Council (1998) *Maintaining Good Medical Practice*. General Medical Council, London.
14 Ministry of Justice (1993) Directie Voorlichting: Act amending Act on the Disposal of the Dead. Staatsblad, cited in van der Wal G and Dillman RJ (1994) Euthanasia in the Netherlands. *BMJ.* **308**: 1346–9.
15 Public Law 101–239, the Omnibus Reconciliation Act 1989. In: M Field and K Lohr (eds) (1990) *Clinical Practice Guidelines: directions for a new program*. National Academy Press, Institute of Medicine, Washington, DC.
16 Human Fertilisation and Embryology Authority (1991) *Code of Practice*. Human Fertilisation and Embryology Authority, London.
17 Maisonneuve H, Codier H, Durocher A and Matillon Y (1997) The French clinical guidelines and medical references programme: development of 48 guidelines for private practice over a period of 18 months. *J Eval Clin Pract.* **3**: 3–13.
18 Durand-Zaleski I, Colin C and Blum-Boisgard C (1997) An attempt to save money using mandatory practice guidelines in France. *BMJ.* **315**: 943–6.
19 *Bolam v Friern Hospital Management Committee* [1957] 2 *All ER* 118–28.
20 *Cranley v Medical Board of Western Australia (Sup Ct WA)* [1992] 3 *Med LR* 94–113.
21 *Crits v Sylvester* [1956] *OR* 132, 1 *DLR* (2d) 502, affirmed [1956] *SCR* 991, 5 *DLR* (2d) 601.
22 Harpwood V (1994) NHS reform, audit, protocols and standards of care. *Med Law Int.* **1**: 241–59.
23 Stern K (1995) Clinical guidelines and negligence liability. In: M Deighan and S Hitch (eds) *Clinical Effectiveness: from guidelines to cost-effective practice*. Earlybrave Publications Ltd, Brentwood.

24 Grilli R, Magrini N, Penna A, Mura G and Liberati A (2000) Practice guidelines developed by specialty societies: the need for a critical appraisal. *Lancet*. **355**: 103–6.

25 *Pierre v Marshall* [1993] AJ No. 1095.

26 McDonagh RJ and Hurwitz B (2003) Lying in the bed we've made: reflections on some unintended consequences of clinical practice guidelines in the courts. *J Obstet Gynaecol Can*. **25**: 139–43.

27 Woolf, Lord (1997) Medics, lawyers and the courts. *J R Coll Phys Lond*. **31**: 686–93.

28 Haines A and Jones R (1994) Implementing findings of research. *BMJ*. **308**: 1488–92.

29 *Bolitho v City & Hackney Health Authority* [1997] 3 *WLR*: 1151–61.

30 Hurwitz B (2003) Medico-legal issues. In: R Jones, N Britten, L Culpepper *et al*. (eds) *Oxford Textbook of Primary Medical Care. Volume 1*. Oxford University Press, Oxford.

31 Schantz SJ (1999) *Developing and Implementing Clinical Practice Guidelines: legal aspects*. American Medical Association, Chicago (cites Rosoff AJ (1995) The role of clinical practice guidelines in health care reform. *Health Matrix*. **5**: 369, 390).

32 Whitty P, Eccles M, Woolf SH *et al*. (2003) Using and developing clinical guidelines. In: R Jones, N Britten, L Culpepper *et al*. (eds) *Oxford Textbook of Primary Medical Care. Volume 1*. Oxford University Press, Oxford.

33 Newdick C (1995) *Who Should We Treat?* Clarendon Press, Oxford.

34 Hurwitz B (1998) *Clinical Guidelines and the Law: negligence, discretion and judgment*. Radcliffe Medical Press, Oxford.

35 *Caparo Industries plc v Dickman and others* [1990] 1 *All ER* 568–608.

36 National Health and Medical Research Council (1995) Legal implications of guidelines. In: *Guidelines for the Development and Implementation of Clinical Guidelines*. Australian Government Publishing Service, Canberra.

37 NHS Executive (1996) *Clinical Guidelines*. NHS Executive, Leeds.

38 National Collaborating Centre for Mental Health (2002) *Core Interventions in the Treatment and Management of Schizophrenia in Primary and Secondary Care*. NICE, London.

39 Scottish Intercollegiate Guidelines Network and the British Thoracic Society (2003) British guideline on the management of asthma. *Thorax*. **58 (Suppl. 1)**: i1–94.

40 Anonymous (2003) Intravenous magnesium for acute asthma? *Drug Ther Bull*. **41**: 79–80.

41 *McFarlane v Secretary of State for Scotland* [1988] *SCLR* 623–8.

42 Cane P (1992) *An Introduction to Administrative Law*. Clarendon Press, Oxford.

43 NHS Executive (1996) *Clinical Guidelines*. NHS Executive, Leeds.

44 Hawkins K (1992) *The Uses of Discretion*. Clarendon Press, Oxford.

45 Subcommittee of WHO/ISH Mild Hypertension Liaison Committee (1993) Summary of 1993 World Health Organization–International Society of Hypertension guidelines for the management of mild hypertension. *BMJ*. **307**: 1541–6.

46 Ellwood PM (1988) Outcomes management: a technology of patient experience. *NEJM*. **318**: 1549–56.

47 *Wickline v California* [1986] *California Reporter* **228**: 661–7.

48 McPherson K (1990) Why do variations occur? In: TF Anderson and G Mooney (eds) *The Challenge of Medical Practice Variations*. Macmillan, London.

49 Hampton JR (2000) The National Service Framework for coronary heart disease: the emperor's new clothes. *J R Coll Phys Lond*. **34**: 226–30.

50 Black D (1998) The limitations of evidence. *J R Coll Phys Lond*. **32**: 23–5.

51 Taylor J (2003) Tough talk from the NICE man. *MedEconomics*. **November**: 44–6.

52 Jones J (1999) Influenza drug to undergo 'fast-track' assessment by NICE. *BMJ*. **319**: 400.

53 NHS Executive (1999) *Health Service Circular*. NHS Executive, Leeds.

54 *R v Secretary of State for Health ex parte Pfizer Ltd* [1999] Case No CO/4934/98 High Court of Justice, Queen's Bench Division, May 1999 at 20–25.

55 NHS Executive (1998) *Sildenafil (Viagra)*. NHS Executive, Leeds.

56 *National Health Service (General Medical Services) Regulations 1992 SI 1992/635 (as amended).*

57 Hyams AL, Brandenburg JA, Lipsitz SR, Shapiro DW and Brennan TA (1995) Practice guidelines and malpractice litigation: a two-way street. *Ann Intern Med.* **122**: 450–5.

58 *W v Egdell* [1990] Ch 359.

59 Hurwitz B (2000) Clinical guidelines, NICE products and legal liability? In: A Miles, R Hampton and B Hurwitz (eds) *NICE, CHI and the NHS Reforms: enabling excellence or imposing control?* Aesculapius Medical Press, London.

60 Samanta A, Samanta J and Gunn M (2003) Legal considerations of clinical guidelines: will NICE make a difference? *J R Soc Med.* **96**: 133–8.

Chapter 18

Risk management and freelance GPs

Judith Harvey and Richard Fieldhouse

Key learning points

- Being a freelance GP is a high-risk job, and employing a freelance GP involves managing risks.
- All of the risks will ultimately affect patients.
- Freelance GPs have an obligation to reduce their isolation, maintain their skills, recognise their limitations and work within practice systems.
- Enforced under-performance is a major problem. Practices have an obligation to provide safe working environments. They need to be explicit about their expectations and to enable freelance GPs to meet them.
- PCOs have the opportunity to support freelance GPs, and it is in their interests to do so.

More than 25% of GPs are freelance non-principals, rather than partners in a practice, and their number continues to grow. Most work full-time or part-time as freelance GPs. Yet the profession as a whole has not recognised this development. The structures that protect principals from risks do not extend to freelance GPs. Patients ultimately pay the price for cultural lag – the exclusion of freelance GPs from the GP establishment.

The following is an example of the freelance GP's nightmare:

> I arrived at a strange practice to find that no one knew how to log me on to the computer. Their *Good Locum Guide* was written five years ago, and since then all that has been done is to shove in bits of paper about pathology service cover during the millennium holiday and outbreaks of meningitis in 1998. The consulting rooms were so untidy it took ages to find anything, and the only way to discover how to organise a test or make a referral was to phone another doctor – if there was one in the building. I remember searching a whole building to find a peak-flow meter.

It's tricky, being a freelance GP. In a year a freelance GP may work in 100 different consulting rooms in dozens of practices in several PCOs, using five different computer systems and referring to 50 different hospitals. Each practice has its own way of working, each hospital has its own forms and referral pathways, each doctor's consulting room is a homage to individuality, and for a freelance GP every patient is likely to be a new patient.

Most complaints and negligence claims involve system failures and communication problems. Freelance GPs are marginalised. At best they are semi-detached members of practice teams, and at worst they are regarded as an unfortunate necessity, only grudgingly acknowledged. However competent they are, ultimately freelance GPs are only as safe as the workplace allows them to be. Forty years ago, it was considered sufficient to scrawl 'URTI – Amoxyl' in the notes. Raised expectations, the increasing complexity of clinical management, protocols, guidelines, quality targets, computerisation and all the paraphernalia of modern general practice are not necessarily well managed by principals. Freelance GPs daily find themselves in a position of enforced under-performance when practices do not provide the tools and information necessary to enable them to make the best use of their clinical skills.

Freelance GPs are professionally isolated. They may have little contact with other doctors in their day-to-day work. Trying to continue their education involves a multiple whammy. They forgo paid work, pay for childcare, have no organisation to subsidise course fees and under the old GMS contract were ineligible for the PGEA. Freelance GPs now receive a copy of the *BNF*, but find it difficult to get on the circulation lists of many publications that are available automatically to principals. Until non-principals have prescribing numbers they will be unable to identify their prescribing and audit it through PACT. Too many practices log all freelance GPs on to their computer systems under 'locum or freelance GP' rather than by name, making consultation audit even more difficult, and giving no audit trail to be followed in the event of a complaint. Even if freelance GPs collect information about their own referrals, they may find it difficult to review it with colleagues.

Up to a third of the consultations in a PCO's area may be with freelance GPs. PCOs could address many of the inherent clinical governance and risk management issues, but as yet few are doing so. Freelance GPs are a crucial and neglected part of the GP workforce, and the more attention they, their employers and the PCOs pay to reducing their risks, the better the care patients will receive.

What freelance GPs can do to reduce their risks

> When I started out as a freelance GP, I realised that my training had prepared me for being a GP principal. I knew nothing about being self-employed. I learned the hard way about setting money aside for sickness and tax bills, about responding quickly and clearly to practices, about handing over after surgeries, and about my own limitations.

It is essential that freelance GPs understand what is required of them as self-employed and freelance professionals. This starts with the ability to work independently. Most freelance GPs start out with no previous experience of working outside an organisation. Presenting a professional approach to practices, negotiating and keeping to agreements, managing tax matters and ensuring reliable childcare are responsibilities which need to be discharged efficiently. The National Association of Sessional GPs (NASGP) (previously the National Association of Non-Principals) (www.nasgp.org.uk) offers advice to doctors who are planning to do freelance GP work, and frequent articles in the press reinforce the information for each new generation of non-principals.[1]

> The practice rang up and asked me to do a surgery. I arrived on my bike and was well into the list before the receptionist told me I was duty doctor and there was an urgent visit for me to do. Now I check exactly what 'doing a surgery' means.

> The receptionist rang me and asked why I wasn't making the urgent phone calls to patients she was e-mailing me about. The answer was that I hadn't been told I was down to take calls, and I didn't know about the email system.

Freelance GP work has traditionally been arranged casually, and is often a response to an emergency. Misplaced assumptions about what the practice expects of the freelance GP lead to dissatisfaction on both sides, and this can have an impact on patients. Freelance GPs can encourage a professional approach by insisting on a written or email contract.

There are now more than 80 support groups run by and for non-principals (also known as freelance, sessional or portfolio GPs).[2] These groups reduce professional isolation, offering education events, significant event auditing and informal exchange of ideas and experience. Some develop into virtual practices.

Freelance GPs need to make the effort to explore educational opportunities in their area, and practices and PCOs can pass on information.

> I get flyers about educational events through the email in one practice. I have picked up on several useful study days, though if I am there only occasionally, it takes a lot of time to go through 150 emails to find the half dozen which are relevant to me and still current.

Preparation for appraisal will provide guidance and a framework for those who are not already working through a personal development plan. The opportunity to review practice and skills with an appraiser will be particularly valuable to doctors who are professionally isolated. Appraisal of freelance GPs will take into account the nature of sessional GPs' work.[3]

Freelance GPs need to consider how they manage their particular risks at the workplace. Most serious incidents involve problems with transfer of information. Freelance GPs may need to set up their own systems within practices to ensure safe hand-over.

> I am on the practice intranet, and I use it for hand-over, for alerting the secretary to referrals I have dictated, and for queries.

> I dictated an urgent referral letter. When I next came in 6 weeks later I found the letter waiting for me to sign. The typist was a locum, too. Now I always say at the start of a tape that I am a freelance GP, and sign the letter 'freelance to Dr X', so Dr X signs the letter and the recipient writes back to the partner.

> I work in a rural area and there may be a visit which I can do on my way home. I have worked out various secure ways, depending on the practice's technology, of ensuring that I have the information I need to

do the visit and can update their records afterwards. The alternative is that they pay for an extra 40-mile round trip.

GP training is still based on the philosophy of cradle-to-grave continuity of care. Freelance GP work requires a different approach.

> When I started doing freelance work I had to adjust to not providing continuity of care. I evolved a new approach to consultations to make my 10 minutes with the patient as useful as possible. It is different, but equally rewarding.

Good clinical records are essential for patient safety.

> I write longer notes than the partners, but I think it is important to demonstrate that I was thorough by recording negative findings, and to make it clear to the next doctor what I said to the patient and what management plan was agreed.

Freelance GPs can mitigate the risks associated with their isolation. They need to cultivate independence and self-sufficiency, while making opportunities to interact with principal and non-principal colleagues. They need to understand their role and to cultivate good communication. Like all doctors, they need to ensure that they are safe.

What practices can do for freelance GPs

> Sometimes the receptionists aren't expecting you. Other times you hear them saying 'you can't see the doctor today – only the locum'.

For many freelance GPs, enforced under-performance starts the moment they walk through the practice door. What patient is going to have confidence in a consultation with someone who has been sold to them as second-rate?

> Undervalued people do not perform well. We make sure that each freelance GP has a nameplate for the consulting-room door, and freelancers we use regularly help us write a handout telling patients about themselves. And we ensure that they join us for coffee so that they get a break and can talk with staff.

Practices naturally want to get the most out of an expensive hired hand. A principal's absence leaves work to be done, and the more a freelance GP can do, the less has to be taken on by the remaining partners. However, both sides need to understand what can safely be expected of a freelance GP.

> We do try to steer the heartsinks away from freelance GPs. It isn't a good use of their time. Inevitably they are less able to resist the pressure to investigate or refer because they are more at risk if they don't, and the patients come back to see their regular doctor anyway. But if we can't avoid it, we do try to brief them.

> I often lose the struggle to keep to time, but I realise now that I need the time to be safe, and I have stopped feeling bad about it.

For a freelance GP, every patient can be a new patient. A freelance GP who is consulting safely is likely to take longer than a principal. Continuity of the notes helps, but requires that the previous GP has written notes in a way that recognises that the next consultation may not necessarily be with themselves. Finding information in unfamiliar computer systems takes time, and so does understanding a complex history. A new doctor may need to spend more time negotiating with a patient than the doctor who has known the patient for months or years. Giving a freelance GP a little more time is not just an investment in safety – a patient who is satisfied with their consultation is less likely to book another appointment on the way out.

> We don't expect freelance GPs to sign scripts for long-term benzodiazepines or to do diabetic clinic checks, but I do think it is reasonable that they should see new patients and check hypertensives' blood pressure. It may not be ideal, but these are the patients who need seeing, and a freelance GP who will only see coughs and colds is not much use.

> I see a lot of patients who are running out of tablets, who have been told they can't have any more without seeing the doctor. They know they shouldn't go without them, there's a 2-week wait to see 'their' doctor, and they come to me. Unless I am following a clear management plan, I am uncomfortable making significant changes to the long-term medication of someone else's patient. For instance, is a patient with angina not taking aspirin because it has been forgotten about, or is there a good reason but I can't find it recorded in the notes?

> Patients are often asked to see the doctor about test results, and being anxious they want an urgent appointment, so they see the freelance GP. But I didn't order the test and I don't know what was in the doctor's mind, or the patient's. Slightly abnormal results are a particular problem when one doesn't know the context.

Freelance GPs need to be aware of their limits and to ensure that the patient has a safety net. Safe hand-over of concerns to a partner is crucial. Freelance GPs also need to know when to say no, and practices need to respect the doctor's professional judgement. If the practice feels that a freelance GP is being unreasonably restrictive, the problem should be discussed at a suitable time. There may be a need for education and support, and the practice may be able to help the freelance GP regain confidence.

Signing repeat prescriptions is a chore for which freelance GPs seem ideally suited (but practices need to be aware that MPOs advise that freelance GPs should not be doing this). Any freelance GP who is prepared to sign these prescriptions should have adequate time to check patients' notes carefully before signing, and the practice should accept their decision if they decline.

> We've had embarrassments and misunderstandings, such as a freelance GP who would not refer women for termination of pregnancy. We now use a freelance GP booking form and have added a list to it so that we can check on conscientious objections and whether freelance

GPs have the skills and the willingness to insert coils, inject joints and deal with substance misuse, etc.

Agreement on expectations should be clarified in writing. Using a freelance GP booking form such as that produced by the NASGP ensures that both sides understand what is expected of them.[4]

> Frankly, finding anything is an archaeological exercise. Digging through heaps of papers and cupboards full of junk and tugging at locked drawers for basic tools of the trade really winds me up. It reflects badly on the practice as well as on me, and is such a waste of time.

In any job, lack of standardisation is a source of error. Principals use the same consulting room day after day and arrange it to suit their own way of working. Freelance GPs often use a different room every day. A doctor who is distracted and pressed for time is at increased risk of missing something clinically important, cutting corners or making a mistake. Some freelance GPs end up carrying every item of equipment they might need, and take their own laptops and printers so that they are not dependent on the practice for referral forms and patient information leaflets. This is costly, and it is not practicable for every freelance GP. Practices have an obligation to provide employees with a safe working environment. They can help by providing freelance GPs with a folder of forms and certificates, and by standardising the equipment provided in consulting rooms, and laying it out in a similar way as far as this is possible. If each room has a list of equipment, less time is wasted on fruitless searching. A notice giving the whereabouts of resuscitation equipment, and clear instructions in large print on each item, can save lives.

> We give every freelance GP a named contact. If the contact doesn't know the answer to a query, it's their responsibility to find someone who does. Freelance GPs are too expensive to pay them to run round the building finding prescription forms.

> Learning about practices' procedures takes time. In whose time should it be done? I do try, but working irregularly in a number of different practices makes it difficult, and few practices invest in giving freelance GPs proper training. I would feel worse about it if the partners followed their own protocols, but it's obvious they don't.

What practices expect of freelance GPs goes beyond hours of work and rates of pay. It includes use of the practice computer systems and following protocols and guidelines. Most freelance GPs will quickly become sufficiently familiar with a new computer system to record basic consultations adequately, but they cannot be expected to make Item of Service claims or to use Read-code quality markers if they don't know how these are done, or follow protocols if they cannot find them on the system. Initial training is needed, and so is a source of reference for the freelance GP whose next engagement at the practice may not be for several weeks.

I work mostly in one PCT but do the odd session in another county and know the area quite well. I saw a baby with what I suspected was acute meningococcal septicaemia. I injected him immediately with penicillin and told the parents to take the child straight to the paediatric hospital 20 minutes away. I received a rather terse call the next day from the practice manager saying that the patient's parents had complained. The paediatric hospital had closed down 2 months ago and all such admissions should go to the general hospital 2 minutes away. Using a retrospectoscope I should have called an ambulance – at least they would have known about the relocation. However, I felt that there should be a mechanism whereby freelance GPs – no matter how sporadically they work – should be involved in a process that allows them to be kept in the information loop.

I've been working here for 2 years and I have only just discovered that all the referral forms are in a Word folder and can be printed off in the consulting room.

A skilled clinician needs local knowledge if the patient is to benefit from those skills. A freelance GP pack with information about services within and outside the practice will save freelance GPs and new doctors a great deal of time and many mistakes, but it must be kept up to date. Easy online access to hospital websites, the availability of referral forms to hand or at the press of a button, and lists of preferred providers all help. It may be worth paying a freelance GP to collect and collate the information, and principals may find that there is a lot they did not know.

We decided not to put freelance GPs on our intranet, but our system does have electronic 'Post-it' notes, and we use those to keep free-lancers informed. But not systematically, I admit.

One freelance GP wrote an important hand-over note and asked the receptionist where to leave it so Dr X would see it. Unfortunately the receptionist didn't tell her that Dr X was on holiday for 3 weeks. The patient suffered and I feel it was our fault. We now have a hand-over book which the duty partner checks.

A freelance GP is not a partner. Practices which recognise, respect and capitalise on freelance GPs' skills will get the most out of them. Practices which are well organised and have reliable two-way communication systems will find that all clinicians can provide safer care.

Freelance GPs and performance

Employers are responsible in law for the acts and omissions of their employees. Thus providers (those who have signed a practice contract with a PCO) are responsible for the actions of employed performers, including freelance GPs. Providers are obliged to ensure that deputies are suitably qualified, so they should check freelance GPs' indemnity and their GMC registration details, and not expect them to undertake tasks outside their sphere of competence. A provider facing a complaint involving a freelance GP would probably wish the freelance GP to participate in the procedure, as would their MPO, but in the absence of a contract to that effect, the freelance GP is not obliged to co-operate.

Providers are only relieved of their responsibility if freelance GPs are themselves providers, or if the freelance GP faces criminal charges, investigation by the GMC, a coroner's investigation or litigation for clinical negligence.

Feedback on performance is crucial to risk management, but is not always easy for freelance GPs to achieve. They cannot benefit from feedback on prescribing through PACT, and standard practice-based audits rarely help them. Practices can help by supporting freelance GPs with audit.

> I felt that I ought to know if the tests and X-rays I arrange for patients are worthwhile. I asked the partners if they could circulate the results of the tests I ordered to me after they had checked them, perhaps with comments on the outcome. They don't always remember, but it does help me audit my performance.

> We decided to pay regular freelance GPs to come to our significant event meetings. We benefit because they learn more about us, and they have different experience to feed into debate.

Audit mechanisms suitable for isolated doctors are being developed, and the inclusion of non-principals in appraisal will encourage freelance GPs to put them into practice.[3]

> In the past, if a locum upset a patient or appeared to be clinically unsound, we just didn't employ them again. But we realise now that we have to tackle it.

When things go wrong, practices have an obligation to deal with poor performance.[5] If necessary they can ask the PCO or the LMC for advice and support.

Table 18.1 Enforced under-performance: causes, effects and remedies

Risk Area	Problem	Effect on patient	Effect on GP	Solution
Reception	Receptionist conveys to patient that freelance GP is second-best	Low expectations of GP and consequent dissatisfaction	Dysfunctional consultation and poor performance	Staff training; freelance GP information leaflet for patients
Consulting room	Haphazard work environments; inadequate provision of information, forms and medical equipment	Reduced level of care; reduced trust in GP and practice	Frustration; wasted time; medico-legal risk; reduced ability to formulate diagnoses and management plans	Practice/PCT policy on consulting-room equipment; freelance GP packs and electronic information and forms
Consultation	Unfamiliarity with systems	Impaired confidence in freelance GP; less likely to accept management plan; likely to rebook appointment with principal	As above; lack of professional satisfaction	Standardised practice induction pack
Computer systems	Unfamiliarity with system; no personal log-in name	Impaired access to medical records, inaccurate recording; problems with prescribing	High risk for GP; no audit trail	Training; unique secure passwords/ usernames
Paperwork	Inadequate procedures for dealing with results, referral letters and handover of clinical information	Delayed care; substandard care; break in continuity of care; possible misdiagnosis	Medico-legal risks; professional dissatisfaction; lack of audit	Good practice systems and clear guidance on how paperwork and results are handled
Visits	Freelance GP not aware that visits are expected; equipment not available	Reduced quality of care; reduced confidence in unknown doctors	Increased risk; demoralisation	Booking form and practice induction pack; ID card
Out of hours	Poor induction	Reduced quality of care; lack of confidence in doctor and in co-op/provision of out-of-hours care	Increased risk; demoralisation	Standardised induction pack and initial support/ buddying systems
Feedback of critical events	Freelance GPs not informed of practice procedures or involved in significant event reviews	Poor resolution of complaints	Loss of learning opportunity	Feedback on freelance GPs' performance; freelance GPs involved in significant event audits

How freelance GPs can help practices

A practice that takes the trouble to explore the opportunities can gain more from freelance GPs than just a few surgeries and visits.

> A freelance GP told us about the slip another practice gives patients telling them how to chase their hospital appointments. It has proved a really useful tip.

> We found a freelance GP who is really keen on minor surgery, and invited him back to do a list. It works very well, and we hope to finance extra training for him so that he can provide the enhanced minor operations service for us.

Practices can make use of a freelance GP's specialised experience, and can tap freelance GPs for ideas. Freelance GPs can also contribute more directly to risk management.

> As a former principal, I have the experience of risk managing a practice. As a freelance GP, I see the things people who are there every day don't see, like tiny ankle-breaking stools to reach the examination couch, sphygmomanometers that haven't been checked since 1994, and no soap and towels in consulting rooms. The practice manager is very grateful for feedback.

> We had a freelance GP who was a CHI reviewer. We paid him to give us a mini-review.

Rarely, freelance GPs will see fundamental and serious problems in a practice. They have an obligation to report these.[5]

PCOs and freelance GPs

A major risk for PCOs is unfilled doctor vacancies. These have a knock-on effect, resulting in more strain on existing GPs, more illness, early retirement, and fewer GPs offering additional and enhanced services. A reputation for being a difficult area in which to work further depresses recruitment. The PCO's workload increases and the quality of services provided for patients decreases. Yet PCOs have the opportunity to engage non-principals and to foster a freelance GP workforce.

In 2001, supplementary lists were introduced to protect the public from dangerous doctors. Ten-page application forms requiring unrealistic references and originals of all manner of documents, including passports, with no arrangements for their safe and speedy return, have not proved a good screening mechanism and deter doctors from applying.[6]

> Nowhere [in the process of application for the supplementary list] were there any questions about possible drug or alcohol abuse. . . . There was certainly nothing to give any protection to the public from mad or bad doctors.

Government ministers say they want retired GPs to contribute to the NHS, [but] I am being prevented from working by them [the system] at every step.

Registering non-principal GPs on PCO performer lists gives the potential to provide a channel of communication which can benefit both doctors and the PCO. Only a few are even beginning to exploit this opportunity.

When I moved, I contacted the nearest PCT to find out about the area. No one seemed to know what a sessional GP was. I got nowhere. So I went to an adjacent PCT. They have a named point of contact for sessional GPs and she knows all about everything. Their application process for the supplementary list is streamlined, they have an induction pack for doctors new to the area, they circulate information about educational events, clinical developments and jobs electronically, and they are setting up a secure chatroom. It was like chalk and cheese.

Concerns were expressed to the PCT about unknown doctors visiting patients. After consultation with sessional GPs and the LMC, we are planning to provide all freelance doctors with photo-identity cards.

The PCT required my CV for the supplementary list. They list refugees as one of their targets. If they looked at it, they might decide they could make use of the particular experience I have in working with refugees.

Today's freelancer is tomorrow's GP with a special interest, appraiser, assistant or principal. PCOs that provide a good service and support for sessional GPs have a larger and higher-quality workforce.

Acknowledgements

The authors would like to thank Dr Jane Harrison and Dr Steve Nickless for their help in preparing this chapter.

References

1   O'Connell S (ed.) (1999) *Handbook for Non-Principals in General Practice*. National Association of Non-Principals; www.nasgp.org.uk/handbook
2   National Association of Sessional GPs; www.nasgp.org.uk
3   Martin D, Harrison P and Joesbury H (2003) *Extending Appraisal to All GPs*; www.nasgp.org.uk/cpd/appraisal
4   National Association of Sessional GPs; www.nasgp.org.uk/booking
5   RCGP Quality Unit (2001) *Toolkit for Managing GPs Whose Performance Gives Concern*; www.rcgp.org.uk/rcgp/quality_unit/toolkit/index.asp
6   Royal College of General Practitioners (2002) *Supplementary Lists: an analysis of the non-principal experience*; www.nasgp.org.uk/lists

Chapter 19

Clinical risk management in out-of-hours primary care

Julie Price, Paul Wilding and Mark Davies

Key learning points

- Implementing risk management strategies within new organisational and service delivery models is paramount to providing and maintaining a quality and safe service to patients.
- A comprehensive, facilitated risk assessment, in partnership with all service providers, is vital to identify out-of-hours (OOH) service risks. This should be an integral stage of each new service development.
- OOH providers must deliver risk management in the context of comprehensive clinical and corporate governance frameworks that meet all national requirements.
- The adoption of skill mix and development of new clinical workforce roles (e.g. emergency care nurses and paramedics) present risk management challenges and demand a particular risk management focus.
- Organisations that provide OOH services must ensure that they have appropriate medical indemnity provision to cover potential liabilities arising from work undertaken by their employees.
- OOH providers should ensure that there are specific policies and procedures pertaining to high-risk patient groups including, for example, children, mental health presentations and palliative care.
- OOH providers should draw up a policy relating to multiple contacts for one care episode, particularly with regard to patients with communication and learning difficulties, for example. Repeat contact triggers a face-to-face assessment (raise awareness of the risk of false reassurance when a patient has already been reviewed by one or more colleagues during a care episode).

Introduction

Around 70% of the week is designated as OOH, i.e. the weekly hours outside normal GP surgery opening times (18.30–08.00 on weekdays, as well as weekends, bank and public holidays). From 31 December 2004, delivery of primary care OOH services has become the responsibility of PCOs as the new GMS contract, which came into force in April 2004, allows GPs to choose to opt out of providing an OOH service. The responsibility for ensuring that services to their population are maintained will be held by PCOs.

This represents a huge strategic change in the NHS, as well as a challenge to maintain a high quality of OOH service provision. Implementing risk management strategies (i.e. identifying and assessing the risks within new organisations and ways of delivering service) is paramount for providing and maintaining a quality and safe service to patients.

The development of the OOH services follows on from the Carson Report *Raising Standards for Patients: new partnerships in out-of-hours care*,[1] published in October 2000, which contains 22 recommendations. As a result of these recommendations, quality standards for organised providers of OOH were introduced in November 2002.[2] However, with the introduction of the *Standards for Better Health*[3] (July 2004), that apply to all services provided to NHS patients, these OOH standards have been replaced by the *National Quality Requirements in the Delivery of Out-of-Hours Services*[4] (October 2004). All providers of OOH services (including GP practices that do not transfer their responsibility for OOH service) must now comply with these Quality Requirements (as from January 2005) and from April 2005 must comply with the *Standards for Better Health*.[3]

PCOs need to be certain that OOH services (commissioned or provided in-house) are underpinned by robust corporate and clinical governance systems and processes and meet the *National Quality Requirements*.[4] In the future it is anticipated that OOH providers will be inspected by the Healthcare Commission against these requirements as well as *Standards for Better Health*.[3]

There are numerous published papers and websites containing information relating to the changes to OOH provision. The purpose of this chapter is not to delve into the history of OOH or changes to the service, but to examine the risks associated with an OOH service regardless of who is providing that service.

Models of care

Assessing and identifying risks would be simpler if there was one common model of OOH provision implemented across the country as to how these services are to be provided. However, there are various ways of delivering the services that PCOs are currently considering or in some cases have already implemented. It is important to note that at the time of writing the OOH reform is in its infancy. In the future, primary OOH care will become one component of a locality urgent care network, with additional challenges to apply risk management across care pathways.

What are the immediate options for OOH service provision?

1 PCOs run or commission an NHS organisation to provide the OOH services (i.e. they form an NHS unit, providing the service in-house). Some PCOs work with existing GP co-operatives, transferring staff to ensure that capability and experience are continued.
2 The PCO commissions an OOH provider to deliver the service. This may be in the form of:
   • a commercial organisation

- a GP co-operative that continues in its current form as a Company Limited by Guarantee (with revised articles of association):
  - the company is registered at Companies House, with each member GP being liable for a nominal share, which is only called upon in the event of the winding up of the company. No dividends are paid on their shares. The company exists for the benefit of the members who elect the board which runs the company.[5]
- a Community Benefit Society:
  - the society is registered at the Financial Services Authority, and although it has members, the company is run for the benefit of the community by a council which may be drawn from wider elements of the community (e.g. ambulance, NHS Direct, mental health, patient and public representatives and staff).
3 There may be some GPs across the country, particularly in rural areas, who do not opt out and who continue to provide OOH services as before the reform.

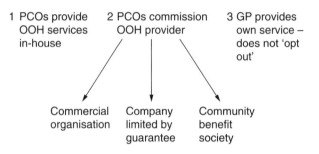

Figure 19.1 Out-of-hours services.

This is a period of extreme change, which is not uniform across England, Wales, Scotland and Northern Ireland. However, irrespective of the provider arrangements, the aims are the same, namely *to promote a quality service for patients and to provide a system that meets the needs of all patients.*

David Carson states the aim in the foreword to the OOH *Accreditation Handbook*:[6]

> the same high-quality out-of-hours service will be available to all NHS patients in England, regardless of where they live, or the GP practice with which they are registered.

The system then has to be streamlined, easy to use and patient friendly.

Clinical risk management

Clinical risk management is an activity aimed at reducing the rate of medical accidents and their cost (both financial and human). Clinical risk management also helps to improve the quality of care provided, and is closely allied to the process of clinical audit and quality assurance. Developing risk management strategies can identify and remedy deficiencies in practice.

So what about risk in the OOH service? Are there significant risks? Can these be prevented? A picture of the risks can be obtained by examining research studies undertaken by MPOs.

Review of complaints and claims relating to OOH services

Complaints

The Medical Defence Union (MDU) has undertaken a series of studies analysing complaints notified to the MDU by GP members. In a 1997 study[7] it was reported that 7% of the complaints notified to the MDU between April and December 1997 involved OOH providers, GP co-operatives and deputising services.

The most common reason for complaints against GP co-operatives was failure to visit (46% of cases). The MDU reported that the large number of complaints relating to failure/delay in visiting was unsurprising, as there was a higher expectation by the patient, at that time, of a visit when a problem occurred out of hours.

Examples of complaints from the study include the following:

> An elderly woman with multiple sclerosis and multiple bed sores fell out of bed at a nursing home. The nurse contacted the co-operative requesting a visit. The GP declined to visit, giving telephone advice. The home, on behalf of the patient, made a complaint.

> A pregnant patient with abdominal pain and vomiting complained that the co-operative GP was reluctant to visit, opting to offer telephone advice only.

In the same study, the reasons for a complaint involving deputising services were as follows:

- failure of delay in diagnosis (38%)
- failure to delay in visit (26%)
- inadequate treatment/management (13%).

A more recent survey, undertaken by the MDU in September 2003,[8] revealed that out-of-hours complaints have risen over the past 7 years, and in 2003 accounted for 10% of all complaints notified to the MDU by its members. It is reported that the rise in complaints relating to OOH services could be due to the change in the way that these services are provided. Over the last few years more GPs have been switching to OOH co-operatives or deputising services. This means that patients will often be seen by, or talk to, a doctor who is not their usual GP and so may not know their medical history.

Hoyte,[9] when discussing the factors relating to the rise in litigation suggests that 'the doctor/patient relationship may be an important factor in the rise of litigation.' He goes on to explain that 40 years ago most general practices were single-handed and the GP was seen as a trusted and highly valued individual, which would make embarking on a litigation suit more psychologically stressful. Since then, partnerships have become established with three to four GPs on average, as well as single-handed GPs and large groups with ten or more GPs. Night and weekend cover is now very often undertaken by consortium groups of doctors, such as GP co-operatives, so that the visiting doctor very often has no medical history and clinical records of the patient: 'The trusting doctor/patient relationship has therefore been eroded over the years.'[9] A patient may then feel more confident about making a complaint against an OOH provider than against their own GP or practice.

This is a risky area of practice. At the time of writing, in most cases the doctor assessing a patient out of hours will not know the patient and not have access to their medical records. Taking and documenting a detailed history is of paramount importance in reducing this risk. The implementation of the electronic care record should help to decrease this risk.

Claims

Dr Nicolas Silk, a research fellow for the MPS, analysed 1000 negligence claims registered against GPs.[10] He noted that 7.7% of the claims identified were associated with OOH contact, and 66% of these involved a co-operative or deputising service.

Further examination of these claims reveals the reasons for them.

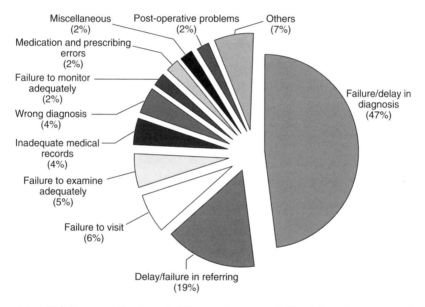

Figure 19.2 Relative contribution of different factors to OOH claims, from an analysis of 1000 negligence claims against GPs.

Extremes of age

- 19% of these claims involved children under the age of 10 years, of which 53% related to failure/delay with regard to diagnosis of meningitis.
- 12% of the claims involved patients over the age of 65 years. Failure to diagnose was the main reason for the claims, relating to conditions such as pneumonia, chest pain, and fractured ribs following a fall.

Box 19.1 Examples of cases and risk management advice

Case

A mother telephoned the local co-operative on a Sunday morning requesting a visit for her 5-year-old child with learning disability complaining of vomiting and abdominal pain. A doctor visited and diagnosed gastroenteritis. The child subsequently died from appendicitis and associated peritonitis

A 59-year-old woman collapsed at home. Her husband telephoned the local OOH co-operative. The call handler passed the patient's details to the duty doctor. Due to the number of calls received, the doctor did not review this patient's details for over an hour. When the doctor finally telephoned the patient, the line was engaged. The doctor forgot to telephone again, and no visit was made. The patient died of a myocardial infarction 3 hours after the original telephone call was made

A 73-year old patient called the deputising service twice during one night complaining of orthopnoea and dyspnoea. Two different doctors visited, but neither admitted the patient to hospital. The patient was later admitted as an emergency suffering from a myocardial infarction. The patient had a past history of ischaemic heart disease

Self-care advice was given over the phone to a patient who telephoned the OOH provider complaining of stomach pains. The patient was subsequently admitted to hospital with acute appendicitis

A mother requested an out-of-hours visit for a child with vertigo, headache and vomiting. Advice was given. The patient was subsequently admitted to hospital where they were diagnosed as diabetic

A doctor for the deputising service failed to visit a child who was later diagnosed with meningitis

A patient suffering from an acute asthmatic attack requested a visit from the local deputising doctor. The visiting doctor did not have the necessary equipment to treat the patient (i.e. nebuliser, oxygen or drugs). An ambulance was called and paramedics subsequently treated the patient

Risk management advice

- In the absence of a patient's medical records, ensure that a detailed account of their past medical history and medication is obtained
- If a decision is taken not to visit a patient, a detailed history should be taken so that a reasonable clinical judgement can be made
- Ensure that an adequate examination is performed
- Make a note in the medical record of all telephone advice given
- Record the visit consultation contemporaneously with the visit
- Ensure that there is an effective and reliable system for passing information from the call handler to the on-call doctor, including a system for prioritising calls
- Ensure that all calls are communicated to the patient's own GP
- Ensure that there is good communication between all staff to aid the smooth running of the OOH service
- Extremes of age:
  - Ensure that there are specific policies and procedures pertaining to paediatric care, which include guidelines for home visiting
  - Draw up a policy relating to multiple contacts for a single care episode, particularly patients with communication and learning difficulties. Train staff to be aware of these risks, and the risks of making assumptions and of false reassurance from a previous contact with a clinician
  - Undertake audits, particularly relating to multiple contacts, diagnosed meningitis, chest pain and falls
- Ensure that all doctors visiting have up-to-date equipment and drugs in their cars. Ensure that all equipment is regularly checked and in working order
- Ensure that clear 'safety-netting' instructions are given and documented (i.e. what the patient should look out for that would necessitate their recontacting the service)

Identifying and assessing OOH risks

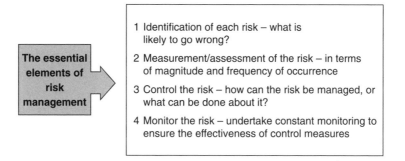

Figure 19.3 Risk management.

To identify the risks, we shall now track the patient through the OOH system using a simple model, based on the Carson Report,[1] to follow their pathway through the system and examine the inherent risks along that pathway. The recommendations are based on the defined set of Quality Requirements.[4] At the time of writing these standards are being revised.

Again, for the purpose of this chapter focus will be generically on OOH services, and not specifically on individual organisations such as NHS Direct or Walk-in Centres, which should conduct their own in-house risk assessments. The risks discussed are not exhaustive, but illustrate some of the risks that can be identified by a facilitated risk assessment provider.

We suggest that a full risk assessment in partnership with all service providers should be undertaken, and that it should be repeated with each new service development.

A risk assessment is a careful examination of what could cause harm, its significance, and what precautions are needed to eliminate the risk or reduce it to an acceptable level.

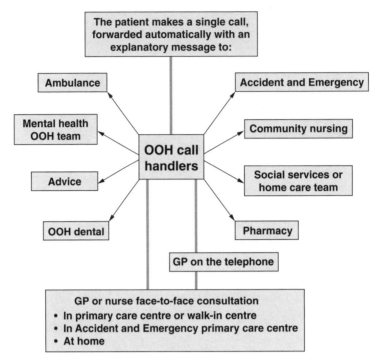

Figure 19.4 Contact with OOH provider.

Organisational or pre-patient-contact risks

Even before the patient makes contact with the OOH provider and enters the OOH system, there are potential risk areas that need to be considered.

OOH providers must deliver risk management in the context of comprehensive clinical governance and controls assurance frameworks that meet all national standards. These include the following:

Complaints procedure
Risk management advice can be summarised as follows.

- Implement a complaints procedure and provide information to service users about how to make comments formally and informally. All staff should be trained in how to handle complaints. A single person within the organisation should be responsible for overseeing the handling of complaints.
- Comply with the OOH Quality Requirement[4] number 6 relating to complaints.

Patient safety incident reporting system (learning from events or near misses)
The GMC document *Good Medical Practice*,[11] states in paragraph 12 that '. . . you must . . . take part in confidential enquiries and adverse event recognition and reporting to help reduce risk to patients'.

A patient safety incident (or adverse incident) reporting system should be established as a principle of clinical governance. This system will ensure that lessons are learned when errors occur, and will thus reduce the risk of the error recurring. The events should be analysed and risk management recommendations and proposed changes fed back to all staff. Staff should be encouraged to participate in the system. The NPSA has set up the National Reporting and Learning System (NRLS),[12] launched in February 2004, which will 'draw together reports of patient safety errors and systems failures from health professionals across England and Wales'. Once the interface between OOH providers and the NPSA has been defined, the NPSA will collate information on reported incidents and, after analysing trends, will issue risk management recommendations.

Risk management advice can be summarised as follows.

- Introduce a patient safety incident reporting system.
- Ensure that reported incidents are analysed and that any changes/findings are reported back to staff.
- Comply with *Standards for Better Health*[3] Core Standard 1, relating to learning from patient safety incidents and other reportable incidents.

Protocols and systems

It is vital to have robust operational systems and protocols in place. Protocols define areas of responsibility and provide documentary evidence of the standard of care provided.

- The OOH provider needs to agree clinical and administrative protocols and ensure that these are regularly reviewed, dated and signed.
- Protocols should be drawn up and discussed by the team involved in the procedure, regularly reviewed, signed and readily available for all staff.
- Out-of-date protocols need to be stored for at least 8 years, because litigation can occur many years after an event.
- Ensure that there are Patient Group Directions for medicines administered by nurses as outlined in the *Health Service Circular HSC 2000/026*,[13] – for example, vaccines, medicines used for minor ailments, etc.

Other policies that need to be developed include the following.

- A policy for the use of chaperones in accordance with GMC advice, ensuring that the OOH centre can offer a chaperone.[14] Patients should be made aware of the policy and the availability of a chaperone (e.g. by means of a poster in the waiting room and details in the OOH provider information leaflet).
- a policy on how to deal with violent or aggressive patients in the home and at the OOH centre.

Communication with GP practices

Good communication between the OOH provider and the patient's GP is important for maintaining continuity of care. An effective messaging system will provide vital communication between the GP and the OOH provider, which will help to ensure continuity of care and reduce the risk of harm to patients. The GMC guidance document *Good Medical Practice*[11] states in paragraph 45 that 'if you provide treatment or advice for a patient, but are not the patient's GP, you should tell the GP the results of the investigations, the treatment provided, and any other information necessary for the continuing care of the patient unless the patient objects.'

Risk management advice can be summarised as follows.

- Develop clear policies on the hand-over of information to the patient's GP, in accordance with GMC regulations and OOH quality standards.
- Develop a system to ensure that practices pass information to the OOH provider about special needs patients (e.g. those receiving palliative care).
- A hand-over form for high-dependency patients should be supplied to all practices, and practices should be encouraged to regularly update the OOH provider with changes to patients' care management plans. This system must comply with the laws and guidance relating to the Data Protection Act 1998.[15]
- Ensure that this information is available to all staff, including triage and visiting clinicians.
- Develop communication lines with other OOH providers, including social services, NHS Direct, dentists, community pharmacists, community nurses and ambulance services.
- Comply with the OOH Quality Requirements[4] 2 and 3, relating to exchange of information and communication.

Record keeping
A system for record keeping needs to be developed.

- Ensure that all consultations, whether by telephone or face to face, are recorded contemporaneously in the patient's record.
- Develop a protocol for handling computerised data and protecting patient information, including procedures for computer access, back-up and off-site archiving.
- Ensure that a copy of the back-up tapes is stored off site, and that these are valid back-ups (i.e. they are able to rebuild data).
- Arrange a systematic audit of a sample of case records to assess them for adequacy and completeness. This monitors the standard of clinical information that is being recorded as well as the quality of case management processes and flow of information within the organisation.
- Ensure that the time of triage call, time of transfer to the doctor and time of visit or appointment are always recorded.
- Develop a system to ensure that calls are tape recorded consistently and in line with GMC guidance,[16] ensuring that patients are always informed that the call will be recorded (through telephone messaging and promotional literature).
- Draw up a protocol for the retention and storage of records, in line with the *Health Service Circular HSC 1998/217*.[17] Include procedures for the retention and storage of tape-recorded calls.
- Comply with *Standards for Better Health*[3] Core Standard 9, relating to clinical records.

Staffing
The move towards workforce modernisation and skill mix in OOH care introduces specific management challenges.

- When employing new staff members, ensure that references are taken up and that relevant statutory obligations are complied with – for example, that all staff have an induction programme.
  - For doctors, this will involve checking that they are on a Primary Medical Performers List and the GMC register, and have appropriate medical indemnity. The GMC document *Good Medical Practice*,[11] paragraph 33, states 'In your own interests, and those of your patients, you must obtain adequate insurance or professional indemnity cover for any part of your practice not covered by an employer's indemnity scheme.'
  - For nursing staff, check their NMC registration and advise them that indemnity should be taken, in accordance with the NMC *Code of Professional Conduct* published in January 2003.[18] The NMC recommends 'that a registered nurse or midwife or health visitor, in advising, treating and caring for patients/clients, has professional indemnity insurance. This is in the interests of clients, patients and registrants in the event of claims of professional negligence.'
- Introduce a formal staff appraisal process and link training requirements to the appraisal.
- Ensure that all staff members have a contract of employment, an explicit job description and a definition of their role, and that they have signed a confidentiality statement which extends to cover staff when they no longer work for the organisation. The need for explicit role definition for staff in extended roles is paramount.
- Implement a training programme for staff to include the following:
  - confidentiality
  - complaints procedure
  - Data Protection and Caldicott
  - management of violent/difficult/aggressive patients
  - health and safety
  - annual resuscitation training
  - telephone skills.
- Ensure that the same standard of care is delivered in the 'twilight hours' between midnight and 7am (i.e. that staff who are working these hours receive the same training and development as other staff).
- Compile a staff handbook for all members of staff, detailing practice procedures, policies, rules and regulations.
- Monitor and manage the performance of all clinical members of staff. Produce performance and quality improvement frameworks (e.g. in line with the approach taken by NHS Direct).
- Comply with *Standards for Better Health*[3] Core Standards 10, 11 and 20, relating to staff working in OOH services.

GP registrars

GP registrars (GPRs) need to continue to receive training in out-of-hours care, by working sessions for OOH providers, even if their training practices have opted out.[19] PCOs will need to:

- discuss arrangements for this training with the local GP Postgraduate Deanery

- ensure that the OOH provider can provide the training and that the provider has been approved to undertake the training by the Director of Postgraduate GP Education
- ensure that the GPR's supervising clinician has received the necessary training to fulfil this role
- check indemnity (see below).

Medical indemnity

OOH service providers will need to ensure that they have appropriate medical indemnity provision to cover potential liabilities arising from work undertaken by their employees (e.g. GP registrars, nurses, healthcare assistants, call handlers). PCO OOH service providers are likely to have NHS indemnity, but private/commissioned OOH service providers may need to take out indemnity (e.g. with a MPO).

Information and communication technology (ICT)

It is important to work with ICT system suppliers to ensure that system interfaces are robust and include red-flagging of failed transfer of data and/or user error.

Health and safety

All providers should consider the health and safety of their staff, visitors and patients[20] (health and safety issues, infection control, etc. are beyond the scope of this chapter). A full risk assessment should be undertaken.

Operational risk

Having looked at organisational risk, what are the operational risks for the OOH service? The following are examples of scenarios that could result in harm to a patient. Risk management strategies are included. Let us follow a fictitious patient, Mrs Jones, through the model pathway.

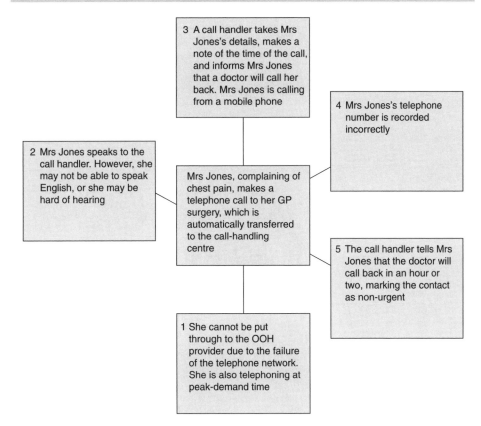

Figure 19.5 Scenario 1: contacting the out-of-hours provider.

Risk management advice

1 Ensure that the provider has a back-up system in the event of failure of the telephone network, which can be activated as a contingency if such failure occurs. The provider must ensure that contingency arrangements are in place to match demand with capacity.

2 Ensure that the provider commissions an interpretation/translation service.

3 Ensure that there is a policy giving details of what to do in the event of failure to make contact with the patient (e.g. due to failure of the telephone network, no mobile phone battery charge, etc.).

4 Voice-recording facilities should be installed on all operational telephones. Ensure that there is a process for rapid retrieval of all records. Patients should be advised to call again if they are not contacted by a clinician within a given timescale.

5 Do not allow a call handler to make unsupported clinical decisions about the urgency of the calls. Ensure that the centre has a robust validated call prioritisation process that includes emergency calls (e.g. a patient with chest pain).

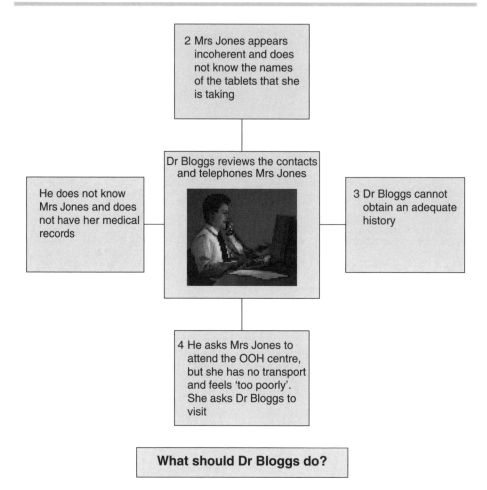

Figure 19.6 Scenario 2: Dr Bloggs' review.

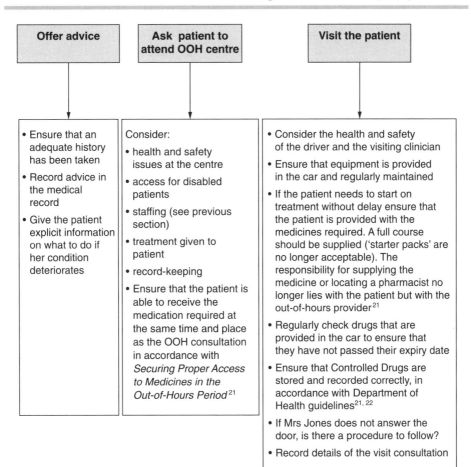

Offer advice	Ask patient to attend OOH centre	Visit the patient

• Ensure that an adequate history has been taken • Record advice in the medical record • Give the patient explicit information on what to do if her condition deteriorates	Consider: • health and safety issues at the centre • access for disabled patients • staffing (see previous section) • treatment given to patient • record-keeping • Ensure that the patient is able to receive the medication required at the same time and place as the OOH consultation in accordance with *Securing Proper Access to Medicines in the Out-of-Hours Period*[21]	• Consider the health and safety of the driver and the visiting clinician • Ensure that equipment is provided in the car and regularly maintained • If the patient needs to start on treatment without delay ensure that the patient is provided with the medicines required. A full course should be supplied ('starter packs' are no longer acceptable). The responsibility for supplying the medicine or locating a pharmacist no longer lies with the patient but with the out-of-hours provider[21] • Regularly check drugs that are provided in the car to ensure that they have not passed their expiry date • Ensure that Controlled Drugs are stored and recorded correctly, in accordance with Department of Health guidelines[21, 22] • If Mrs Jones does not answer the door, is there a procedure to follow? • Record details of the visit consultation

Figure 19.7 Choice of actions for Dr Bloggs, with risk management advice.

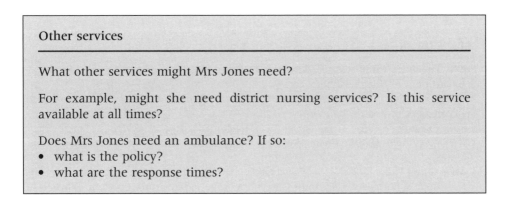

Other services

What other services might Mrs Jones need?

For example, might she need district nursing services? Is this service available at all times?

Does Mrs Jones need an ambulance? If so:
• what is the policy?
• what are the response times?

Mrs Jones is finally treated in her own home with a satisfactory outcome.

The doctor makes a record of the visit consultation. He requests that the visit details are faxed to the GP surgery the following morning, in accordance with the organisation's policy.

OOH strategic direction

NHS reforms are rapidly leading to alternative organisational and service delivery models for OOH care. The OOH providers of tomorrow will operate at scale and across the 24-hour divide as part of an integrated network of unscheduled care providers. Core functions of these integrated care networks are likely to include network co-ordination as well as clinical service delivery (multi-disciplinary clinical assessment and diagnosis by telephone and face to face) and the delivery of call-centre services.

The adoption of skill mix and the development of new clinical workforce roles (e.g. emergency care nurses and paramedics) present risk management challenges, including the need for performance frameworks in line with the approach taken by NHS Direct as well as clarity in role definition. NHS Direct have adopted the *Balanced Scorecard* approach,[23,24] using a mix of qualitative and quantitative approaches and indicators to assess and improve the performance of staff in service delivery roles.

Technology, in particular the adoption of integrated ICT systems across whole health economies and the proposed national care records service,[25] as part of the national programme for IT, will enable the care pathway approach to service delivery. *Increasingly, risk management will need to focus on end-to-end patient care pathways with organisations working in partnership to improve the safety and quality of pathways, in place of the current focus on individual organisations.* Clinical decision-support and knowledge-management systems will be widely available and accessible via desktop computers. Such systems will play an important role in supporting the safe and effective delivery of changing workforce roles and clinical services.

Acknowledgements

The authors would like to thank Logie Kelman, Manager of the National Association of GP Co-operatives, for his help in the preparation of the chapter. Paul Wilding is supported by the Health Foundation.

References

1 NHS Executive (2000) *Raising Standards for Patients. New partnerships in out-of-hours care.* Department of Health, London; www.doh.gov.uk/pricare/oohreport.htm
2 NHS Executive (2002) *Quality Standards in the Delivery of GP Out-of-Hours Services.* Department of Health, London.
3 NHS Executive (2004) *Standards for Better Health*. Department of Health, London.
4 NHS Executive (2004) *National Quality Requirements in the Delivery of Out-of-Hours Services.* Department of Health, London.
5 Mills C and Hunt P (2004) *Delivering Care on Call. An implementation guide for PCOs and GP co-ops.* National Association of GP Co-operatives and Mutuo, London.
6 NHS Executive (2002) *Accrediting Providers of Out-of-Hours Care. A system for improving patient care and assuring quality.* Department of Health, London; www.doh.gov.uk/pricare/accredhandbook.htm
7 Green S and Price J (1998) Complaints. *Pulse.* **Special Report 63**.
8 Medical Defence Union (2003) *Complaints in General Practice 2001–2002;* www.the-mdu.com

9 Hoyte P (1994) Medical negligence litigation, claims handling and risk management. *Med Law Int.* **1**: 261–75.

10 Silk N (2001) What went wrong in 1000 negligence claims. *Healthcare Risk Report.* **7**(3): 13–15.

11 General Medical Council (2001) *Good Medical Practice.* General Medical Council, London; www.gmc-uk.org

12 National Patient Safety Agency (2004) *The National Reporting and Learning System.* National Patient Safety Agency, London; www.npsa.nhs.uk

13 NHS Executive (2000) *Health Service Circular HSC 2000/26. Patient Group Directions.* Department of Health, London; www.doh.gov.uk

14 General Medical Council (2001) *Intimate Examinations.* General Medical Council, London; www.gmc-uk.org

15 Data Protection Act 1998, Chapter 29; www.hmso.gov.uk/acts/acts1998

16 General Medical Council (2002) *Making and Using Visual and Audio Recordings of Patients.* General Medical Council, London.

17 NHS Executive (1998) *Health Service Circular HSC 1998/217. Preservation, retention and destruction of GP General Medical Service records relating to patients.* Department of Health, London.

18 Nursing and Midwifery Council (2003) *Code of Professional Conduct.* Nursing and Midwifery Council, London; www.nmc-uk.org

19 Committee of General Practice Education Directors (COGPED) (2004) *Out-of-Hours Training for GP Registrars.* COGPED, London.

20 Health and Safety at Work Act 1974; www.hse.gov.uk

21 NHS Executive (2004) *Securing Proper Access to Medicines in the Out-of-Hours Period.* Department of Health, London.

22 National Prescribing Centre (2004) *A Guide to Good Practice in the Management of Controlled Drugs in Primary Care (England). Preview edition.* Department of Health, London; www.npc.co.uk

23 Kaplan R and Norton D (1996) *The Balanced Scorecard: translating strategy into action.* Harvard Business School Press, Boston, MA.

24 Kaplan R (1996) *What is a balanced scorecard?* www.balancedscorecard.org

25 Department of Health (2003) *Every Patient to Get an Electronic Patient Record. National Programme for IT announces contracts to run NHS care records service;* www.dh.gov.uk

Chapter 20

Health and safety

John Jeffries

Key learning points

- Places of work can be dangerous: more than 500 people in the UK are killed each year in workplace accidents.
- The Health and Safety at Work Act 1974 is the guiding piece of legislation placing responsibilities on employers and employees, with commensurate sanctions.
- All practices need a health and safety policy with clearly allocated responsibilities.
- Practices can start by having an effective procedures manual dealing with controls for substances hazardous to health, moving and handling, fire precautions, violence, workplace equipment, the environment and first aid.
- The Health and Safety at Work Act requires all employers to carry out risk assessments.

Introduction

Work is dangerous and can be bad for your health. Even visiting places where work is being done can be risky. These are not the observations of a dedicated idler. They are the inevitable conclusions of any study of the statistics that are collected by the Health and Safety Executive.

Despite the fact that obviously unhealthy and dangerous occupations such as coal mining, foundry working and deep-sea fishing have virtually ceased to exist, we still manage to kill over 500 people every year in UK workplace accidents. When you consider the number of buses, lorries, taxis, sales reps' cars, fire engines, ambulances and police cars that attempt to rush through our crowded traffic every hour, you can easily see that we have invented modern ways of replacing the older, more dangerous occupations.

Statistics for the 2 million people who are registered as suffering from occupation-related illnesses show an equal reluctance to improve. The incidence of 'modern' stress-related conditions has made them second only to the perennial 'back problems' in the count of days lost through illness.

So this is serious business with very real costs. There are economic costs for the nation's productivity, for the employer's profitability and for sick or injured people's short- and long-term earning capacity. There are the legal costs of the often long process of apportioning blame and agreeing compensation, and there are the moral costs paid by everyone who knows that their act or omission has resulted in the death or serious injury of a colleague, friend or innocent bystander.

The Health and Safety at Work Act (1974)

This Act is the central piece of Health and Safety legislation in the UK. It incorporates all previous safety legislation, and provides a framework for the development and issue of regulations, including many EU directives. What distinguishes this Act from its predecessors is that it allocates absolute responsibility. It is not sufficient to comply with the regulations – the Act requires us all to be responsible for our own safety when at work. It also makes us individually responsible for other people who may suffer illness or injury because of our work.

The employer who plans, organises and equips us with the premises, plant and procedures for our work will normally bear the bulk of the responsibility.

The Act lists the employer's duties.

The responsibilities

It shall be the duty of every employer to ensure so far as is reasonably practicable, the health, safety and welfare of all his/her employees. To achieve this obligation the employer shall provide:
1   a safe place of work with safe access and egress (exit)
2   safe plant and equipment
3   safe systems of work
4   a safe working environment with adequate facilities and arrangements for the employees' welfare
5   safe methods for handling, storage, use and transport of articles and substances
6   adequate information, training and supervision
7   consultation with employees
8   a written statement on Health and Safety and the organisation's arrangements for carrying out that policy.

In addition, every employee has three main obligations:

1   to take reasonable care with regard to the health and safety of themselves and of other persons who may be affected by their acts or omissions at work
2   to co-operate with their employer (or any other person) so far as it is necessary to enable any duty or requirement under the Act or relevant legislation to be performed or complied with
3   not to interfere with anything provided in the interests of health, safety or welfare.

GP surgeries: the practicalities

General practice has its share of dangerous equipment, lethal substances, work practices and personal safety issues that affect those who work in it. What makes it particularly demanding from a Health and Safety perspective is that it mainly provides its service to people whom it has invited to attend its place of work, namely the surgery. A sizeable proportion of those people will be infirm, troubled and vulnerable. Add to this the fact that a good number of them will be children, and you can see the need for extraordinary vigilance.

It is important that everyone in the practice appreciates that the Health and Safety at Work Act is criminal legislation, and that the employer and/or any employee can be prosecuted, fined and even imprisoned if they fail to meet their obligations. It is not necessary to show that anyone was injured or became ill for these sanctions to be imposed.

To ensure that the employer and every member of the team understands the full extent of these obligations there needs to be full communication on all matters regarding Health and Safety, and that communication must be regular and comprehensive.

The first requirement is that the organisation publishes and communicates its general policy to all staff. It is a good idea to communicate it to anyone else who could be at risk, too, and it should be kept simple. Box 20.1 shows a perfectly adequate document which could be displayed in the waiting room and office. Note that this is signed by the GP with nominated overall responsibility. That responsibility cannot be delegated, but it is recommended that the individual duties are delegated to other members of the staff.

Box 20.1 Example of a Health and Safety policy document

Nutwood Surgery

General Statement of Policy

Our policy is to provide and maintain safe and healthy working conditions, equipment and systems of work for all our employees, our primary care organisation employees on site, our patients and particularly their children.

We will provide employees with all the information, training and supervision that they need to ensure their personal health and safety and to enable them to discharge their responsibility to others.

We also accept our responsibility for the health and safety of other people who may be affected by our activities.

The particular arrangements that we have made to implement this policy are set out in the appropriate section of our *Health and Safety Manual.*

The allocation of duties and responsibilities for safety matters and the Safe Operating Procedures are listed below.

This policy will be kept up to date, particularly as the practice develops. To ensure this, the policy and the way in which it has operated will be reviewed at the end of each quarter. We welcome any suggestion that will help us to improve our Health and Safety arrangements.

Signed:

(GP with practice Health and Safety responsibility)

Date:

Allocating roles

The Act requires that organisational arrangements for the implementation of the policy (who does what, and when) are clearly set out and understood by all employees. Box 20.2 shows the key roles in a format suitable for display.

It is important that everyone is completely clear about what their duties are. Box 20.3 sets these out in detail.

It is useful to keep a schedule of 'when' these duties should be performed as, for example, is shown in Table 20.1.

Box 20.2 List of post-holders

Nominated competent person with
overall responsibility

Appointed person with responsibility
to the above for the control of
first-aid provision

Qualified first aiders

Fire officer

Safety representative

Safety Committee members

Box 20.3 Post-holder duties

Nominated competent person with overall responsibility
1 Ensure that the Risk Assessment is reviewed annually.
2 Appoint staff to undertake the offices listed below and to ensure that they discharge their responsibilities rigorously.
3 Establish written procedures for the safe performance of all tasks.
4 Establish procedures to safeguard the health of all staff.
5 Ensure that all staff receive adequate information, training and supervision to enable them to carry out all assigned duties safely and without risk to their health.
6 Carry out quarterly reviews of the Health and Safety arrangements within the practice.

Appointed Person (first-aid provision)
1 Ensure that first-aid kits are readily available at all surgeries.
2 Ensure that the first-aid kits are fully stocked at all times (including eye wash equipment).
3 Call emergency services when required.
4 Make recommendations on the training of first aiders.
5 Record all injuries and near misses in the accident book.
6 Report all qualifying accidents or occupation-related diseases.

Qualified first aiders
1 Give emergency treatment in those areas for which they are trained.

Fire officer
1 Ensure that the practice maintains up-to-date Fire Authority approval.
2 Arrange the regular maintenance of fire alarm systems.
3 Ensure that regular maintenance of fire extinguishers takes place.
4 Carry out routine checks on fire evacuation systems (obstructions, signage, etc.).
5 Plan and action a fire drill for all staff at least once a year.]

Safety representative
1 Inform all staff that any concerns about the Health and Safety arrangements or practice should be reported to them in the first instance.
2 Bring the concerns of staff to the attention of the person with overall responsibility for Health and Safety (the nominated competent person).

Safety Committee members
1 Participate in the quarterly practice review of Health and Safety arrangements.
2 Represent the interests of nominated members of staff.

Table 20.1 Schedule of routine checks/procedures

Item	Daily	Weekly	Monthly	Quarterly	6-monthly	Yearly
Fire-alarm Test						FO
Fire extinguishers						FO
Fire evacuation routes	FO					
Fire drill						FO
Handling violent behaviour			CP			
Safe storage procedures				CP		
Portable appliance testing						CP
Fire prevention safe practice check			FO			
Clinical waste collection	CP					
Sharp bin collection	CP					
Workstation comfort				SR		
Floor, steps, ramps				CP		
Boiler maintenance						CP
Environment				CP		
Intruder alarm system						CP
CO_2 detector					CP	
Vaccine fridge service						AP
Autoclave maintenance						AP
Ear-syringe service					CP	

CP, competent person; AP, appointed person; FO, fire officer; SR, safety representative.

Setting standards

Planning for Health and Safety can be daunting because of the many different types of dangers in the workplace. Where should one start? In general practice it is useful to break down the dangers and the consequent obligations into 10 sections as follows.

1 Management
2 Control of Substances Hazardous to Health
3 Moving and handling
4 Fire precautions
5 Violence
6 Provision and use of workplace equipment
7 Workplace
8 Recording and reporting
9 First aid
10 Risk assessment.

Use these as the framework for your procedures manual. In each of the sections set down the minimum acceptable standard of performance and explain the way in which that standard is to be achieved and maintained.

Management

Table 20.2 shows an example of management standards, the second column indicating how the practice makes sure that those standards are maintained.

Table 20.2 Management responsibilities

Minimum standard	How standard is achieved and maintained
The practice must have a written Health and Safety policy which complies with current legislation	Signed copy of Health and Safety policy published Organisational arrangements for implementation set out in manual List of relevant procedures
The policy must be reviewed quarterly	Quarterly management meeting agenda Minutes of meetings (Minutes file)
Each member of the practice team must be made aware of the policy	Noticeboard copy Induction training programme
The practice must have a nominated competent person who is responsible for Health and Safety within the practice	List of organisational arrangements
The nominated competent person must carry out a systematic risk assessment of workplace risks and prioritise any measures required	Risk assessment papers Action Plan
The practice must display the employer's liability insurance certificate in a public place	Current certificate displayed in main office
The practice must display the statutory Health and Safety notice	Displayed in main office
The practice must ensure that all staff receive regular and adequate Health and Safety Training	Training record

Control of Substances Hazardous to Health (COSHH)

Recommended minimum standard

- There are policies and procedures for controlling drugs, medicines, syringes, etc.
- There are policies and procedures for the safe use, handling, storage and transport of 'articles and substances' which are inherently or potentially dangerous.
- The practice must display notices warning of the hazards arising from the use, handling, storage and transport of inherently or potentially dangerous substances.
- The practice must maintain a file of data sheets on substances in use which have been identified as hazardous to health.

Moving and handling

Recommended minimum standard

- There are policies and procedures for the safe use, handling, storage and transport of 'articles and substances' which are inherently or potentially dangerous.
- Staff must receive adequate training in the moving and lifting of all hazardous loads including, particularly, patients.

Fire precautions

Recommended minimum standard

- The practice's safety policy must address fire safety and cover fire prevention and fire procedures.
- There must be a Fire Certificate or written evidence of approval of the Local Authority Fire Officer.
- There must be a nominated fire officer.
- There must be regular fire training and evacuation drills for staff (at least once a year).
- There must be a procedure for ensuring that fire exits are unobstructed at all times.
- All fire exits must be clearly marked.
- There must be regular testing of fire warning systems.
- There must be sufficient and appropriate fire-fighting equipment available and maintained on a maintenance contract.

Violence

Recommended minimum standard

- Where doctors and/or staff consider themselves to be at risk from violent behaviour, there must be evidence that discussions have taken place about this issue and that appropriate training has been considered.

Provision and use of workplace equipment

Recommended minimum standard

- The practice must provide equipment which is safe and without risks to health.
- All equipment must conform to current Health and Safety requirements.
- Proper and regular maintenance of all appropriate equipment must be organised.
- Staff must receive appropriate training before being allowed to use any tools or equipment.

Workplace

Recommended minimum standard

- The practice premises must be maintained in a safe and risk-free condition.
- Safe methods of access and egress must be maintained at all times.

- The practice must maintain a safe and healthy working environment.
- There must be adequate welfare facilities and arrangements.
- The practice must display notices warning of any particular hazards.

Recording and reporting

Recommended minimum standard

- The practice must record all incidents and near misses.
- The practice must notify the Health and Safety Executive of all serious accidents or occupationally related diseases.

First aid

Recommended minimum standard

- The practice must have a first-aid box readily accessible, including eye-wash equipment.
- The practice must have an appointed person with responsibility for first-aid arrangements.
- The practice must ensure that first-aid treatment is available to staff during working hours.

Risk assessment

Recommended minimum standard

- The practice must have written evidence of an up-to-date risk assessment covering all of the above sections.
- The practice must review the risk assessment annually with the co-operation of all staff.

Against each of these sections you need to be able to explain the process by which you maintain the minimum standards listed.

Risk assessment

The Act requires all employers to carry out a risk assessment on all aspects of their work.

The process is straightforward. Identify anything with the potential to cause harm (the *hazards*), evaluate how likely each hazard is to cause harm and how severe that harm might be (the *risks*), and then implement *control measures* to reduce the most dangerous risks.

This chapter ends with a fairly comprehensive list of the hazards to be found in the GP surgery, each accompanied by a description of the kind of harm that could be caused. Do add anything which you have that constitutes an additional hazard (lawn mowers, tropical fish and antique surgical instruments have figured in the hazard list of various surgeries).

The lists are presented as worksheets.

- In column 3, list your existing control measures (the steps that you have already taken to reduce the risk, e.g. locking cupboards or writing protocols).
- In column 4, indicate who might be in danger. Is it the clinical staff? Or all members of staff? Or the patients, too?
- In columns 5 and 6 you must make a judgement and rate the likelihood and potential severity. It is essential to keep this simple. You might want to use the British Standard that has been produced as a result of practical experience in many industries. The BS8800 rating scale (*see* Table 20.3) allows you only three gradations, which is quite adequate.
- Column 7 (score) allows you to record the product of columns 5 and 6. Table 20.3 shows how these scores are categorised to provide suggested courses of action. Any score of 6 or over (the rating scale describes these as 'Substantial' Risks) should cause you to reconsider your existing control measures. A score of 9 ('Intolerable' risks) requires immediate improvements.

Transfer all your 6 and 9 scores, and any others that can be improved, to your Health and Safety Action Plan. This becomes the key agenda item for the quarterly meeting. Use that meeting to canvas everyone's views on the control measures that might be introduced.

The most effective control measure is to remove the hazard. For example, powder-based cleansers with their attendant risk of inhalation of irritants can be replaced by cream-based cleansers. However, this is not always possible and you may need to consider using protective equipment such as masks or spectacles. If you do decide to use these, you will need to enforce their use, so a procedure setting out the requirement will be needed.

Table 20.3 Risk rating using scales from BS 8800

	Slightly Harmful (1)	Harmful (2)	Extremely harmful (3)
Highly unlikely (1)	Trivial risk	Tolerable risk	Moderate risk
Unlikely (2)	Tolerable risk	Moderate risk	Substantial risk
Likely (3)	Moderate risk	Substantial risk	Intolerable risk

Risk level	Action and timescale
Trivial $(1 \times 1 = 1)$	No action is required and no documentary records need to be kept
Tolerable $(1 \times 2 = 2)$	No additional controls are required. Consideration may be given to a more cost-effective solution or improvement that imposes no additional cost burden. Monitoring is required to ensure that controls are maintained
Moderate $(1 \times 3 = 3)$	Efforts should be made to reduce the risk, but the cost of prevention should be carefully measured and limited. Risk reduction measures should be implemented within a defined time period. Where the moderate risk is associated with extremely harmful consequences, further assessment may be necessary to establish more precisely the likelihood of harm as a basis for determining the need for improved control measures
Substantial $(3 \times 2 = 6)$	Work should not be started until the risk has been reduced. Considerable resources may have to be allocated to reduce the risk. Where the risk involves work in progress, urgent action should be taken
Intolerable $(3 \times 3 = 9)$	Work should not be started or continued until the risk has been reduced. If it is not possible to reduce the risk even with unlimited resources, work must remain prohibited

Conclusion

All the effort that you put into completing a risk assessment will be wasted if supervision is lax.

Around 60% of all reported accidents happen because people have ignored the written procedures or failed to wear the protective equipment prescribed. In these instances the employee will always be shown to have been contributarily negligent, but the courts will always question the quality of supervision and the enforcement of agreed procedures.

The duties set out in Box 20.3 must be taken seriously. Health and Safety officials investigating tragic workplace incidents in which people have been grievously injured tire of collecting statements that begin 'He was only . . .' or 'No one bothered usually . . . .'

Accidents can and do happen in general practice. Doctors, nurses, support staff and patients have been killed or seriously injured in recent incidents. Like the lottery, there may be only a remote chance, but remember the lottery's slogan – 'it could be you'. Less serious injuries are correspondingly more common.

Useful contacts

*   Royal College of General Practitioners, 14 Princes Gate, Hyde Park, London SW7 1PU. Tel: 0207 581 3232. Website: www.rcgp.org Publishes a very practical guide, *Health and Safety: Guidance for General Practitioners* (this includes a model alcohol policy!).
*   Health and Safety Executive; www.hsebooks.co.uk Gives easy access to a host of relevant Health and Safety publications, many of which are free and very useful for staff training.
*   Ergonomos Ltd, 11 St John's Road, Richmond, Surrey TW9 2PE. Tel: 0208 8040 7939. Publishes probably the best guide to safety advice for computer users, *14 Steps to Safe and Comfortable Computer Use.*
*   The Royal Society for the Prevention of Accidents; www.rospa.com/CMS/index.asp Gives access to training, signs, posters, consultation, videos, multi-media and more. It is probably more appropriate as a PCT contact rather than for individual practice.

Appendix 20.1: Risk assessment – working papers

Table A1 Substances hazardous to health – clinical

Hazard	Risk identified	Control measure	Category at risk	How likely	How severe	Score	Action plan ref.
1 Controlled drugs	Misuse		A, B				
2 Vaccines	Deterioration/child consumption		B				
3 Medications	Child consumption		B				
4 Sterilising liquid	Child consumption						
5 Methylated spirits	Child consumption/misuse						
6 Samples – blood – body fluids	Infection through handling Infection through handling						
7 Clinical waste	Infection through spillage/handling						
8 Accidental discharge – blood – body fluids	Infection through handling Infection through handling						

Category at risk: A, staff; B, public.

Risk assessment – working papers

Table A2 Substances hazardous to health – cleaning

Hazard	Risk identified	Control measure	Category at risk	How likely	How severe	Score	Action plan ref.
1 Disinfectants	Child consumption /user injury		A, B				
2 Bleach	Child consumption/ User injury		A, B				
3 Aerosols – Polish – Air freshener	Child consumption/user injury Child consumption/user injury		A, B				
4 Polish wax	User injury		A				

Category at risk: A, staff; B, public.

Risk assessment – working papers

Table A3 Substances hazardous to health – other

Hazard	Risk identified	Control measure	Category at risk	How likely	How severe	Score	Action plan ref.
1 Tippex correcting fluid	Misuse		A, B				
2 Glues/solvents	Misuse		A, B				
3 Toner for copiers	Inhalation of dangerous fumes/user skin or eye injury/unsafe disposal		A,B				

Category at risk: A, staff; B, public.

Risk assessment – working papers

Table A4 Violence

Hazard	Risk identified	Control measure	Category at risk	How likely	How severe	Score	Action plan ref.
1 Patient/intruder violence in waiting area	Personal physical injury/nervous disorders		A, B				
2 Reception office violence	Personal physical injury/nervous disorders		A, B				
3 Consulting room violence	Personal physical injury/nervous disorders						
4 Treatment room violence	Personal physical injury/nervous disorders						
5 Outpatient visits – doctors	Personal physical injury/nervous disorders						
6 Outpatient visits – practice nurse	Personal physical injury/nervous disorders						

Category at risk: A, staff; B, public.

Risk assessment – working papers

Table A5 Fire

Hazard	Risk identified	Control measure	Category at risk	How likely	How severe	Score	Action plan ref.
1 Unsuitable storage of flammable materials	Cause of ignition						
2 Smoking	Cause of ignition						
3 Faulty fire-fighting equipment	Uncontrolled fire						
4 Electrical faults	Cause of ignition						
5 Blocked exits	Personal injury						
6 Faulty alarm systems	Slow evacuations/personal injury						
7 Inefficient slow evacuations	Personal injury						
8 Inadequate signage	Slow evacuations/personal injury						
9 Faulty detection systems	Undetected fire						

Risk assessment – working papers

Table A6 Moving and handling

Hazard	Risk identified	Control measure	Category at risk	How likely	How severe	Score	Action plan ref.
1 Handling needles	Infection						
2 Lifting and moving patients	Personal injury						
3 Moving furniture	Personal injury						
4 Moving portable equipment	Personal injury						
5 Lifting/carrying files, boxes	Personal injury						
6 Using step ladders/stools	Personal injury						
7 Using trolley	Personal injury						

Risk assessment – working papers

Table A7 Plant and equipment – clinical

Hazard	Risk identified	Control measure	Category at risk	How likely	How severe	Score	Action plan ref.
1 Autoclave	Inefficient sterilisation/Infection/						
2 Sharps Needles Syringes	Personal injury Personal injury Personal injury						
3 Scales	Unstable/personal injury						
4 Screens	Unstable/personal injury/finger traps						
5 Ear syringes	Infection						
6 Examination beds	Hand trap						
7 Mercury blood pressure sphygmomanometer	Poisonous if broken						

Risk assessment – working papers

Table A8 Plant and equipment – office

Hazard	Risk identified	Control measure	Category at risk	How likely	How severe	Score	Action plan ref.
1 Electrical – Computers and associated equipment – Photocopier – Fax – Video recorder – Televisions – Electric fans – Radio/tape/CD player	Source of ignition/shock/eye strain/ migraine/repetitive strain injury Source of ignition/shock Source of ignition/shock Source of ignition/shock Source of ignition/shock Source of ignition/shock Source of ignition/shock						
2 Scissors	Personal injury						
3 Staplers	Personal injury						
4 Hole punchers	Personal injury						
5 Scales	Personal injury						
6 Workstations – Desks – Chairs – Foot rests	Discomfort leading to muscular disorders						

Risk assessment – working papers

Table A9 Plant and equipment – other

Hazard	Risk identified	Control measure	Category at risk	How likely	How severe	Score	Action plan ref.
1 Kitchen – Kettles – Cooker/hob – Cutlery – Cups/mugs – Plates – Water – Heater	Fire/shock						
2 Portable electric fan heaters	Fire/shock						
3 Portable fans	Fire/shock						
4 Plant – Central heating boiler – Immersion heater – Radiator – Storage heaters – Hot-air hand dryers – Fixed extraction fans	Fire/shock						

Risk assessment – working papers

Table A10 Electricity

Hazard	Risk identified	Control measure	Category at risk	How likely	How severe	Score	Action plan ref.
1 Overload sockets	Source of ignition						
2 Trailing cables	Tripping/source of ignition						
3 Contact – Faulty wiring – Equipment	Source of ignition Source of ignition						

Risk assessment – working papers

Table A11 Premises/environment – reception

Hazard	Risk identified	Control measure	Category at risk	How likely	How severe	Score	Action plan ref.
1 Storage/shelving	Collapse						
2 Floors – condition	Trips/falls						
3 Doors	Traps						
4 Steps/stairs	Trips/falls						
5 Windows	Opening difficulty						
6 Lighting	Eye strain						
7 Ventilation	Breathing						
8 Heating	Discomfort						

Risk assessment – working papers

Table A12 Premises/environment – toilets/washroom/kitchens

Hazard	Risk identified	Control measure	Category at risk	How likely	How severe	Score	Action plan ref.
1 Doors	Traps						
2 Floors – condition	Trips/falls						
3 Light switches	Shock						
4 Shelving	Collapse/falling objects						
5 Storage	?Collapse/strain to reach						
6 Steps/stairs	Trips/falls						
7 Lighting	Eye strain						
8 Heating	Discomfort						
9 Ventilation	Discomfort						
10 Water temperature	Scalding						
11 Sanitary arrangements including: – Towels – Soap – Disposals, etc.	Contamination Infection Infection Infection						

Risk assessment – working papers

Table A13 Premises/environment – offices

Hazard	Risk identified	Control measure	Category at risk	How likely	How severe	Score	Action plan ref.
1 Workstations – Chairs – Desks – Tables – Layout	Posture injury						
2 Office layout – Cabling – Shelving – Stacking – Doors – Flooring – condition – Steps/stairs	Trips/falls Strains						
3 Heating	Discomfort						
4 Ventilation	Discomfort						
5 Lighting – General – Local	Eye strain						
6 Space per person	Collision/discomfort						

Risk assessment – working papers

Table A14 Premises/environment – consulting rooms

Hazard	Risk identified	Control measure	Category at risk	How likely	How severe	Score	Action plan ref.
1 Layout – Steps – Floors – Doors	Trips						
2 Seating/work area – Desks – Equipment	Discomfort/strain		B				
3 Practice security systems – Alarms – Panic buttons	Non-functioning						
4 Environment – Working space – Control of natural light	Overheating Lack of ventilation Inadequate central heating Inadequate local lighting						

Category at risk: A, staff; B, public.

Risk assessment – working papers

Table A15 Premises/environment – Stairs, gangways and corridors

Hazard	Risk identified	Control measure	Category at risk	How likely	How severe	Score	Action plan ref.
1 Surface condition	Trips/falls						
2 Safe usage	Trips/falls						
3 Signage	Misdirection to prohibited areas						

Risk assessment – working papers

Table A16 Premises/environment – access and regress

Hazard	Risk identified	Control measure	Category at risk	How likely	How severe	Score	Action plan ref.
1 Car/pedestrian division	Falls/collisions						
2 Paving/road surface	Trips						
3 Ice/snow	Falls						
4 Lighting	Trips/falls						
5 Signage	Misdirection to dangerous areas						

Section 3

Chapter 21

Communication and risk: some answers

Malcolm Thomas

Key learning points

- Changing learners' communication behaviour requires a skills-based approach.
- The key elements are direct observation, feedback, reflection and rehearsal of alternatives.
- This is in common with other areas of skills acquisition (e.g. sports coaching).
- The communication skills related to risk are outlined in Chapter 8. Improvement in most can be achieved by targeting three areas of the consultation:
  - openings
  - getting the full story
  - explanations.
- We offer skills – based exercises for you to use, which cover the three target areas.

Introduction

In Chapter 8 we looked at the evidence linking communication behaviours with outcomes. In this chapter we shall explore the 'best buy' skills and offer a framework in which you can work to improve them.

An analogy with improving skills in other contexts might be helpful. I am writing this as the Wimbledon tennis tournament draws to a close and Tim Henman has been defeated, after flying the flag on his own for the UK for a week. Picture him planning to do better next year. He will want to review several key games by looking over recordings of the matches. He will have the help of a skilled coach. Together they will try to decide just which areas of his game to work on. They will devise a timetable for doing this, and they will also have a clear idea of the focus ('2 weeks on forehand ground strokes', '1 month on serve placement', etc.). Then he will practise as planned, getting feedback, reflecting, possibly looking at more recordings of what he is doing and refining the plan.

Compare this with the norm for doctors who decide to try to do something about their communication skills. They might generate the idea from a problem they have had, or perhaps from reading the report of a medico-legal case or heeding the words of a respected colleague (e.g. a 'Doctors need to listen more' headline). They will often then try to make a change immediately in consultations, and it is unlikely that many of the elements of the above approach will have been implemented. It is a bit like asking Tim Henman to change his performance by reading the coaching manual and then being able to do it in his very next match.

This analogy works for other sports, or for learning a musical instrument. It even matches quite well with the normal method of learning technical skills in medicine (e.g. palpating a spleen, acquiring a new surgical technique). So we know that doctors can do this – observation, reflection and feedback, planning, rehearsal. In this chapter we offer the most important skills packaged in a way that should allow learners to practise them and obtain useful feedback.

Background

I first read the coaching analogy in a book by Roger Neighbour[1] (an enjoyable and informative read). The coaching approach to skills development is now increasingly being adopted. In Australia the Cognitive Institute[2] and in the USA the Bayer Institute[3] both have programmes of skills-based training. In the UK, MPS Risk Consulting[4] and Effective Professional Interactions[5] offer such training involving the editors of this book. The Calgary–Cambridge authors have published a scholarly work supporting effective learning in this area.[6] What follows is informed by all of these sources, filtered through my own experience.

There is direct research evidence to show that communication training can affect the outcome of the consultation. The work of Maguire and colleagues indicated that skills-based interview training improved the amount and accuracy of information gathering, and that the benefits persisted.[7] Around the same time, two other studies confirmed that structured, skills-based interventions improve outcomes.[8,9]

On the other hand, there are studies that fail to demonstrate any improvement resulting from skills-based training.[10] What, then, are the elements that we need in order to succeed with the skills-based approach?

The Toronto consensus statement[11] contains a useful list of relevant references confirming, among other things, that observation (ideally video or audio tape) and rehearsal of skills (using role play or simulated patients) are crucial ingredients of effective interventions.

Understanding is still deepening. A recent example concerns the value of training in the detection of cues (called 'clues' in the paper) – that is, non-verbal and paraverbal information ('paraverbal' referring to the way things are said rather than the actual content of speech).[12] This is a major part of the rationale for using videotaped evidence of a doctor's own consultations as the central plank of effective training.

The 'disease–illness' model concisely summarises the communication task.[13] Developed by McWhinney, it underpins most skills-based training (*see* Figure 21.1).

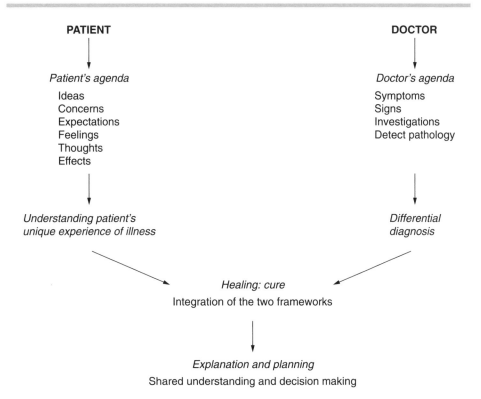

Figure 21.1 Disease–illness model (after McWhinney[13]).

The skills

What we have learned so far is that the ideal intervention for a doctor to develop his or her communication skills is regular, personalised coaching based on direct observation of performance (i.e. videotape). Since we cannot do that for you in this book, we propose a number of structured exercises that in some cases could be attempted alone, but are usually achieved with two and are ideally designed for three people. This approach characterises the training offered by, for example, MPS Risk Consulting and Effective Professional Interactions.

The skill areas that we are targeting are as follows:

* openings
* getting the full story
* acceptance
* explanations.

We shall explain the reason for the exact construction of the exercises as we go along.

Openings

The goals of the opening include the following:

* greetings and introductions
* listening to the patient's opening remarks effectively

- connecting with the patient (first impressions count)
- getting the full agenda
- agenda setting.

Ideally, by the end of this phase the patient will be thinking 'This doctor has understood where I am coming from', and the doctor will be thinking 'Now I know how many problems the patient has and what we are going to have to cover today'. However, as we know from the work of Beckman and Frankel onwards, this is rarely the case in practice.[14,15]

Some helpful observations

Beckman and Frankel's work shows that even echoing back or asking for clarification deflects the patient's opening statement.[14] It is best to remain as silent as possible, while paying attention to what the patient is saying. 'I see' or 'Go on' are the longest phrases that *do not* deflect the patient's opening remarks.

A brief summary at the end of the opening statement shows that you have been listening and want to make sense of what the patient has said. It lets the patient correct you quickly if you are way off the mark, and it is a potentially efficient thing to do.

A brief statement of empathy then shows that you have understood the patient's distress. We are looking for the smallest effective dose of empathy here (e.g. 'That must have given you a fright'). The empathetic response is available to anyone and does not depend on sympathy or a highly sensitive nature.[16] It consists of the following:

- identifying the emotion
- identifying the source of the emotion
- demonstrating to the patient that you have made the link between the two.

Let us put this together. If a patient presents with a story involving chest discomfort and breathlessness, then the response at the end of the opening statement might go along the following lines: 'So you had this aching in your chest, felt terribly breathless and were concerned that you might be going to die from a heart attack, like your dad did. That sounds pretty scary.'

The patient confirms your hunch. Next it is time to find out if there are any other agenda items. Something like this seems to work: 'Just before we sort out the chest pain, can I check if there was anything else you wanted to talk about today?'. Reflection will confirm to you the findings of research, namely that patients in general practice often bring more than one problem to a consultation, even to a consultation that has been set up as a review appointment.

The patient might bring up another point, in which case you should take it in and ask again, repeating until the patient replies 'no' to the question. 'Anything else?'. This might involve saying something like this: 'So that's the chest pain, the mole and your mum's repeat prescription. Anything else?'.

Finally, introduce a doctor agenda item if this is relevant (e.g. 'When you were last here we talked about your blood pressure. Would it be okay to touch on that as well?').

Now you might want to try the 'Openings' exercise in Box 21.1.

Box 21.1 Exercise: openings

There are three roles in this exercise – *patient*, *doctor* and *observer*.

The goal is for the *doctor* to achieve four tasks.

Please look at the four tasks, and the observer checklist below, before proceeding.

1 Greetings and introductions.
2 Listening without interruption to the whole of the *patient's* opening statement.
3 Connecting with the patient, with a very brief summary and brief empathetic comment.
4 Checking with the patient for further agenda items.

If you have three learners, quickly rotate the roles and repeat twice, giving everyone a chance to play every role. This is more effective than prolonged discussion of the feedback.

A is the *patient*. He or she brings a real or imagined story from a patient, which should be realistic.

B is the *doctor*. He or she is trying to achieve the four tasks listed above, using the skills listed below.

C is the *observer*. He or she ticks off each skill that has been achieved, using the following recording sheet (please feel free to photocopy this list for your own use).

Allow *2 minutes* for the exercise and *2 minutes* for the feedback.

The goal is for the observer to give factual feedback about the points on the list. If they try to do more than this, cut them short!

Observer record – please tick if skill is achieved

- Greets
- Maintains eye contact
- Uses encouraging body language and posture
- Listens to the end of the opening statement without interrupting
- Uses a short summarising statement
- Makes a brief empathetic comment
- Asks for any other agenda items

Getting the full story

Now that you have agreed the agenda, it is time to begin exploring the first problem to work on. Doctors often feel relatively comfortable at this point, at least as far as soliciting the medical aspect of the story is concerned.

In our experience, it is common for doctors (especially those in early training) to narrow down quickly into a symptom-questionnaire approach. In fact, experience and research point to a gradual closing down of the agenda as the strategy most productive of information. This involves asking the patient to start out in their own words, and then using increasingly closed prompts to fill in any gaps. Closed questions are certainly allowed, and are particularly necessary to flush out significant negatives (e.g. 'Can you tell me if there was blood in the spit?').

So the series of prompts might go as follows:

> 'We agreed to start with this chest pain and breathlessness – can you tell me more?'
>
> 'Tell me more about that pain.'
>
> 'How would you describe that pain?'
>
> 'How long exactly did the pain last?'

This approach is mentally tougher for the doctor. Instead of having your checklist and working through it methodically, it is necessary to pay close attention to what the patient is saying, making an effective mental note of areas that you will need to return to for further elaboration.

We can list possible prompts along a spectrum ranging from most open to most closed (*see* Box 21.2). This is sometimes called the open-to-closed cone. An interesting facet of this approach is that you can go from a more open to a more closed prompt quite easily (e.g. from silence to encouragement, to a question). However, it is difficult to revert to a more open prompt once a closed one has been used. Therefore attentive silence is recommended as the default option if the patient is showing signs of contemplation. The famous advice is 'Don't just say something, sit there!'.

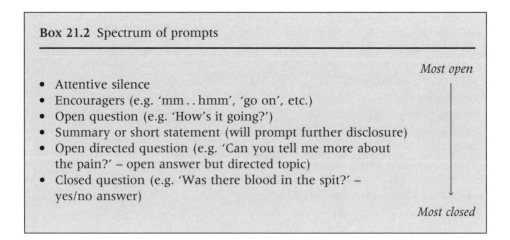

Box 21.2 Spectrum of prompts

Most open

- Attentive silence
- Encouragers (e.g. 'mm .. hmm', 'go on', etc.)
- Open question (e.g. 'How's it going?')
- Summary or short statement (will prompt further disclosure)
- Open directed question (e.g. 'Can you tell me more about the pain?' – open answer but directed topic)
- Closed question (e.g. 'Was there blood in the spit?' – yes/no answer)

Most closed

Thus the key behaviour to practise is that of active listening – paying close attention to what the patient is saying and monitoring their face and tone of voice for cues to things that are of significance to them.

The exercise in getting the full story (*see* Box 21.3) is designed to practise the skills of active listening. It is quite fun and, if achieved, will get the doctor out of the role of 'fixer' into that of understanding. It has been pointed out that this could be described as 'listening like a woman'. Certainly there is evidence that women are more likely to engage in this behaviour. Deborah Tannen, in a very readable book entitled *That's Not What I Meant*,[17] calls this 'rapport talk'. We can all learn to do this.

Box 21.3 Exercise: getting the full story

There are three roles in this exercise – *talker*, *listener* and *observer*.

The talker is talking about a non-medical topic.

The goal of the exercise is for the listener to achieve three tasks.

Please look at the three tasks, and the observer checklist below, before proceeding.

1 Listen attentively, using encouraging prompts.
2 Understand and demonstrate this understanding to the listener.
3 *Avoid* offering solutions.

If you have three learners, quickly rotate the roles and repeat twice, giving everyone a chance to play every role. This is more effective than prolonged discussion of the feedback.

A is the *talker*. He or she brings a topic that is meaningful to him or her. A hobby or pastime is ideal. There should be an element of challenge (e.g. never enough time, inability to master some technique), but it should not be medical or emotionally charged.

B is the *listener*. He or she encourages the story to emerge, attempting to achieve the tasks listed above and to utilise the skills noted below.

C is the *observer*. He or she ticks off each still that has been achieved, using the following recording sheet (please feel free to photocopy this list for your own use).

Allow *4 minutes* for the exercise and *2 minutes* for the feedback.

The goal is for the observer to give factual feedback about the points on the list. If they try to do more than this, cut them short!

Observer record – please tick if skill is achieved
• Maintains eye contact
• Uses encouraging posture and body language
• Listens attentively – not interrupting and allowing pauses
• Uses encouraging words or short phrases
• Paraphrases (e.g. 'So what you are saying is . . .')
• Seeks clarification (e.g. 'What did you mean when you said that . . . ?')
• Uses summaries
• Avoids offering solutions

The acceptance response

This skill is so important that it will be given a section to itself. The successful deployment of the acceptance response will help you to avoid fruitless arguments and can allow you more successfully to be true to yourself, without losing the confidence of the patient (with its attendant clinical and medico-legal risks).

The acceptance (or accepting) response is attributed to Briggs and Banahan by the Calgary–Cambridge collaborators.[18] The goal is to accept the patient's thoughts or feelings, without engaging them yourself. This means *avoiding* the following:

- giving reassurance
- argument
- agreement (perhaps surprisingly).

The point is that it is too early in your relationship to engage in these activities. You need to build trust first, not least by finishing gathering the medical information and then completing a physical examination.

So the key steps are as follows, with an illustrative example.

- Acknowledge the patient's thought or feeling. Use statements, paraphrasing or brief summarisation (e.g. 'So you have been coughing for 5 days, it's still coming up green and you thought it was time to come for an antibiotic – is that right?').
- Acknowledge the patient's right to have this thought or feeling (e.g. 'It sounds like this is still a problem for you').
- Deploy attentive silence. You might hear something like 'Yes, I have to go on a business trip next week and I just have to be better by then.'
- *Avoid* reassurance, argument or agreement, and *especially avoid the words 'yes, but . . .'.*
- Factor the patient's view into your plan (e.g. 'We'll take a careful look at that').

You should note that the acceptance response does not denote agreement. It is possible to use acceptance in very disagreeable situations without compromising your integrity (e.g. 'So you were found guilty of sexually abusing two children and have been jailed for seven years. Now you are being harassed by some fellow inmates and it seems unfair to you, is that right?', 'That's about it, doc', 'I can see that must be hard for you').

The research shows that it is feeling heard which most helps the patient to trust the doctor enough to value their advice. We have not yet packaged this skill into an exercise. Feel free to photocopy this page so that you can have it to hand in your consulting room. Very few consultations pass without an opportunity to practise acceptance.

Explanations

The training I received in communication at medical school focused on history taking. I believe this to have been typical until relatively recently. Perhaps it is not surprising, then, that poor or absent explanations are an area of frequent complaint by patients, leading to clinical and medico-legal risk (as we saw in

Chapter 8). This is the reason for making this our fourth and final priority skill area.

Most doctors are giving the wrong amount (and often level of detail) of explanation to most patients most of the time. Several studies have shown that patients can be divided into information seekers (80%) and information avoiders (20%).[18] In general, 'seekers' want more information than doctors usually give them, and 'avoiders' are happy with a minimum amount.

Unfortunately, doctors tend to have rather stereotypical information delivery patterns. How often have you caught yourself in the middle of a favourite mini-lecture noticing that the patient has switched off?

The simple tactic of asking the patient if they actually want an explanation will screen out the 'avoiders' and save time in 20% of your consultations. The next step should be a negotiation with the 'seeker' patient over the agenda for the explanation. It makes sense to ask the patient what information they would like and to check their starting point. Clearly, the appropriate explanation for an illiterate and unschooled patient about the cause of angina is likely to be different to that for a graduate, for example. Doctors should be wary of making assumptions here. Your own experience will doubtless furnish examples of having got this level completely wrong – research backs up just how poor doctors are at judging what explanation patients want in the absence of having made a specific enquiry.

You can also make sure that you find out early on whether you are off track. This skill has been called 'chunking and checking', and most people do it instinctively to some extent. It simply refers to the technique of giving your information in bite-sized portions and looking at the patient for cues confirming that they are receiving it. There is a range of accessible cues (e.g. attentive body language, nodding, facial expressions confirming understanding so far).

There is much research to inform the delivery of information. Many non-medical fields require skill in this area, an obvious example being the pharmaceutical representative. They will often try to find out the doctor's starting point ('Have you heard anything about Novacure?'), and will then deliver an organised explanation, in appropriate language and backed up by written material (words and/or pictures), with a parting invitation to make contact if more information is needed.

These elements (listed below) would serve a doctor well:

- organisation (shared with the patient)
- summarisation, with repetition of important points
- keeping the language appropriate – avoiding jargon
- writing things down – written words or pictures.

With regard to the last point, the basic message from research seems to be that new words or pictures created by the doctor with the patient present have the greatest impact, followed by pre-printed material that the doctor writes on (e.g. 'This is your heart and I'm ringing the blood vessel that is blocked'). Simply handing over pre-printed material is in general less effective, and having a smorgasbord of leaflets in the waiting room is least effective of all.

Finally, since you have now devoted three or four minutes to explaining things to your patient, it might be efficient to find out whether the patient has benefited from your explanation. Explicit checking of the patient's understanding is a behaviour that I have never spontaneously observed in any of the doctors with whom I have worked. It seems to require a conscious decision to adopt it.

Perhaps some doctors have been put off by being unable to find a form of words that does not imply 'Listen carefully, there will be a test at the end.' We suggest that it could be reflected back to the patient along the following lines: 'Now that I have told you a few things about angina, it would help me to know how well I have done. Can you say the most important things that you have taken from what we have been saying?'.

In summary, it seems to be the degree of personalisation of the elements of the explanation that holds the key to its effectiveness. The final exercise (*see* Box 21.4) gives you an opportunity to practise an explanation that incorporates these ideas.

Box 21.4 Exercise: explanations

There are three roles in this exercise – *patient*, *doctor* and *observer*.

The goal is for the *doctor* to demonstrate the skills in the checklist below.

The *doctor* and the *patient* agree a scenario, based on the *doctor's* real-life practice. Some suggestions are made below for GP patients.

If you have three learners, quickly rotate the roles and repeat twice, giving everyone a chance to play every role. This is more effective than prolonged discussion of the feedback.

Possible scenarios
- A 54-year-old manual worker with a new diagnosis of angina.
- A 75-year-old female hypertensive non-smoker – it is now time to recommend medication.
- A patient who wants to know why they need to take warfarin after their pulmonary embolus.
- A patient who wants to know why they need to be on antidepressants for so long.

A is the *patient*. They have has their own perspective on what they want from the explanation.

B is the *doctor*. They are trying to demonstrate the skills on the checklist below.

C is the *observer*. They tick off each skill that has been achieved on the following recording sheet (please feel free to photocopy this list for your own use).

Allow *4 minutes* for the exercise and *2 minutes* for the feedback.

The goal is for the observer to give factual feedback about the points on the list. If they try to do more than this, cut them short!

Observer record – please tick if skill is achieved
- Asks if the patient wants an explanation, and if so, what they want explained
- Asks for any other information needs
- Actively discovers the patient's starting point
- Chunks and checks (looks at the patient and makes sure that they are 'getting it')
- Organises the explanation, with signposting of the process ('firstly . . . , secondly . . . , then . . .)
- Summarises
- Repeats important points
- Uses simple language, avoiding jargon
- Uses *pictures* or *written text* to amplify points
- Explicitly checks the patient's understanding

Where next?

In GP training in the UK, it has for many years been normal for trainers to review videotapes of learners' consultations. This represents the gold-standard learning procedure, but it is not without risk.

The main problem is that without effective acceptable feedback for the learner, plus a chance to try out alternatives, this can come over as unhelpful (fatuous positive global judgements) or even harmful ('Carry on like that and you'll never pass summative assessment').

We shall not try to define the need any further in this book. Kurtz and colleagues have done it masterfully,[6] and we refer you to their book. We recommend that you find a doctor with experience of using their method to help you, as it is almost impossible to master the elements of the method without seeing it in action, even *with* their book beside you. The Cambridge course[19] is an obvious place to start. The author's company[5] runs two-day courses designed to equip participants with a good grasp of the elements involved in their method. Most directors of postgraduate GP education should be able to put you in touch with suitably skilled teachers. A full list of their contact details can be found on the website of the Joint Committee for Postgraduate Training for General Practice (JCPTGP).[20]

If you do decide to progress to videotape review of your consultations, you will need to obtain the consent of your patients. For this we refer you to the GMC website, where you can find up-to-date advice on how to go about it and obtain consent.[21]

Another possible route to feedback is through questioning patients after their consultations. This is less direct than observing yourself in action, but it is much easier to do and can give you sufficient evidence to make a useful start, as well as providing practical confirmation of your judgements if you have videotaped evidence available.

The most widely used assessment tool for this purpose in the UK is an instrument called the Doctors' Interpersonal Skills Questionnaire (DISQ).[22,23] This was developed in general practice in New Zealand and Australia. It is short and has been well tested for reliability and validity. It is easy for patients to complete, and my experience is of a high response rate by patients.

Summary

Improving your medical communication skills is feasible. It has strong parallels with learning a musical instrument or improving in a technical sport. It is a potentially lifelong task that requires regular effective reflection and practice.

In this chapter we have presented a number of exercises that provide opportunities for practice and feedback of skills that should make a difference both to the outcome for patients (clinical risk) and to your chances of being sued (medico-legal risk). Finally, we have offered suggestions as to where you might go in terms of continuing to reflect on and develop your skills.

References

1 Neighbour R (1987) *The Inner Consultation*. MTP Press, Dordrecht.
2 www.cognitiveinstitute.com.au
3 www.bayerinstitute.org
4 www.mps-riskconsulting.com
5 www.effecitveprofessionalinteractions.co.uk
6 Kurtz S, Silverman J and Draper J (1998) *Teaching and Learning Communication Skills in Medicine*. Radcliffe Medical Press, Oxford.
7 Maguire P, Roe P, Goldberg D *et al.* (1978) The value of feedback in teaching interviewing skills to medical students. *Psychol Med.* **8**: 695–704.
8 Hutter MJ, Dungy CI, Zakus GE *et al.* (1977) Interviewing skills: a comprehensive approach to teaching and evaluation. *J Med Educ.* **52**: 328–33.
9 Carroll JG and Monroe J (1979) Teaching medical interviewing: a critique of educational research and practice. *J Med Educ.* **54**: 498–500.
10 Brown JB, Boles M, Mullooly JP and Levinson W (1999) Effect of clinician communication skills training on patient satisfaction. A randomized, controlled trial. *Ann Intern Med.* **131**: 822–9.
11 Simpson M, Buckman R, Stewart M *et al.* (1991) Doctor–patient communication: the Toronto consensus statement. *BMJ.* **303**: 1385–7.
12 Levinson W, Gorawara-Bhat R and Lamb J (2000) A study of patient clues and physician responses in primary care and surgical settings. *JAMA.* **284**: 1021–7.
13 McWhinney I (1989) The need for a transformed clinical method. In: M Stewart and D Roter (eds) *Communicating with Medical Patients*. Sage Publications, Thousand Oaks, CA.
14 Beckman HB and Frankel RM (1984) The effect of physician behaviour on the collection of data. *Ann Intern Med.* **101**: 692–6.
15 Marvel MK, Epstein RM, Flowers K and Beckman HB (1999) Soliciting the patient's agenda: have we improved? *JAMA.* **281**: 283–7.
16 Buckman R (2002) Communications and emotions: skills and effort are key. *BMJ.* **325**: 672.
17 Tannen D (1992) *That's Not What I Meant!* Virago, London.
18 Silverman J, Kurtz S and Draper J (1998) *Skills for Communicating with Patients*. Radcliffe Medical Press, Oxford.
19 www.easterngp.co.uk
20 www.jcptgp.org.uk
21 General Medical Council (2002) *Making and Using Visual and Audio Recordings of Patients*; www.gmc-uk.org
22 Greco M, Cavanagh M, Brownlea A and McGovern J (1999) Validation studies of the Doctors' Interpersonal Skills Questionnaire. *Educ Gen Pract.* **10**: 256–64.
23 www.cfep.net

Chapter 22

Risk assessment

Keith Haynes

Key learning points

- There are a number of tools in the risk management armoury, including risk assessment, significant event audit, root cause analysis and reviewing complaints and claims.
- Risk assessment is a prospective and proactive tool.
- A structured approach to risk assessment involves the identification, measurement and control of risks.
- Risk assessment is a powerful tool that enables practices to fix problems before they occur.
- Risk assessment is a useful technique for teambuilding.

Introduction

What is in the clinical risk management armoury that might help practices to identify and manage their risks more effectively?

There are a number of tools, some of which can be used prospectively (before the event has occurred) and others that can be used retrospectively (trying to learn from the event once it has happened). They include the following:

- risk assessment
- significant event audit
- root cause analysis
- reviewing complaints and claims.

In this chapter and the next (Chapter 23) we shall look at two of these tools, namely risk assessment and root cause analysis.

Risk assessment and root cause analysis:
two important tools

Generally speaking, most of the tools are retrospective in their application. However, risk assessment is prospective and proactive – it offers a practice the opportunity to identify, evaluate and manage their risks before something goes wrong. Because it is prospective in its application, it has the potential to generate for the practice an operational plan of things that need to be fixed.

On the other hand, root cause analysis is a retrospective technique. It helps us to understand the 'root causes' of an incident. As a technique, it helps to confirm that we should be reviewing systems when things have gone wrong, rather than the direct 'symptoms' of an incident.

Carrying out a risk assessment: an approach

Risk assessment is based on the core elements of risk management (*see* Chapter 5), namely:

* the identification of risk
* measurement of the identified risk in terms of consequence and frequency of occurrence
* the control or the way in which the risk is managed
* constant monitoring to ensure the effectiveness of control measures.

These core elements combine to provide the definition of effective risk management.

Practices may want to use the core elements of risk management to enable them to carry out a risk assessment. MPS Risk Consulting has done this, and to date has carried out risk assessments in over 200 practices in the UK. A key benefit of this approach is that it gets the whole practice team involved and convenes a half-day workshop.

In advance of the workshop, and in order to identify potential risks and weaknesses in current systems, the practice manager and one of the general practitioners may wish to complete the assessment questionnaire (*see* Appendix 22.1). On its own, the questionnaire will begin to identify areas for further enquiry for the practice.

Step 1: workshop preparation

Participants should be asked to consider, as pre-work before the workshop, the risks which may threaten their area of operation. For each of these risks they should also be asked to identify the potential causes and consequences of the risk event occurring.

Step 2: identify risks

At the beginning of the workshop, participants should be asked to identify the key risks that they have identified both in their specific area of work and within the practice more generally. You should give participants a few minutes to do this, and you should ask them to record each risk that they identify on a 'Post-it'® note. Participants should be asked to discuss the risks that they identify with their colleagues. You may also find it helpful to provide the participants with a definition of risk (e.g. the possibility of loss, injury or adverse consequence for a patient, member of staff or even the reputation of the practice). Providing the participants with some specific risks may be helpful, and for this you may want to draw on the list given in Chapter 6.

Step 3: determine the consequences of a risk occurring

Participants should be asked to describe the consequences associated with each risk. At this stage the question is hypothetical – that is, having identified a potential risk, what might its consequences be if it were to occur?

For example, one of the risks identified may relate to equipment malfunction. The causes may include any of the following:

- inadequate maintenance
- operator error
- poor operator training, etc.

The following consequences may be identified as flowing from the risk of malfunctioning equipment:

- injury/harm to patients
- injury/harm to staff
- death
- damage to reputation.

A rating is then assigned to each risk based on the consequences described and categorised as follows:

- insignificant
- minor
- moderate
- major
- catastrophic.

Not surprisingly, many consequences of risks in healthcare are likely to be at the more severe end of the scale.

Step 4: determine likelihood

Participants should then be asked to determine the likelihood of the risk occurring.

The likelihood ratings are as follows:

- almost certain
- likely
- moderate
- unlikely
- rare.

If the risk has already occurred, then it is 'almost certain', while the likelihood that other risks may occur is so remote that they will be categorised as 'rare'.

Step 5: determine a risk rating

The consequence and likelihood ratings are then used to determine the risk rating for each risk, as shown in Table 22.1.

Table 22.1 Determining a risk rating

Likelihood	Consequences				
	Insignificant	*Minor*	*Moderate*	*Major*	*Catastrophic*
Almost certain	Significant	Significant	High	High	High
Likely	Moderate	Significant	Significant	High	High
Moderate	Low	Moderate	Significant	High	High
Unlikely	Low	Low	Moderate	Significant	High
Rare	Low	Low	Moderate	Significant	Significant

The above table is based on one contained in the Australia/New Zealand standard 4360, and is reproduced here with the kind permission of Standards Australia.

Step 6: identify and determine the effectiveness of the controls

Participants should then be asked to identify the controls which currently exist for managing the risks. The 'control' is the defence that is in place to reduce the risk to prevent it from occurring in the first place. 'Controls' are the systems, policies and procedures that the practice has in place.

In order to assess the effectiveness of the control, the following ratings should be used:

* *satisfactory* – controls are strong and operating properly, providing a reasonable level of assurance that the risks are being managed and objectives met
* *some weaknesses* – some control weaknesses/inefficiencies have been identified. Although these are not considered to present a serious problem, improvements are required to provide reasonable assurance that the risks are being managed and objectives met
* *weak* – controls do not meet any acceptable standard, as many weaknesses/ inefficiencies exist. Controls do not provide reasonable assurance that the risks are being managed and objectives met.

Step 7: determine the overall risk rating

At this stage the participants will want to have some meaningful debate about how effective the controls are for managing each risk that they have identified. The initial risk rating can then be evaluated against the effectiveness of the control as shown in Table 22.2.

Table 22.2 Overall risk rating

Control effectiveness	Risk rating			
	Low	*Moderate*	*Significant*	*High*
Weak	Moderate	Significant	High	High
Some weaknesses	Low	Moderate	Significant	High
Satisfactory	Low	Moderate	Moderate	Significant

Step 8: agreeing an action plan

This is what the process has been about – identifying and agreeing an action plan for addressing those risks that have been identified as 'high', and perhaps later those that are 'significant'. If 'risk' has been defined in broad terms, then the action list that emerges may well form the operational plan for the practice over the coming period. Having identified these potential risks, it also enables the practice to be proactive in fixing them. It should enable a practice to anticipate and fix the risks rather than 'fire-fighting' them, which may have been the case in the past. What may have started out looking like a sterile management technique offers the potential to change the way in which many practices have traditionally managed. Moreover, the whole practice team has been involved in the process and identified solutions to improve the quality and safety of current practice. Why not try it?

For example, with regard to the risk of malfunctioning equipment, and in particular our steriliser, after discussion in the workshop the following was agreed:

Consequences = major	May lead to injury/harm to patient as a result of inadequately sterilised medical device, and impact upon the reputation of the practice
Likelihood = unlikely	During the workshop there was a keen discussion about the unlikely likelihood of this being a problem. The practice nurses thought that the current maintenance schedule was satisfactory and so the risk was unlikely
Risk rating = significant	
Review of controls = weak	The participants agreed that the controls for managing this risk were as follows: • regular maintenance • review and recording of decontamination cycle • compliance with national and local guidance on decontamination During the workshop interval the practice manager reviewed the equipment maintenance file and noticed that the last service was two years ago, and that the maintenance contract had not been renewed The practice nurses were also unable to produce any records relating to the cycle temperature The practice concluded that they should take some immediate action
Overall risk rating	*High*
Agreed action	• Arrange for immediate service and set up regular service contract • Review and implement national and local decontamination guidance • Discuss and review arrangements with PCT Control of Infection Adviser

Risk assessment: some benefits

Carrying out a risk assessment in this way enables the practice to deal with potential risks before they occur. 'It has been useful for our practice to learn that the steriliser is not being regularly maintained' – they can now do something about it!

The approach that we suggest also offers the potential to bring the whole practice team together to share in the identification and improved control of the risks.

Appendix 22.1 Pre-risk Assessment Practice Questionnaire

A	Your appointment system
A1	What is your appointments frequency? *Please state as a rate per hour.*
A2	How many appointments are booked in a typical surgery?
A3	Is the appointment system computerised?
	YES ☐ NO ☐
A4	How far in advance can appointments be made?
A5	On average, how many extra appointments might be added on to a typical surgery?
A6	Do surgeries overrun?
	YES ☐ NO ☐
	If Yes, by how long typically?
A7	What are your arrangements for seeing urgent patients at the surgery? *For example, added on to surgery, duty doctor system, emergency surgery, and so on.*
A8	Is there telephone triage for urgent appointment requests?
	YES ☐ NO ☐
	If Yes, who deals with it?
A9	What is the waiting time for booked appointments generally?
	Same day ☐ 2–3 days ☐ 4–5 days ☐
	5–7 days ☐ 1 week ☐ 2 weeks ☐
	If it varies with different doctors (or for other reasons), please give the range of waiting times:
A10	Does the practice nurse see urgent patients?
	YES ☐ NO ☐
	If Yes, how easy is it to get in?
A11	What arrangements, if any, are in place for follow-up appointments?
	Are there protected appointments for follow-up patients?
	YES ☐ NO ☐
A12	In general, are patients followed up by the same doctor?
	YES ☐ NO ☐

B	Record-keeping

B1 How are consultations recorded?

On computer ☐   By hand ☐   Mixture of both ☐

B2 If you use paper records, are they Lloyd George or A4?

Lloyd George ☐   A4 ☐

B3 Are all handwritten records legible?

Yes ☐   No ☐

B4 Are the notes in chronological order, both continuation cards and correspondence?

Yes ☐   No ☐

B5 Are individual records summarised?

Yes ☐   No ☐

B6 If you keep computer records, how are incoming letters and reports recorded?

B7 Is there an audit trail for computerised records?

Yes ☐   No ☐

B8 Do notes go missing?

Yes ☐   No ☐

If Yes, how often? *Please describe frequency in your own terms:*

B9 Is there a tracker system for manual records?

Yes ☐   No ☐

B10 How quickly does filing generally get done?

Same day ☐   Next day ☐

Next week ☐   More than a week later ☐

B11 Are manual records taken on home visits?

Yes ☐   No ☐

Are computer records taken on home visits?

Yes ☐   No ☐

If you use computer records, are home visits subsequently recorded?

Yes ☐   No ☐

B12 How would a note be made in the patient records about an out-of-hours phone call and/or visit?

B13 How well do you think staff understand the provisions of the Data Protection Act (DPA) 1998?

Very well ☐   Well ☐   Not very well ☐

It varies ☐   Don't know ☐

Is anyone acquainted with the rules on disclosure?

Yes ☐   No ☐   Don't know ☐

C	Test results
C1	Are there clear instructions for the staff about the safe collection, handling and storage of specimens?
	Yes ☐ No ☐
C2	Are results obtained online or by paper?
	Online ☐ Hard copy ☐ Mixture ☐
C3	To whom can results be given?
	How do you ensure confidentiality?
C4	Please describe how results may be given to patients:
C5	Is a record kept of tests ordered?
	Yes ☐ No ☐
	Are checks made to ensure that results have been received back?
	Yes ☐ No ☐
	Please describe the systems in place:
C6	Are patients routinely told if multiple tests are being done?
	Yes ☐ No ☐
C7	If patients ask for their results, would staff always know if multiple tests had been done?
	Yes ☐ No ☐
C8	How are test results monitored and actioned?
	Please describe what happens:
C9	Are test results easily identifiable during a consultation?
	Yes ☐ No ☐
C10	Is there a significant period between results being received and being filed?
	Yes ☐ No ☐

D	Repeat prescribing
D1	**Please describe your system for repeat prescribing:**
D2	**Do you accept telephone requests?** Yes ☐ No ☐
D3	**By whom are prescriptions signed?** Patient's usual doctor ☐ Registered doctor ☐ Any doctor ☐
D4	**Are patients on repeat prescriptions easily identifiable during a consultation?** Yes ☐ No ☐
D5	**What arrangements are there for monitoring a patient on repeat prescriptions?**
D6	**Is there a system for reviewing repeat prescriptions that have not been collected?** Yes ☐ No ☐
	If yes, please describe it:
D7	**Is there a system to monitor those patients who fail to maintain their medication/attend for review?** Yes ☐ No ☐
	If yes, please describe it:
D8	**Do you have protocols for repeat prescribing?** *For example, length of each prescription, number of repeats before review, and so on.* Yes ☐ No ☐
	Please state your protocols:

E	Complaints

E1 Is there a practice complaints procedure?

Yes ☐   No ☐

Is the procedure written down for staff?

Yes ☐   No ☐

If Yes, please attach a copy of the procedure or outline it in the space provided here:

E2 Is there written guidance for patients on how to make a complaint?

Yes ☐   No ☐

E3 Is there a notice in the waiting room about complaints?

Yes ☐   No ☐

E4 Does a nominated person deal with complaints?

Yes ☐   No ☐

Who is it (*by job title please*)?

E5 Are all staff and doctors aware of the complaints procedure?

Yes ☐   No ☐

E6 Typically, how many complaints are received each year?

How many proceed to a formal written response?

F	Referrals

F1	**How are patient referrals done?**
	Is there a formal protocol for this arrangement?
	Yes ☐ No ☐

F2	**Is there a system to ensure a referral is sent?**
	Yes ☐ No ☐
	If Yes, please describe it.

F3	**Are all referral letters typed?**
	Yes ☐ No ☐
	Is a copy kept in the patient's record, either manual or computerised?
	Yes ☐ No ☐

F4	**Are any checks made to see that an appointment has been made or the patient has been seen?**
	Yes ☐ No ☐

F5	**Are medication lists sent with referrals?**
	Yes ☐ No ☐

F6	**What is the incidence of GPs forgetting to make referrals?**

G	Confidentiality

G1	Can patients at the reception desk be overheard by others?
	Yes ☐ No ☐

G2	Can waiting patients overhear staff on the phone?
	Yes ☐ No ☐

G3	Are all staff aware of their obligation to maintain confidentiality?
	Yes ☐ No ☐
	Is there a clause about this in their contracts of employment?
	Yes ☐ No ☐

G4	Is somewhere specially provided for patients who wish to discuss a matter in private?
	Yes ☐ No. ☐
	Are patients aware that this facility exists?
	Yes ☐ No ☐
	Please describe what this facility is:

G5	Are computer screens or surgery lists visible to patients at the front desk?
	Yes ☐ No ☐

G6	Are screensavers used at the front desk and in the surgeries?
	Yes ☐ No ☐

G7	Are the surgeries soundproof?
	Yes ☐ No ☐

G8	How are patients called from the waiting room to their appointment?

H	Telephones
H1	How many telephone lines do you have?
H2	How many dedicated lines are there? *For example, one for emergencies, one for appointments, and so on.*
H3	How many staff answer phones?
H4	Are your phone lines often engaged, or does it often take a long time to answer a ringing phone?
	Yes ☐ No ☐
H5	Is there a protocol for passing on messages?
	Yes ☐ No ☐
	If Yes, please describe it:
H6	Is someone responsible for checking that messages have been passed on?
	Yes ☐ No ☐
H7	Do patients have to call in at certain times for particular things? *For example, repeat prescription between 2 and 4pm.*
	Yes ☐ No ☐

I	Staffing
I1	Do new staff have induction training?
	Yes ☐ No ☐
	If Yes, please describe your arrangements briefly:
I2	How often are staff meetings held?
	Who attends?
I3	Have individuals got specific management responsibilities? *For example, a staff partner.*
	Yes ☐ No ☐
	Does everyone in the practice know who is responsible for what?
	Yes ☐ No ☐
I4	Is anyone ever alone in the building?
	Yes ☐ No ☐
I5	Are there panic alarms?
	Yes ☐ No ☐
	If Yes, is there a protocol to respond to them?
	Yes ☐ No ☐
I6	Has anyone been physically attacked or threatened with physical attack?
	Yes ☐ No ☐
	If Yes, describe in what way:
	Do you consider it a real risk?
	Yes ☐ No ☐
	If Yes, describe in what way:
I7	Have staff had training in the handling of difficult/violent patients?
	Yes ☐ No ☐
I8	Are locums employed?
	Yes ☐ No ☐
	If Yes, are they typically regular locums, who know the practice and are known by it?
	Yes ☐ No ☐
I9	Are locums given written instructions or inducted into practice protocols and ways of working?
	Yes ☐ No ☐

J	Consent

J1	Is minor surgery performed at the surgery?
	Yes ☐ No ☐

J2	Is written or verbal consent obtained before the surgery is carried out?
	Yes ☐ No ☐
	If Yes, by whom:
	Is verbal consent recorded in the patient's record?
	Yes ☐ No ☐

J3	Are warnings of potential risks or outcomes given to the patient?
	Yes ☐ No ☐
	If Yes, is the advice recorded in the patient's record?
	Yes ☐ No ☐

J4	Is an information leaflet about the procedure to be performed given to the patient?
	Yes ☐ No ☐

K	Equipment

K1	Is there an inventory of surgery equipment?
	Yes ☐ No ☐

K2	Is a designated person responsible for maintaining and checking practice equipment?
	Yes ☐ No ☐

K3	Are staff trained in the use of the equipment?
	Yes ☐ No ☐

K4	What medical equipment is available in the practice? *For example, ECG, defibrillation, autoclaves.*

L	Health and safety
L1	Does the practice have an up-to-date, written health and safety policy?
	Yes ☐ No ☐
L2	Has the policy been brought to the attention of all staff?
	Yes ☐ No ☐
L3	Has a health and safety risk assessment of the workplace been carried out?
	Yes ☐ No ☐
	If Yes, were the findings acted on?
	Yes ☐ No ☐
L4	Is there an accident book?
	Yes ☐ No ☐
L5	Is there a procedure for reporting accidents?
	Yes ☐ No ☐
L6	Are there arrangements for first aid?
	Yes ☐ No ☐
L7	Is there a written procedure for what to do in the event of a fire?
	Yes ☐ No ☐
L8	Do you hold fire drills regularly?
	Yes ☐ No ☐
L9	Has a Control of Substances Hazardous to Health (COSHH) assessment been carried out?
	Yes ☐ No ☐
L10	Have measures been taken to prevent, or at least control, exposure to substances hazardous to health?
	Yes ☐ No ☐
L11	Do you train employees in the safe handling procedures and control measures they should use when in contact with substances hazardous to health?
	Yes ☐ No ☐
L12	Is the hepatitis B vaccination given to anyone at risk of contamination with body fluids?
	Yes ☐ No ☐
L13	Are all hazardous substances kept out of reach of children?
	Yes ☐ No ☐
L14	Are sharps containers kept out of reach of children?
	Yes ☐ No ☐
	Do you always dispose of the containers when they are two-thirds full?
	Yes ☐ No ☐
L15	Is there a procedure for the safe handling, storage and disposal of clinical waste?
	Yes ☐ No ☐
L16	Does the practice have employer's and public liability insurance?
	Yes ☐ No ☐

M	Controlled drugs
M1	Are controlled drugs stored on the practice premises?
	Yes ☐ No ☐
M2	If Yes, is there a person responsible for ensuring that their storage and control complies with current regulations?
	Yes ☐ No ☐
	Who is it *(by job title please)* ?
M3	Is there a procedure for the disposal of controlled drugs?
	Yes ☐ No ☐
M4	Are controlled drugs carried by individual GPs?
	Yes ☐ No ☐
M5	If Yes, are they aware of the regulations concerning the recording of stocks and administration?
	Yes ☐ No ☐

Chapter 23

Root cause analysis

Keith Haynes

Key learning points

- Root cause analysis (RCA) helps us to understand the 'root causes' and not just the immediate 'symptoms' of an incident.
- To err is human, and so in requiring us to look at systemic failures RCA helps us to move beyond individual blame.
- RCA as a technique helps us to understand what has happened and why, and enables us to put in place corrective actions.
- There are a number of useful techniques that can be used to carry out an RCA.
- The expectation is that full-blown RCAs will be carried out infrequently in primary care, but the taxonomies that are available can be used to review many incidents.

Demystifying root cause analysis

> I keep six honest serving-men (they taught me all I know). Their names are what and why and when and how and where and who.
>
> (Rudyard Kipling, *Just So Stories*)

RCA as a tool has only recently been introduced into the UK healthcare system, largely as a result of the NPSA, which has developed a very useful toolkit that can be found on their website (www.npsa.nhs.uk/rcatoolkit).

RCA is an important technique which helps us understand the 'root causes' of an incident. As a technique, it helps to confirm that we should be reviewing systems when things have gone wrong, rather than the direct 'symptoms' of an incident which will involve human beings. It helps us to move away from a culture of blaming individuals and towards looking at the bigger picture associated with systems issues. A lot is currently being made of this tool, but essentially it is probably best encapsulated in the Rudyard Kipling quotation above.

RCAs systematically search out latent system failures that underlie adverse events or near misses. Some commentators have observed that they are limited by their retrospective and inherently speculative nature, often influenced by hindsight bias.[1] Shojania and Wald go on to suggest that there is insufficient evidence in the medical literature to support RCA as a proven patient safety practice, although:

> it may represent an important qualitative tool that is complementary to other techniques employed in error reduction. When applied appropriately, RCA may illuminate targets for change and, in certain healthcare contexts, may generate testable hypotheses. The use of RCA merits more consideration, as it lends a formal structure to efforts to learn from past mistakes.[1]

Taylor-Adams and Vincent[2] in the revised and updated version of their original 'Protocol for the Investigation and Analysis of Clinical Incidents' (now called 'The London Protocol') emphasise the proactive and forward-looking nature of RCA. They suggest that finding out what happened and why is only a 'way station' in the analysis and that 'the real purpose is to use the incident to reflect on what it reveals about the gaps and inadequacies in the healthcare system.'

The Joint Commission on Accreditation of Healthcare Organisations (JCAHO) defines RCA as 'a process for identifying the most basic or causal factor or factors that underline variation in performance, including the occurrence of an adverse sentinel event.'[3]

JCAHO defines 'sentinel event' as 'an unexpected occurrence involving death or serious physical or psychological injury, or the risk thereof'.[3]

Another organisation which provides training and support in RCA, namely Systems Improvement: TapRoot (www.taproot.com), defines RCA as:

> The most basic cause(s) that can reasonably be identified, that management has control to fix and when fixed will prevent (or significantly reduce the likelihood of) the problem's recurrence.

Already, then, we are limiting the occasions on which it might be appropriate to carry out an RCA. After all, as you will see, conducting an RCA will be a resource-intensive exercise.

The premise is that correcting problems, symptoms and apparent causes will not prevent the recurrence of an unwanted event. *Only finding and resolving the root causes of an event can do this.*

Before we consider RCA further, we need to understand something about *human error theory.*

An introduction to human error theory

James Reason has been particularly influential in aiding our understanding of human error.[4-6] He defines human error as a generic term to encompass 'all occasions in which a planned sequence of mental or physical activity fails to achieve its desired outcome', and proposes an algorithm that distinguishes between unintentional actions (slips or lapses) and intentional but mistaken actions (mistakes). A further distinction can be made between these causes of error and violations.[7]

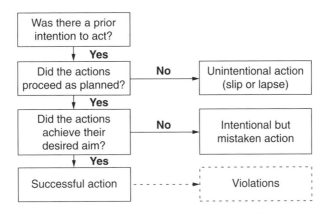

Figure 23.1 Intention–action algorithm (adapted from Reason[7]).

Slips and lapses occur when the plan is appropriate but there is a failure of execution. This may occur when the individual is distracted while performing some routine task and so deviates from what was intended.

Mistakes also occur when the action(s) go entirely as planned, but the 'rule' or 'knowledge' that is being applied to the problem is inappropriate. This could include the application of a 'good' rule in the 'wrong' circumstances, or performing a procedure for which there is contradictory or weak evidence.

Violations are deliberate deviations from procedures, guidelines or rules – not errors. They may or may not result in an adverse outcome.

While to err is human, Reason's work goes on to suggest that although human error theory starts with the individual (the person approach), we should also be looking at systems (the system approach).[6] The person approach focuses on the unsafe acts (errors and violations) of those at the sharp end, and views these unsafe acts as arising primarily from aberrant mental processes. In these circumstances it is all too easy to blame the individual healthcare professional. Traditionally, this is how healthcare organisations have approached error – by blaming individuals in a 'naming and shaming' culture.

Reason offers us a more mature view in his 'system approach'. The basic premise of this approach is that humans are fallible and therefore errors are to be expected, even in the best organisation. According to this model, errors are consequences rather than causes, having their origin in an 'upstream' systemic failure.

Developing this model, Reason describes 'active failures' (the operator's error, the impact of which is often immediate, obvious and the focus of attention) and 'latent conditions' (those factors that are normally outside the control of the operator, including the significant but often subtle contribution of poorly structured and managed organisations). Reason described the latent conditions as the 'resident pathogens' within the system which arise from those who manage the organisation. Latent conditions can translate into error-provoking conditions within the local workplace (e.g. time pressure, understaffing, inadequate equipment, fatigue, inexperience, etc.), and they can create longstanding holes or weaknesses in the defences (poor or unworkable procedures, design deficiencies, etc.). These latent conditions may lie dormant for a long time, but when they combine with the active failure of the operator they give rise to an incident (*see* Figure 23.2).

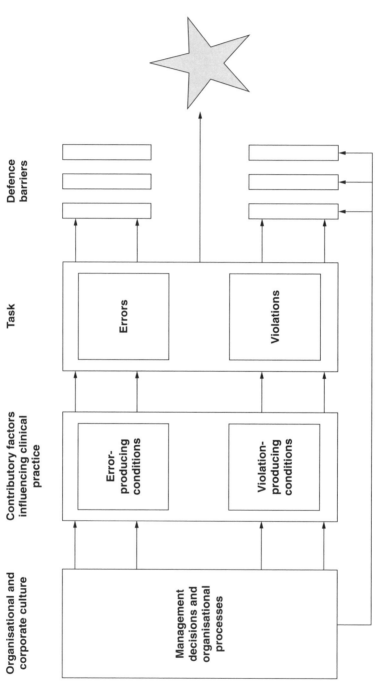

Figure 23.2 Stages of development of an organisational accident (adapted from Reason[7]).

We have explored this in detail because it is important to understand something of the theory associated with human error which underpins RCA. The latter requires that we look at the root causes which will lie in the systemic failures (the latent conditions) of an organisation.

Now we shall consider in more detail how to carry out an RCA.

Carrying out a root cause analysis

Simply put, conducting an RCA involves the following:

- the *incident* – identifying what has happened
- the *root causes* – identifying why it has happened
- the *corrective action* – identifying what can be done to prevent if from happening again.

The first stage will be to identify the chronology of events. This may be a painstaking process in which you have to piece together the facts from incident reports, medical records, witness statements, etc. Clearly this needs to be done as soon after the event as possible. Any evidence (e.g. equipment, medical devices, etc.) should also be preserved. Photographic evidence may also be helpful.

The key players involved in the incident will also need to be interviewed. Handling the interview in an appropriate and sensitive manner will be critically important. The last thing that the investigator wants to do is convey the impression that the process is about identifying an individual who can be blamed. After all, this is about finding the root causes!

Once the investigations have been carried out, the starting point is to develop a chronology of events. A 'cause-and-effect' (or fishbone) diagram may be helpful in cases where there has been one 'effect' or incident (e.g. wrong site surgery). However, if there has been a multi-factorial incident, it will be more appropriate to use a flowchart-type diagram. TapRoot® use a tool called SnapChart® which is a flow diagram on which the event is plotted at the top and the conditions below. Within the conditions are the underlying causal factors which will enable the root causes to be identified, and these are marked ▲ as shown in Figure 23.3.

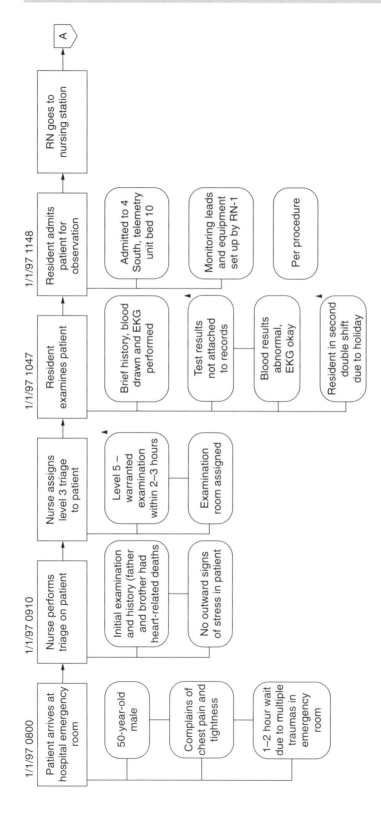

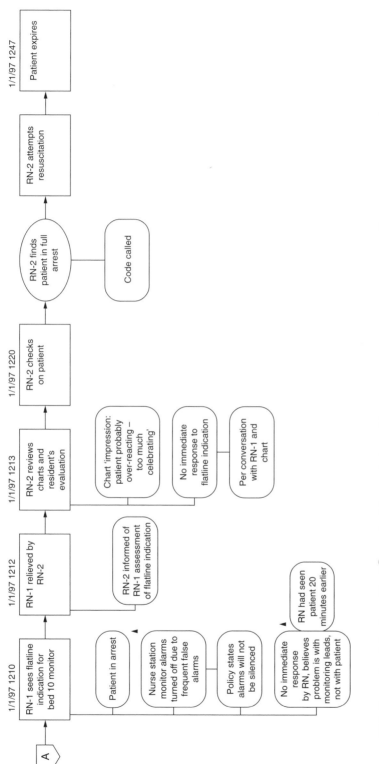
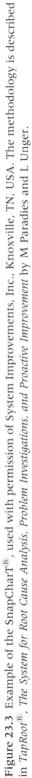

Figure 23.3 Example of the SnapCharT®, used with permission of System Improvements, Inc., Knoxville, TN, USA. The methodology is described in *TapRoot®, The System for Root Cause Analysis, Problem Investigations, and Proactive Improvement* by M Paradies and L Unger.

Identifying the root causes

Once the possible causes of the incident have been identified, you need to identify the root causes. You will need a taxonomy to enable you to do this, and there are several in use.

The Veterans' Affairs National Centre for Patient Safety has a set of triggering and triage questions (www.patientsafety.gov/concepts.html). JCAHO also has a *Framework for a Root Cause Analysis and Action Plan in Response to a Sentinel Event* (www.jcaho.org/accredited+organizations/ambulatory+care/sentinel+events/index.htm).

A preferred taxonomy is probably that developed jointly by University College London and the Association of Litigation and Risk Managers (ALARM), namely the *Protocol for the Investigation and Analysis of Clinical Incidents*[8] (www.patient safety.ucl.ac.uk/CRU-ALARMprotocol.pdf). This is a very useful publication and it provides a very helpful taxonomy for the investigation of clinical incidents (*see* Box 23.1).

Box 23.1 Taxonomy for the investigation and analysis of a clinical incident

Cause category	Possible causal factors	Sub-components underpinning causal factors
Patient	• Condition	• Complexity • Seriousness
	• Personal issues	• Personality • Language • External support • Social and family circumstances
	• Treatment	• Known risks associated with treatment
	• History	• Medical • Personal • Emotional
	• Staff–patient relationship	• Good working relationship
Individual (staff)	• Competence	• Verification of qualifications • Verification of skills and knowledge
	• Skills and knowledge	• These are possibly the same as for competence
	• Physical and mental stressors	• Motivation • Mental stressors (e.g. the effects of workload, etc. on the individual's mental state) • Physical stressors (e.g. the effects of workload, etc. on the individual's physical state)
Team	• Verbal communication	• Communication between junior and senior staff • Communication between professions • Communication outside the ward/department, etc.

Box 23.1 *Continued*

Cause category	Possible causal factors	Sub-components underpinning causal factors
Team (*continued*)	Verbal communication (*continued*)	• Adequate hand-over • Communication between staff and patient • Communication between specialties and department • Communication between staff of the same grade • Voicing disagreements and concerns • Communication between staff and relatives/carers
	• Written communication	• Incomplete/absent information (e.g. test results) • Discrepancies in the notes • Inadequately flagged notes • Legibility and signatures of records • Adequate management plan • Availability of records • Quality of information in the notes
	• Supervision and seeking help	• Availability of senior staff • Responsiveness of senior staff • Willingness of junior staff to seek help • Responsiveness of junior staff • Availability of junior staff
	• Congruence/consistency	• Similar definition of task between professionals • Similar definition of task between different grades of staff • Similar definition of task between same grade of staff
	• Leadership and responsibility	• Effective leadership • Clear definitions of responsibility
	• Staff colleagues response to incidents	• Support by peers after an incident • Support by staff of comparable grades across professions (e.g. senior nurse and junior doctor)
Task	• Availability and use of guidelines and protocols	• Procedures for reviewing and updating protocols • Availability of protocols to staff • Use of protocols • Availability of specific types of protocol (e.g. Health and Safety, etc.) • Quality of information included in the protocol • Accident and investigation procedures
	• Availability and accuracy of test results	• Tests not done • Disagreement regarding the interpretation of the test results • Need to chase up test results

Continued

Box 23.1 *Continued*

Cause category	Possible causal factors	Sub-components underpinning causal factors
Task (*continued*)	• Availability and use of decision-making aids	• Availability, use and reliability of specific types of equipment (e.g. cardiotacograph, CTG) • Availability, use and reliability of specific types of tests (e.g. blood testing) • Availability and use of a senior clinician
	• Task design	• Can the specific task be completed by a trained member of staff in adequate time and correctly?
Work environment	• Administration and systems design and operation, including notes/records	• Ease of running and review of general administration systems • Notes handling
	• Building, including design for functionality	• Maintenance management • Functionality (ergonomic assessment, e.g. lighting, space, etc.)
	• Environment	• Housekeeping • Control of the physical environment (e.g. temperature, lighting, etc.) • Movement of patients between wards/sites
	• Equipment/supplies	• Malfunction/failure/reliability • Unavailability • Maintenance management • Functionality (e.g. ergonomic design, fail-safe, standardisation)
	• Staffing availability	• (Un)availability
	• Education and training	• Induction management's influence on training • Process • Refresher training • Provision of training (in general)
	• Workload/hours of work	• Regular rest breaks • Optimal workload (neither too high nor too low) • Involved in non-job-related duties
	• Time factors	• Delays
Management and organisation	• Leadership • Organisational structure	• Strategic emphasis on patient safety • Hierarchical arrangement of staff within the organisational context • Span of control • Levels of decision making

Box 23.1 *Continued*

Cause category	Possible causal factors	Sub-components underpinning causal factors
Management and organisation (*continued*)	• Policy, standards and goals	• Mission statement and objectives of management arrangements (function) • Contract services • Human resources • Financial resources/constraints • Information services • Maintenance management • Task design • Education and training policy • Policies and procedures • Facilities and equipment • Risk management (e.g. incident reporting, adverse event investigation and analysis) • Health and Safety management (e.g. fire safety, waste management, infection control and occupational health) • Quality improvement
	• Risks imported/ exported	
	• Safety culture	Is invoked via the other organisational processes and management factors • Attitude to work, safety and others in the workplace • Provision of support mechanisms by management for all staff
	• Financial resources and constraints	
Institutional context	• Economic and regulatory context • Department of Health, Social Services and Public Safety policy and requirements • Clinical Negligence Scheme for Trusts requirements • Links with external organisations	

From the *Protocol for the Investigation and Analysis of Clinical Incidents*, reproduced with the kind permission of the Clinical Risk Unit, University College, London and the Association of Litigation and Risk Managers.

Summary

The real point of all of this is to agree some corrective actions which will flow from the root causes that have been identified. For many healthcare organisations, carrying out RCAs will be resource-intensive, as will implementing the corrective actions. The incidents that are going to be investigated will need to be chosen with care. In primary care it is to be hoped that in reality there will be few incidents that require an RCA. It will probably suffice for many incidents or near misses to be subjected to a significant event audit. However, even when carrying out a significant event audit it may be worth drawing on the University College London/Association of Litigation and Risk Managers taxonomy (*see* Box 23.1) to help to identify a wider set of issues.

References

1 Shojania KG and Wald H (2001) Root cause analysis. In: KG Shojania (ed.) *Making Health Care Safer: a critical analysis of patient safety practices*. Agency for Healthcare Research and Quality, Rockville, MD.
2 Taylor-Adams S and Vincent C (2004) *Systems Analysis of Clinical Incidents. The London Protocol*; http://csru.org.uk
3 Joint Commission Resources (2003) *Root Cause Analysis in Health Care: tools and techniques* (2e). Joint Commission Resources, Chicago, IL.
4 Reason J (1990) *Human Error*. Cambridge University Press, Cambridge.
5 Reason J (1995) Understanding adverse events: human factors. In: CA Vincent (ed.) *Clinical Risk Management*. BMJ Publications, London.
6 Reason J (2000) Human error: models and management. *BMJ.* **320**: 768–70.
7 Reason J (1993) The human factor in medical accidents. In: CA Vincent (ed.) *Medical Accidents*. Oxford Medical Publications, Oxford.
8 Clinical Risk Unit, University College London and Association of Litigation and Risk Managers (1999) *Protocol for the Investigation and Analysis of Clinical Incidents*. ALARM Secretariat, London; www.patientsafety.ucl.ac.uk/CRU-ALARMprotocol.pdf

Useful resources

• http://csru.org.uk
• www.npsa.nhs.uk/rcatoolkit/
• www.patientsafety.gov/concepts.html
• www.jcaho.org
• www.patientsafety.ucl.ac.uk/CRU-ALARMprotocol.pdf
• Dineen M (2002) *Six Steps to Root Cause Analysis*; www.consequence.org.uk

Chapter 24

Significant event audit

John Sandars

Key learning points

- Learning from significant events is familiar to most GPs.
- Significant event audit can be regarded as a mini-incident-reporting system involving the identification and rectification of threats to patient safety.
- The realisation of the potential of significant event audit requires an efficient process and effective group leadership skills.
- A particular strength of significant event audit is the building of a practice safety culture.

Introduction

Learning from *significant events* (*critical events*) is a concept familiar to most GPs, being enshrined in the case-based discussions of which everyone is aware in medical education. However, a recent estimate is that less than 20% of practices regularly use this process as part of clinical governance.[1] Significant event audit has been enthusiastically promoted as an important part of the quality improvement programme in any practice, and also as a method for identifying learning needs in the development of personal development plans, a cornerstone for CPD and accreditation. It also has great potential for improving patient safety in primary care.

Background

The role of significant event audit in patient safety is to view the process as a 'mini'-incident-reporting system in which adverse incidents are identified and made sense of, and then actions are taken to prevent similar occurrences in the future.

The basic process of significant event audit can be undertaken in a series of steps as follows:

1 consideration of identified events
2 collection of data on these events
3 holding a meeting to discuss the events
4 documentation.

There has been an intuitive acceptance of this by many doctors, and many PCOs have placed significant event audit on their clinical governance agenda.

The process of significant event audit

The process follows a well-described stepwise procedure.[2]

1 Consideration of significant events

The definition is wide-ranging – 'any event thought by anyone in the team to be significant in the care of patients or the conduct of the practice'. All practice members are encouraged to identify significant events, including those that have positive aspects in addition to those that have adverse aspects. It has been suggested that practices begin with a core list of events, including the areas of preventive care, acute care, chronic disease management and practice organisation. A useful way for a PCT to encourage practices to start undertaking significant event audit is to begin by using the latter to capture events and near misses that might have occurred as a result of poor communication from secondary care.

2 Data collection

Mechanisms for identifying and reporting significant events are developed in the practice. This is usually achieved by the completion of a pre-designed form.

3 Significant event meetings

It is recognised that the heart of significant event auditing is the meeting held to discuss events. The meeting allows discussion of what happened and why, and considers the implications of the event for the quality of care being provided by the practice, but most importantly of all there is the development of a clear action plan. The result may be that there is no change to current practice or procedures required, and congratulations may be due to the team, or a conventional audit may be required to ascertain the extent of the problem, or immediate action may be required to prevent the event from occurring again. Subsequent follow-up is clearly a feature if the process is to be regarded as an audit, rectifying identified shortfalls in care.

4 Documentation

Keeping a record of the salient points and the action plan is considered to be a key component of significant event audit. This record is usually regarded as confidential and anonymous. If agencies outside the individual practice require information (e.g. for clinical governance or CPD), only minimal information is provided.

> **Box 24.1** The suggested main steps involved in performing a significant event audit
>
> 1 Consider significant events for audit.
> 2 Collect data on these events:
>   • identification of events for analysis
>   • recording details of cases.
> 3 Hold a meeting to discuss the events:
>   • implications of events
>   • discussions of cases
>   • decisions about cases:
>   – immediate action
>   – no change in practice
>   – congratulations
>   – perform conventional audit
>   • follow-up of cases.
> 4 Documentation.

The benefits of significant event audit

The big question is whether significant event audit improves patient safety. The available evidence demonstrates that there is improved quality of care, with a beneficial impact on both clinical care and practice administration. In a 1-year study of ten practices (both urban and rural), 177 clinical and 109 administrative events were identified.[2] A wide range of topics was covered, and 86% of the decisions made were implemented. Overall, nine of the ten practices were satisfied with the process and benefits of performing significant event audit.

In a single practice case study, significant event audit increased the effectiveness of a primary healthcare team caring for terminally ill patients, improving information exchange between key workers, continuity of care and changes in medication.[3]

Qualitative evaluation of significant event audit consistently identifies the improvements in primary healthcare team functioning that have been reported by practice team members.[2–5] The wide range of benefits is shown in Box 24.2. Overall, there is increased communication and trust within the team.

> **Box 24.2** Reported practice team benefits of significant event audit
>
> • Improved team communication
> • Greater understanding of roles
> • Participation in decision making
> • Opportunity to give and share ideas
> • More cohesive approach to working together
> • Opportunity to receive reassurance

Evaluation following the introduction of significant event audit into a single practice gives some further insights into the process.[4] The main focus of topics was related to the day-to-day running of the practice, especially inter-disciplinary communication issues. The 26 identified issues resulted in 62 separate solutions, of which 21 solutions had been acted upon by the practice. The most common reason for not taking any action was deferment by the group for further discussion.

There is an integral relationship between quality of care and patient safety. Many of the identified events were related to patient safety issues, such as delays in cancer diagnosis.

The difficulties of significant event audit and how to overcome them

All studies have acknowledged difficulties when introducing significant event audit into a practice.[2-5] These are listed in Box 24.3. It is immediately apparent that these identified factors are interrelated.

Box 24.3 Reported difficulties of significant event audit

- Logistics of meeting
  - Time
  - Size
- Confidentiality
- Feeling that it imposed on members of staff
- Conflicts between members of the group
  - Gender
  - Position in practice hierarchy
- Doctor domination as leader
- Lack of congratulations
- Topic no longer of current concern
- Superficial, with lack of decisions
- No follow-through with regard to decisions
- Lack of personal support after meeting

The main suggestions for overcoming these difficulties are related to effective leadership of the process. Suggestions include a fixed structure to the meetings, setting ground rules, variation in time to suit part-time staff, summarising the suggested actions at the end of the meeting, and selection of topics for discussion, as some events may be too emotionally laden and need to be managed effectively.

Developing an evidence-based approach to performing significant event audit

The evidence suggests that for a practice to introduce a successful significant event programme, it is important to consider certain logistic factors before beginning the process. There are no correct solutions, but they need to be thought about and decisions made. Each general practice is different – this is a strength, but it can also make it difficult to follow a guide to practice. Anyone who is planning to introduce significant event audit needs to consider how each factor can be resolved in their practice to ensure that it has the best chance of working.

Leadership issues

The importance of good leadership for the process cannot be over-emphasised. The ideal leader should be a person whom everyone respects and trusts. The person should be enthusiastic about the process but should be careful not to dominate it. The ideal candidate may be an existing practice member, but my personal experience of working with numerous groups has led me to believe that an external facilitator may be the best person for many groups.

Planning to introduce significant event audit

Consider the following factors:

1   time of meeting
2   place of meeting
3   membership of the group
4   length of meeting
5   frequency of meetings.

Time of meeting

It is important to ensure that the meeting takes place at a time that is convenient for all team members. Remember that many practice staff, including GPs, are part-time. It may be worth considering varying the time on a rotational basis. Some practices arrange meetings as part of the regular practice meeting, while others hold separate meetings.

Place of meeting

Many practices do not have a meeting room that is large enough to accommodate all of the practice team.

Membership of the group

The strength of significant event audit is the multi-disciplinary aspect with all of the team present. However, it is important to remember that many practices have a large extended primary healthcare team that includes practice-employed and attached staff.

Length of meeting

Most people have a short attention span, and it is unlikely that more than 30 minutes will be spent presenting and discussing an event.

Frequency of meetings

It is important to decide how often the group should meet.

Planning the process of significant event audit

Consider the following factors:

1 identification of the events
2 collection of the events
3 selection of events
4 discussion of events
5 documentation of events

1 Identification of the events

The definition 'any event thought by anyone in the team to be significant in the care of patients or the conduct of the practice' is important, as it includes apparently trivial events (which may act as precursors to more serious events), and it also encourages the practice to include events that are positive and can be celebrated.

2 Collection of the events

Once the event has been identified by the practice member, it has to be recorded and made available for the subsequent discussion. The recording form (or the form on the computer system) should note the context of the event and sufficient factual details to enable possible causes to be identified. These records need to be placed in a secure place and made readily available for the meeting. Some practices have a 'postbox' in which the reports are placed.

3 Selection of events

It is helpful for the leader to select the events prior to the meeting. This is beneficial for several reasons. It is important that events which the team can celebrate are regularly introduced, especially when the process is first being introduced into a practice and if the group is going through a time when all they appear to be discussing are quite emotive topics. Sometimes the event is no longer 'hot' and has been dealt with prior to the meeting, and sometimes the topic is too emotionally laden, so that it has to be managed sensitively. It is also helpful to ensure that a variety of topics are discussed that reflect the wide context of general practice. A suggested matrix includes both clinical and administrative topics.

4 Discussion of events

This should be a structured process to ensure that important lessons are learned from the event. There may be several outcomes – immediate actions may need to be taken, a conventional audit may need to be performed to find out whether the identified problem is widespread in the practice, or no action may need to be taken and good care may be celebrated.

Sometimes the group process can become no more than a cosy chat, without identifying the real causes and solutions, but equally it can become an inquisitorial session. Neither process is helpful, and skilled group leadership is required.

5 Documentation of events

It is important that the proposed actions are recorded. This allows follow-up to ascertain whether they have indeed been acted upon. People like to see that they have spent their precious time productively.

After the significant event audit meeting

There are still important tasks to be done once the meeting is over. Group members may feel upset and 'emotionally bruised'. The proposed actions have to be acted upon. It is helpful to reflect on the group process before running the next session, considering what worked well and what did not work so well.

Significant event audit and the new GMS contract

The new General Medical Services (GMS) contract for primary care has focused on quality and outcomes, an integral part of which is improving patient safety.[6] GPs are for the first time financially rewarded for achieving various performance targets. There is a practice standard for undertaking significant event review, which is at two levels in the area of education and training (*see* Box 24.4).

Box 24.4 The standards for significant event review in the new GMS contract

Education 2 4 points	The practice has undertaken a minimum of six significant event reviews in the past 3 years
Education 7 4 points	The practice has undertaken a minimum of 12 significant event reviews in the past 3 years which include (if these have occurred): • any death occurring on the practice premises • two new cancer diagnoses • two deaths where terminal care has taken place at home • one patient complaint • one suicide • one section under the Mental Health Act

---

Conclusion

Significant event audit combines the identification of adverse events with analysis and rectification in an easily accessible form. A particular strength of significant event audit is the development of an organisational culture in which safety becomes a focus. Increasingly there is recognition that culture is a major determinant of patient safety and that cultural change is essential to ensure long-lasting patient safety improvements.[7]

Resources for significant event audit

Reporting and recording significant event audit

See Appendices 24.1 and 24.2.

Introducing significant event audit

Practical half-day workshops to help practices introduce significant event audit are available from MPS Risk Consulting. Contact details are as follows:

> MPS Risk Consulting
> Granary Wharf House
> Leeds
> LS11 5PY
>
> Tel: 0845 605 4000 (UK only); +44 (0) 113 243 6436 (all other countries).
>
> Website: www.mps-riskconsulting.com
> Email: riskconsulting@mps.org.uk

There is also an excellent article that describes the basic details:

* Robinson LA, Stacy R, Spencer JA and Bhopal RS (1995) How to do it: facilitated case discussions for significant event auditing. *BMJ*. **311**: 315–18.

References

1 School of Health and Related Research (2002) *Significant Event Audit and Reporting in General Practice*. ScHARR, Sheffield.
2 Pringle M, Bradley CP, Carmichael CM, Wallis H and Moore A (1995) *Significant Event Auditing*. Occasional Paper 70. Royal College of General Practitioners, London.
3 Benett IJ and Danczak AF (1994) Terminal care: improving teamwork in primary care using significant event analysis. *Eur J Cancer Care*. **3**: 54–7.
4 Sweeney G, Westcott R and Stead J (2000) The benefits of significant event audit in primary care: a case study. *J Clin Govern*. **8**: 128–34.
5 Westcott R, Sweeney G and Stead J (2000) Significant event audit in practice: a preliminary study. *Fam Pract*. **17**: 173–7.
6 NHS Confederation and General Practitioners Committee (2003) *Investing in General Practice: the new General Medical Services contract*. British Medical Association, London.
7 Department of Health (2001) *Building a Safer NHS for Patients. Implementing 'An Organisation With a Memory'*. The Stationery Office, London.

Appendix 24.1: Sample incident reporting form for use in significant event audit

ADVERSE INCIDENT REPORT FORM This form should be filed separately from medical records. Write clearly and in black ink.	*PRACTICE STAMP*

PATIENT DETAILS
Surname: Date of birth:

Forename: Sex: Male/female:
Address:

DETAILS OF INCIDENT (what happened, treatment required, what immediate action was taken and any further treatment required):

DATE AND TIME OF INCIDENT:	LOCATION:

PERSONS INVOLVED (specify name and designation of staff involved, and any other persons):

EQUIPMENT, SUBSTANCE OR DEVICE INVOLVED:

Does RIDDOR form need to be completed or does Medical Devices Agency need to be contacted?   Yes/No

RESULT OF ENQUIRY (including details of any preventive actions taken/alterations to systems, etc.)

Name: . . . .   Position: . . . .   Date: . . . .

Signature: . . . .

Appendix 24.2: Sample recording form for use in significant event audit

Significant event analysis

Significant event:

Issues arising from incident and discussion	
Positive points	
Concerns	
Suggestions	
Action	

Chapter 25

Risk management: how to reduce the likelihood of medication errors

Mark Dinwoodie

Key learning points

- Communication between healthcare professionals and between healthcare professionals and patients is of paramount importance.
- A structured approach to *medicines management* should be adopted.
- The new GMS GP contract includes 10 medicines management quality indicators.
- Improving patient concordance can help to reduce medication errors.
- Using computers effectively can help significantly in the risk management process with regard to medication.
- The controlled drugs regulations are complex but important to understand.

There are a number of ways of trying to reduce the likelihood of errors occurring. These range from national initiatives to safer systems within general practice and increased individual responsibility for appropriate prescribing.

The key to reducing medication errors is to understand the underlying cause of the error. Detailed *root cause analysis* (i.e. getting to the bottom of exactly what caused the error) is invaluable. As in other areas of risk management, concentrating on the underlying systems (i.e. the latent errors) is likely to be more productive and beneficial than just looking at the active error made by the individual. This encourages changes to systems to reduce the likelihood of future error. The use of significant event analysis is linked to this. As outlined in the Department of Health's document, *Building a Safer NHS for Patients*,[1] the cause of medication errors is often due to multiple failures in the system. This has commonly been likened to the *Swiss-cheese* model, where for an error to occur, there have to be holes in several layers of defence. Similarly, in order to try to reduce the likelihood of errors, several layers of defence or error traps need to be incorporated into the system.

The Centre for Medication Error Prevention at the University of Derby, established by the European Foundation for the Advancement of Healthcare Practitioners, aims to generate quality data on medication errors, to develop products and systems to reduce error and to raise the profile of medication errors. The website contains useful case examples (www.medication-errors.org.uk/).

Over the last few years a number of Government health organisations have been established that have a significant role in this area in setting standards, monitoring medical error and helping develop initiatives to improve the quality of prescribing. These include the NPSA (www.npsa.nhs.uk) with its national monitoring system for errors, and the NPC (www.npc.co.uk), which has produced (among other things) the resource document *GP Prescribing Support*.[2]

Medicines management

Recently the concept of *medicines management* has evolved. This is a system of processes and behaviours that determines how medicines are used by patients and by the NHS. In September 2000, the Department of Health approached the NPC to co-ordinate a three-year national MMS programme, following the publication of *Pharmacy in the Future: implementing the NHS Plan*.[3] In their publication *Modernising Medicines Management*,[4] the NPC and the National Primary Care Research Centre state that 'Effective medicines management should: improve health; improve patient care and satisfaction; make better use of professional skills; deliver effective clinical governance and maximise use of resources available.'

The Medicines Management Action Team (MMAT), based at the NPC, was established in 2001 with the remit of helping organisations to improve the way in which medicines are managed in primary care using the collaborative methodology. The National MMS collaborative programme started the first wave of its programme in 2001.

It states four aims to support the overall goal of 'optimising prescribing and improving health outcomes and patient experiences when medicines are involved', namely:

1 to identify and address unmet pharmacological need
2 to help patients to make better use of medicines, thereby achieving real improvements in health
3 to develop innovative approaches to medicines management that have the patient's needs uppermost while at the same time improving service efficiency and reducing waste
4 to provide convenient access to a range of MMSs in different environments through multi-disciplinary working which builds on the strengths of pharmacists.

Useful examples of locally developed initiatives can be found at www.npc.co.uk/mms/index.htm

In the initial pilot sites, four global improvement measures were used.

1 The average number of repeat items prescribed for all patients aged 65 years or over who take four or more regular items of medication, *the aim being to reduce unnecessary polypharmacy.*
2 The percentage of requests for repeat prescriptions that do not include all of the regular repeat items for a patient, *the aim being to improve efficiency and reduce waste.*

3 The percentage of patients leaving the GP surgery each month with a prescription for one or more items that do not have specific dosage instructions, *the aim being to improve safety, efficiency and concordance.*

4 The percentage of patients receiving a regular prescription who answer 'Yes' to the question 'Did you experience any problems in ordering or receiving your last supply of medicines?', *the aim being to improve efficiency and service for patients.*

The new GMS GP contract quality indicators

The new contract includes 10 quality indicators under 'Medicines Management', which give some indication of what the Department of Health considers to be important. They are listed below.

- Details of prescribed medicines are available to the prescriber at each surgery consultation.
- The practice possesses the equipment and in-date emergency drugs necessary to treat anaphylaxis.
- There is a system for checking the expiry dates of emergency drugs on at least an annual basis.
- The time interval from requesting a prescription to availability for collection by the patient is 72 hours or less (excluding weekends and bank holidays).
- A medication review is recorded in the notes in the preceding 15 months for all patients who are being prescribed four or more repeat medicines (standard is 80%).
- The practice meets the PCO prescribing adviser at least annually and agrees up to three actions related to prescribing.
- Where the practice has responsibility for administering regular injectable neuroleptic medication, there is a system to identify and follow up patients who do not attend.
- The time interval from requesting a prescription to availability for collection by the patient is 48 hours or less (excluding weekends and bank holidays).
- A medication review is recorded in the notes in the preceding 15 months for all patients who are being prescribed repeat medicines (standard is 80%).
- The practice meets the PCO prescribing adviser at least annually, has agreed up to three actions related to prescribing, and has subsequently provided evidence of change.

In addition there are a few quality indicators relating to medication in the records situation:

- the medicines that a patient is receiving are clearly listed in his or her record
- there is a designated place for the recording of drug allergies and adverse reactions in the notes and these are clearly recorded
- for repeat medicines, an indication for the drug can be identified in the records (for drugs added to the repeat prescription with effect from 1 April 2004).

General principles for reducing the risk of medication errors

A number of strategies at different points in the prescribing, dispensing and administration processes can be introduced in order to try to reduce errors. These include the following.

- *Removing the hazard (including differentiation – separating or identifying similar things).* For example, ensuring that drugs with similar packaging or similar-sounding names are stored in separate areas of a pharmacy or general practice treatment room, removing a drug like penicillamine from the computer database to avoid confusion, as it is very rarely prescribed in primary care, using a compliance aid for a patient with memory problems, discontinuing telephone repeat-prescribing requests.
- *Adding alerts to highlight potential errors (reminders or giving immediate insight into how or why to use or not use something).* For example, computer software warning of potential drug interactions or allergies in general practice, warning labels on drugs that are easily confused due to their names or packaging, adding alert messages to the computer that highlight patients with similar names, overdue review date indicated by changing colour or flashing, alerting clinician to medication that should be prescribed weekly rather than daily (the NPSA has distributed a computer warning alert for methotrexate), pictures indicating inappropriate action (e.g. with a large cross through them).
- *Preventing the action from being completed (constraints).* For example, the computer preventing a prescription for penicillin from being issued for a patient who has an entry for penicillin allergy.
- *Minimising the consequences of error.* For example, having appropriate antidotes available, such as naloxone for opiates or resuscitation equipment and adrenaline for vaccines in the event of anaphylaxis.
- *Increasing the availability of prescribing decision support.* Prescribing should be in accordance with up-to-date evidence and guidance. This includes guidelines regarding the appropriateness of medication [e.g. PRODIGY (www.prodigy.nhs.uk), NICE (www.nice.org.uk), Clinical Evidence (www.nelh.nhs.uk/clinicalevidence) or other recognised authorities, such as the Scottish Intercollegiate Guidelines Network (SIGN) (www.sign.ac.uk), UKMI (www.ukmi.nhs.uk) and the *Drug and Therapeutics Bulletin* (www.which.net/health/dtb)], as well as easier access to and use of community or hospital pharmacists for advice.
- *Encouraging patients to acquire knowledge of and involvement in their medication.* Patients can be a useful source of knowledge about their medication and what they should be receiving. This is being facilitated through the Medicines Partnership Programme (www.medicines-partnership.org). The Expert Patients Programme can also be a useful resource (www.doh.gov.uk/cmo/progress/expertpatient).
- *Considering how compliance and concordance issues could be improved.* For example, through better communication, explanation and use of compliance aids.
- *Improving training and education for healthcare professionals.* Healthcare professionals need to keep up to date in the field of therapeutics and medication and

to ensure that they undergo CPD in this field. A regular meeting with the local PCO Prescribing Advisor is likely to be beneficial.

- *Improving communication between healthcare professionals.* Community pharmacists are a relatively under-utilised resource in many general practices, yet they are likely to have an increasing role in the future following the Department of Health's publication *Pharmacy in the future: implementing the NHS Plan.*[3] Improved communication between orthodox and complementary practitioners would also be helpful.
- *Human factors.* For example, addressing the environmental and situational factors that make individuals more likely to make errors (e.g. distractions, workload, working environment, inadequate management, unsuitable equipment and lack of training), and ensuring that staff have sufficient knowledge and experience to carry out the task they are expected to perform (this relates equally to dispensing and practice staff).
- *Making greater use of reporting and monitoring systems.* CSM (http://medicines. mhra.gov.uk/aboutagency/regframework/csm/csmhome.htm) collates all information supplied to it on adverse drug reactions. Many GPs are familiar with this as the 'Yellow card' system, but sadly most doctors infrequently use it. It is now possible to complete these on-line. The black triangle symbol in the *BNF* identifies newly licensed medicines that are monitored intensively by the CSM and MHRA, who have combined the roles of the old MCA and MDA (www.mhra.gov.uk). The NPSA has rolled out its National Reporting and Learning System (NRLS) across the NHS. NHS staff anywhere in England and Wales are able to report patient safety incidents, including prevented patient safety incidents (known as near misses), that they are involved in or witness. The issue of methotrexate safety is a good example of how the NPSA has responded to an increasing number of adverse events reported about methotrexate, by producing computer software alerts, a patient-held monitoring and dosage record and guidance for the safe prescribing, monitoring and dispensing of methotrexate for both patients and health professionals.
- *Audit.* Consider using audit to maintain clinical governance with regard to prescribing. Reviewing the practice's PACT data can be useful.

Specific prescribing principles for reducing the risk of medication errors

Before prescribing any drug for a patient, check the following.

- The medication is appropriate and indicated for the condition.
- Does the patient have any drug allergies? Ask them, and check the medical record. Computer records may not have been updated from manual records. It is important to ensure that allergies are entered into the computer in a way that prevents the drug from being prescribed to the patient.
- Ensure that you have all of the medical information about the patient before prescribing. This includes past and current medical history (e.g. renal or hepatic impairment). The *BNF*[5] has useful appendices.
- Is the patient pregnant, trying to conceive or breastfeeding? If in doubt, ask

them. The *BNF*[5] has useful appendices, and *Prescribing in Pregnancy*[6] is a useful reference book.

- Does the medication interact with any prescribed or over-the-counter medication that the patient is already taking? With the increasing popularity of complementary and alternative therapy, there are increasing numbers of people taking homeopathic, herbal and over-the-counter preparations. For example, St John's Wort, which is used to treat depression, has a wide range of drug interactions. A useful website is www.mca.gov.uk/ourwork/licensingmeds/herbalmeds/herbalsafety.htm

- Consider giving reduced quantities of medication to patients with mental illness who might be vulnerable to taking an overdose, or who have a history of doing so. It is also worth trying to prescribe a less toxic medication in these circumstances in case an overdose is taken.

- Prescribe *generically* unless *proprietary* prescribing is important due to different formulations (e.g. lithium, theophylline, nifedipine modified-release, diltiazem modified-release, cyclosporin and mesalazine).

- Double-check for drugs with similar-sounding names.

- All prescribing should now occur using rINNs rather than BANs.

- Counsel the patient about possible side-effects, including whether the drug might affect work, operation of machinery or driving, how to take the medication, whether any monitoring is needed and what follow-up is necessary. It is considered appropriate to give the patient as much information about side-effects as you would want to know yourself. It is also worth advising them whether they should avoid taking the medication with alcohol. The language we use in communicating risk is open to misunderstanding such as *common*, *rare* and *unlikely*, with patients tending to overestimate the level of risk.[7]

- Consider reinforcing the instructions and explanation with a drug information leaflet (often available on computer systems). A medicines reminder chart might be helpful. Many patients do not know the purpose of their medication. Including the purpose of the medicine on the label when prescribing (for example *one daily for high blood pressure*) could help patients on multiple medicines to know what each is for and improve concordance.[8]

- Prescribing over the telephone without having seen the patient carries a higher level of risk and is generally best avoided.

Specific dispensing issues

- Consider ways of reducing the likelihood of confusing similar-sounding or similar-looking drugs (e.g. by means of warnings, labels or storing on different shelves).

- Use clearer labelling and packaging to allow better differentiation between similar-sounding and similar-looking medications.

- It is a legal requirement to include the following on the medication label: name of patient; name of dispensing organisation; date of dispensing; directions for use; *KEEP OUT OF REACH OF CHILDREN*; *FOR EXTERNAL USE ONLY* (where appropriate). It is also considered good practice to include: the name and strength of the medication; form of medicine; quantity dispensed; specific dosage instructions; relevant cautionary labels.

- Consider environmental factors (e.g. distractions, lighting and workload).
- Ensure that staff are adequately trained, supervised and sufficiently experienced.
- Use a double-checking procedure.
- Clarify any clinical concerns or administrative problems about a prescription with the prescriber.
- Ensure there is a robust checking system for unsigned prescriptions, unfamiliar medicines and controlled drugs.
- Carry out a risk assessment of dispensing procedures, bearing in mind the factors that contribute to dispensing errors.[9] Produce a dispensing protocol.
- Carry out regular audit and quality control.
- The Royal Pharmaceutical Society,[10] which has a number of useful resources and publications, recommends using the mnemonic **HELP** for dispensing:
  - How much has been dispensed
  - Expiry date check
  - Label checks for the correct patient's name, drug name, dose and warnings
  - Product check (i.e. check that the correct medication and strength are supplied.
- Discuss with the patient or their carer their understanding of the medication.
- Medicines issued OOH by GPs as part of an OOH service or dispensing service are not immune from the regulations regarding labelling. The DoH has recently produced guidance on the availability of medicines OOH.[11]
- With regard to product liability, keep a record of batch numbers and manufacturer and invoices for 11 years.
- There are specific requirements regarding containers, packaging and collection (particularly from remote sites).
- Since January 1999, all medication should be supplied with a patient information leaflet.
- The Dispensing Doctors Association produced dispensing guidelines in 2003 incorporating important legal aspects and good practice in relation to dispensing for dispensing doctors.[12]

Issues relating to concordance and compliance

- Discuss the benefits and risks with the patient before prescribing.
- Involve them in the decision-making process as much as they want to be.
- Use explanation leaflets (e.g. drug information leaflets) to reinforce what has been said.
- Ask the patient to summarise their understanding of the purpose of the medication and how they will take it.
- Assess whether the patient is likely to have any difficulty taking the medication and whether a compliance aid or different formulation would be more appropriate.
- Consider whether the patient is likely to have difficulty remembering to take their medication.

Specific administration principles

- Always double-check the name, dose and expiry date on the vial or container before administering a drug to a patient.
- Always double-check the identity of the patient to whom you are giving the drug, and make sure that there are no contraindications or allergies to the drug.
- Never give an injection that you have not drawn up yourself.
- For dispensed or personally administered items, record details of the drug (dose, quantity and formulation), batch number, expiry date, supplier and manufacturer.
- Where appropriate, ensure that you have appropriate drugs and equipment available in the event of a serious reaction (e.g. adrenaline for anaphylaxis and naloxone for diamorphine use).
- Where appropriate, give clear instructions to a carer or relative about how any medication should be administered. An information leaflet about the medication should be provided by the pharmacist for all medication dispensed in primary care.
- Consider using a compliance aid such as a *dossett box*. Further information is available at www.medicines-partnership.org/medication-review/toolkit.
- A district nurse, community pharmacist or health visitor might be a useful health professional to help monitor whether administration of medicines has been successful in specific circumstances.
- A simple way of trying to reduce the risks of drug administration error involves the *five rights* – right medicine, right dose, right route, right patient and right time.[9]

As mentioned earlier in the chapter, there is clear evidence that patients are not taking medication in the way that it was intended. Although some of this may be a result of a clear decision not to concord with treatment, some will be due to accidental incorrect self-administration of medication, or being given it incorrectly by a carer, relative or healthcare professional. Communication and explanation will play an important part in trying to improve the administration of medication.

There is a useful summary of recommendations for safer prescribing in the Department of Health's publication *Building a Safer NHS for Patients: improving medication safety*.[9] In addition the DoH recently published *Management of Medicines*. It includes useful advice regarding good practice along with useful resources.[8]

Box 25.1 Writing and issuing a prescription

- Write legibly if the prescription is not computer generated.
- Include the patient's name, age or date of birth, and address.
- Write clear unambiguous instructions on dosage, frequency and route of administration. This is particularly important with increasing or decreasing doses (e.g tailing off of steroids, or increasing the dose of an antidepressant).
- Document what has been prescribed and what warnings have been given to the patient in the medical record.
- Re-read the prescription before you hand it to the patient, to check that it is correct.
- Further information is available at the front of the *BNF* (a useful website is: www.BNF.org).[5]

Computers and medication errors

The increased use of computers in primary care will hopefully soon confine the illegible prescription (due to the doctor's poor handwriting) to history. Most people consider that the introduction of computers has helped to reduce the likelihood of some aspects of medication error. Computer software systems have improved the repeat-prescribing process, allowed the highlighting of alerts such as allergies, certain contraindications, drug–drug and disease–drug interactions, and dosage hazards. They have allowed a more systematic approach to audit, facilitating the optimum management of and prescribing for patients with chronic diseases, and they have facilitated audits for ensuring that monitoring of certain drugs (e.g. lithium, thyroxine and amiodarone) has occurred. Formularies can be designed or imported to the system (e.g. listing generic drugs preferentially or an agreed local formulary). Prescribing guidelines can be incorporated into the system.

In the USA there is evidence that computerised prescription entry can reduce the rate of serious medication errors by 55%.[13] The fifth edition of *In Safer Hands* outlines how computers can support patient safety.[14]

The IT abilities of the personnel who are using computers and the quality of the data entered into them can significantly limit their usefulness. Practices therefore need to have a robust system to ensure that patients' notes are summarised, Read-coded and have allergies entered into the computer in an appropriate way. In some practices there is great variation in the level of enthusiasm with which different doctors use computers. Clearly this is likely to make any systems within the practice prone to errors and omissions if the computer is relied upon.

The computer software is by no means perfect, and there are frustrations, for example, that the interaction warnings are over-cautious and may lead to inappropriate under-prescribing. Allergies on one system can be entered in a variety of ways, but only when they are entered in one of these ways will the computer flag up a warning if the clinician tries to prescribe that drug.

To help make the most of your computer in terms of correct data entry, advice can be obtained from PRIMIS at www.primis.nhs.uk.

Controlled drugs (CDs)

Following recent high-profile cases such as that of Shipman, it is not surprising that the prescribing of opiates and their relevant documentation by GPs came under closer scrutiny. A recent article highlighted the fact that many GPs found the CD regulations confusing.[15] The NPC has produced a very useful document *A Guide to Good Practice in the Management of Controlled Drugs in Primary Care (England)*,[16] and readers are recommended to refer to this for up-to-date guidance of good practice regarding all aspects of CDs. They plan to update this as recommendations from the Shipman Inquiry are implemented by the government. It was last updated in November 2004. This also includes a useful audit template; www.npc.co.uk/publications/audit_of_cds2.doc.

Clinical advice on prescribing for drug addicts is beyond the scope of this chapter (*see Drug Misuse and Dependence: Guidelines on Clinical Management*, available from the Department of Health website).[17] However, doctors should use great caution when prescribing drugs that have an addictive potential (e.g. benzodiazepines). The Misuse of Drugs (Supply to Addicts) Regulations 1997 specify that only medical practitioners who hold a special licence issued by the Home Secretary may prescribe, administer or supply diamorphine, dipipanone or cocaine for the treatment of drug addiction.

Many doctors will have had prescriptions for CDs returned by the pharmacist because they have been completed incorrectly. The main legislation covering drugs control is the Misuse of Drugs Act 1971, which prohibits certain activities, in particular the manufacture, supply and possession of CDs, and outlines the penalties according to the following three classes (I have only included the more commonly used drugs; for a full list *see* the *BNF*[5]):

- *class A* – cocaine, ecstacy, lysergide (LSD), (dia)morphine, opium and pethidine
- *class B* – oral amphetamines, barbiturates and codeine
- *class C* – buprenorphine, most benzodiazepines, cannabis and anabolic steroids.

The most important regulations affecting medical practitioners are the Misuse of Drugs Regulations 2001 (MDR), which define the classes of person authorised to supply and possess CDs while acting in their professional capacity, and specify the conditions under which these activities may be carried out. The regulations divide CDs into five categories, each specifying the requirements governing such activities as import, export, production, supply, possession, prescribing and record-keeping.

- *Schedule 1* – includes drugs such as cannabis and LSD. Possession and supply of these drugs is prohibited except in accordance with Home Office authority (e.g. for research).
- *Schedule 2* – includes drugs such as (dia)morphine, pethidine, amphetamine, methadone and cocaine. These drugs may be prescribed, lawfully supplied and possessed when on prescription. They are subject to full CD requirements relating to prescriptions, safe custody, the need to keep registers, etc.
- *Schedule 3* – includes barbiturates, buprenorphine and temazepam. They are subject to special prescription requirements (except for phenobarbitone and

temazepam), but not to the safe custody requirements (except for bupre-norphine and temazepam).

- *Schedule 4* – includes in Part 1 benzodiazepines other than temazepam which are subject to minimal control, and in Part 2 anabolic steroids. Controlled drug prescription requirements do not apply, and they are not subject to safe custody requirements.
- *Schedule 5* – includes preparations of low strength whose only requirement is retention of invoices for 2 years.

Specific issues relating to controlled drugs (CDs)

Writing a prescription

Prescriptions ordering CDs subject to prescription requirements (Schedule 2 and part of Schedule 3) must be signed and dated by the prescriber (a computer-generated date is not acceptable, although a date stamp is) and specify the prescriber's address. The prescription must always state *in the prescriber's own handwriting in ink* (this does not apply to temazepam):

- the name and address of the patient
- the formulation (e.g. tablets or solution)
- the strength (where there is more than one strength)
- the total quantity of the preparation, or the number of dose units, *in both figures and words*
- the dose
- the words 'For dental treatment only', if issued by a dentist.

A prescription may order a CD to be dispensed in instalments, in which case the amount and intervals must be specified. A total of 14 days' treatment by instalment may be prescribed using FP10MDA (currently blue) in England and Wales. In Scotland, GP10 should be used. Clearly legible handwriting is extremely important, as it is an 'offence' to issue an incomplete or invalid prescription. A prescription is valid for 13 weeks for CDs (as opposed to 6 months for ordinary prescriptions).

Phenobarbitone prescriptions can be computer generated, but the date must be entered by hand by the prescriber.

Ordering, possessing and supplying CDs

Doctors, dentists and pharmacists can possess and supply CDs in their professional capacities, and patients can possess them with a prescription, Registered nurses in primary care may administer CDs when these are prescribed by a GP, and community midwives can possess and administer pethidine and pentazocine.

CDs may be obtained by a GP for stock, but any requisition must be signed by the recipient, and state the name, address and profession of the recipient, the purpose for which the drug is required and the total quantity to be supplied. The GP can send a representative to collect the CD, but the requisition must be accompanied by a statement signed by the GP. In an emergency, a GP can obtain a supply immediately, but a signed requisition must be provided within 24 hours.

GPs must not use patient-specific prescriptions for CDs to replace or 'top-up' their 'doctor's bag' or practice stock, even if the stock was used for that patient initially. The stock levels held in a GP practice should be kept to a minimum. Invoices for CD stock received should be kept for longer than the mandatory 2 years, ideally 7 years.[16]

CD register and records

Any person who is authorised to supply CDs must keep a CD register, which must be chronological and be a bound book, not loose-leaf. In addition, entries should be made on the day when the drugs were obtained or supplied or, if this is not practicable, on the next day. Entries must be indelible and must not be altered, cancelled or obliterated. Corrections may be made by way of a footnote or marginal note specifying the date of the correction. The register must not be used for any other purposes, and must be preserved for at least 2 years after the date of the last entry (though good practice would now suggest 7). For CDs received into stock from a supplier, a record of the date, supplier, quantity and name, form and strength of CD should be entered into the register. Wherever possible it would be good practice for two members of staff to check all stock received and removed and both individuals to sign the register. Running balances should be kept, although this is not yet a legal requirement.[16] A separate register, or part of the register, must be used for each class of drug. This applies to drugs in Schedules 1 or 2. Administratively, it is regarded as good practice to use a separate page for each different form and strength of a preparation. The class to which any page relates must be given at the head of the page. If a preparation contains more than one class of drug subject to these requirements, then an entry needs to be made on each page of the register assigned to the different classes of drug involved. No register entries need to be made for CDs returned to a doctor, dentist or pharmacist by patients or their representatives for destruction (see below).

If a practitioner has more than one set of premises, he must keep a separate register for each set of premises at which he keeps a stock of drugs from Schedules 1 or 2. Each register must relate only to drugs obtained at or supplied from that particular set of premises and kept at the relevant premises. Doctors working in groups or partnerships in shared premises should keep a joint register. Good practice would suggest that where a practitioner carries a doctor's bag containing CDs, then a separate CD register should be kept for CD stock held in that bag and that restocking of a doctor's bag should be witnessed by another member of staff.[16]

Dispensing doctors should be aware of the need to retain invoices for a minimum of 2 years (but ideally 7 years or more) for all CDs.

Inspection and verification

Those involved in prescribing and supplying CDs must provide certain materials on demand by the appropriate Secretary of State or persons authorised by him or her in writing (e.g. Home Office inspectors and health authority medical advisers, although not police constables). The materials include the following:

- particulars with regard to the producing, obtaining or supplying by them of any CD or with regard to any stock of CDs in their possession

- any stock of CDs in their possession for the purpose of confirming the above
- any register, book or document required to be kept under the regulations relating to any dealings in CDs which is in their possession.

However, there is no right of access to personal medical records made by a doctor of a patient (alive or dead).

It would be good practice for a GP practice to carry out a stock check of CDs at least monthly.[16]

Destruction of controlled drugs

Any person who is required to keep records with regard to Schedules 1, 2, 3 or 4 of the MDR may not destroy such a drug except in the presence of a person who is authorised to witness its destruction.

The following people in PCTs are now authorised to witness the destruction of CDs:

- a PCT chief pharmacist or pharmaceutical/prescribing advisor who reports directly to the Chief Executive or a Director of the PCT.
- a registered medical practitioner who has been appointed to the PCT Professional Executive Committee on the PCT board with responsibility for clinical governance or risk management.

Others who are entitled to witness the destruction of CDs, depending on the location, include police officers, inspectors of the Home Office Drugs Branch, inspectors of the Royal Pharmaceutical Society of Great Britain, the Chief Dental Officer of the Department of Health or a senior dental officer to whom authority has been delegated, supervisors of midwives appointed by the Local Supervising Authority, senior officers in an NHS trust who report directly to the Trust Chief Executive and who have responsibility for health and safety or risk management matters in the trust, and Chief Executives of NHS trusts.[18]

The Professional Standards Factsheet produced by the Royal Pharmaceutical Society of Great Britain (updated in October 2003) clarifies the position for community pharmacists:[19]

> Any person required by the regulations to keep records of Controlled Drugs, that is Schedule 1 and 2 drugs, may only destroy them in the presence of a person authorised by the Secretary of State either personally or as a member of a class. The latter includes inspectors of the Royal Pharmaceutical Society, police chemist liaison officers and Home Office inspectors. Particulars of the date of destruction and the quantity destroyed must be entered in the register of Controlled Drugs and signed by the authorised person in whose presence the drug is destroyed. The authorised person may take a sample of the drug to be destroyed.

Nothing in this authorises a person to witness the destruction of CDs which have been supplied to him or her or by him or her. Anyone who is directly involved in the practice (e.g. practice pharmacists who have access to CDs in GP premises) or who is authorised to supply CDs from the GP practice (e.g. clinical governance lead working in his or her own GP practice) should not be asked to witness the destruction of CDs in that GP practice, even if they fall within the groups authorised.

CDs returned by patients may be passed on to a doctor or pharmacist for destruction. Although there is currently no requirement that CDs returned by patients should be destroyed in the presence of an authorised person, it is good practice for doctors and pharmacists to have the destruction of these CDs witnessed by an authorised person, and to make a record of their destruction in a separate book specifically for this purpose which should include the following details:[14]

- date received
- name and address of patient they were prescribed for
- name of pharmacy they were dispensed from
- name, quantity and form of CD
- role of person returning CDs
- name and signature of staff receiving CDs
- name and signature of person destroying CDs and date
- name and signature of person witnessing destruction of CDs and date.

It would therefore be prudent for GPs to encourage patients and their relatives to return all unused CDs to a pharmacy. Any CDs in general practice that are out-of-date should only be destroyed in the presence of one of the witnesses described above. This is most likely to be the prescribing advisor from the PCT or the doctor on the Professional Executive Committee of the PCT with responsibility for clinical governance or risk management.

Storage of controlled drugs (CDs)

Drugs in Schedules 1 and 2 and buprenorphine and temazepam from Schedule 3 should be kept in a locked receptacle that can only be opened by the practitioner or someone authorised by him or her. The courts have held that a locked car is not a receptacle for the purpose of this regulation (i.e. it needs to be a *locked receptacle in a locked car*). There are no storage requirements placed on patients. Where CDs are stored on premises, the cabinet should not be portable and a record should be kept of who has keys. Doctors' bags containing CDs (even though locked) should not be left overnight in a car.[14]

Notification of addicts

It is no longer necessary to notify the Home Office, but doctors are expected to report on a standard form available from their local Drug Misuse Database (DMD), details of which are available in the *BNF*.[5]

The Shipman Inquiry and the government's proposals regarding controlled drugs

The Fourth Report of the Shipman Inquiry, chaired by Dame Janet Smith, was published on 15 July 2004.[20] The government responded with the publication of *Safer Management of Controlled Drugs* in December 2004.[21]

A number of recommendations made by the inquiry have been adopted by the government and have resulted in a number of proposed actions. Some of the more relevant ones are briefly summarised below. Clearly, further consultation will need to take place and the practicalities of implementing these recommendations will need further consideration.

1 *Improving the monitoring and inspection of CDs*. A number of recommendations including the requirement of healthcare organisations to nominate a *Proper Officer* who will be responsible for all aspects of the management of CDs within the organisation.

2 *Improving the prescribing of CDs*
   - By strengthening professional and ethical guidance on doctors prescribing CDs to themselves, their immediate family, outside their area of knowledge or expertise and prescribing in circumstances other than a genuine doctor–patient relationship.
   - Considering reducing the validity and quantity supplied for CD prescriptions to 28 or 30 days.
   - Strengthening the system and regulations for those prescribers who have any CD related convictions or restrictions placed on them.

3 *Improving the audit trail*
   - Redesigning prescription forms which will require additional information.
   - The use of a standard form for privately prescribed CDs and a copy of this to be sent to the PPA.
   - Use of a standardised form for practices to requisition CDs, with a copy sent to the PPA.
   - Allow electronic versions of controlled drugs registers (CDRs) in practices and pharmacies, requiring them to keep a running total of each item.
   - Pharmacists to keep ID and name of pharmacist dispensing any CD.
   - Provide a model of best practice for use in NHS and private sectors.
   - Require CDRs to be kept for 11 years.
   - Pharmacists, dispensing practices and secondary care to prepare a patient drug record card (PDRC) to accompany each supply of injectable Schedule 2 CDs dispensed into the community.
   - All healthcare professionals to make a record when administering, removing or destroying any injectable Schedule 2 CD.
   - Review the class of persons entitled to witness destruction of CDs.
   - Issue guidance for PCTs to be responsible for the recovery and safe disposal of any unwanted CDs and associated PDRC after a patient's death or at the end of a course of treatment.

4 *Improving information for patients*
   - Explaining to patients the benefits of allowing information on their condition to be shared with other members of the care team, e.g. pharmacists.
   - Advise patients of the need for safe storage and the return of unwanted medication to pharmacies.
   - Information for patients about the legal status of CDs by pharmacists.

5 *Training and professional development*
   - Review the training at all levels in the safe use and handling of CDs.
   - Ensure that healthcare professionals prescribing CDs are regularly appraised to the extent to which they are up-to-date with clinical and regulatory changes and use this to identify learning needs.

- Ensure training is available for staff who will be involved in monitoring and inspecting CD arrangements.

A timetable for implementation is included in the government document which aims for most recommendations to be implemented by March 2007.

The doctor's bag and emergency medication

There are several references on what should be included in a doctor's bag with regard to medication, but the exact choice will almost inevitably be down to personal preference. The *Drug and Therapeutics Bulletin* published an article on this subject in 2000.[22]

With the development of local GP co-operatives, many of which provide the emergency drugs for doctors, the turnover of medication in the doctor's bag has diminished, and consequently much of it may be out of date when it is needed. Other dangers include running out of certain drugs, incorrect storage allowing heat damage (e.g. in cars),[23] and not having the most appropriate and up-to-date drugs. These problems are discussed in Issue 2 of *In Safer Hands*.[24]

It is worth developing a protocol or system for ensuring that these difficulties are managed. Some practices designate a member of the nursing staff as part of the monthly nursing duties to update all doctors' bags against a checklist in a similar way to checking the emergency drugs. Other practices have one or two emergency bags that everyone shares, but which are predominantly available for the duty doctor. Another solution is to have an arrangement with a local pharmacist on a monthly basis to update the emergency drug box of each doctor.

Prescribing for children

Medication that may be suitable for adults may be unsuitable for children. Some medication doses are linked to a child's age, but it is more accurate to use their weight or surface area. The following is adapted from the MPS guidelines.

- Refer to a paediatric formulary if you are uncertain.
- Prescribe drugs with which you are familiar with regard to dose, side-effects, interactions, contraindications and indications.
- Always put a zero in front of a decimal point. For amounts smaller than 1 milligram, use micrograms to avoid confusion over the decimal points. Never abbreviate micrograms.
- When writing a prescription, include the child's age and write the exact dose in weight (or volume, if liquid) required for administration.
- Counsel the parents about administration and side-effects.
- Consider asking a colleague to double-check your calculations.
- Encourage parents to keep all medicine safely out of children's reach.

Oral anticoagulation

Anticoagulants are one of the commonest drugs associated with fatal medication errors, according to the 1996 MDU report.[25]

Box 25.2 Causes of increased risk associated with the use of oral anti-coagulants in primary care

---

- Increasingly prescribed due to more clinical indications (e.g. atrial fibrillation)
- Narrow therapeutic margin
- Wide range of interactions with other medications (and over-the-counter and herbal products)
- Often the elderly are prescribed warfarin, who may be prone to falling or confusion
- Some patients are particularly sensitive to warfarin
- Significant side-effects (e.g. bleeding)
- Regular monitoring and dose adjustment are required

Practices should have a robust protocol in place for monitoring those patients who are taking warfarin. Good understanding by the patient of their anticoagulant medication is vital. Most patients are issued with an anticoagulant monitoring book which allows the recording of the international normalised ratio (INR) and the appropriate dose. Good communication between the patient and the GP surgery is critical to ensure that appropriate dosage alterations are acted upon quickly in response to the INR, and that subsequent tests can be arranged. In some areas, near patient testing has been introduced, where patients have a fingerprick sample taken, the INR is calculated immediately and the patient is advised on the correct dose of warfarin and the date of the next test there and then through the use of computer software support systems. Patient self-testing is likely to become an option as well, although it is important to have quality-control systems in place.

The British Society for Haematology has published guidelines on oral anti-coagulation.[26] A computer-based decision-support system may well be helpful for standardising dosage regimes.

A special focus on warfarin was produced in the *In Safer Hands* series.[27] Useful websites include www.anticoagulation.org.uk and www.anticoagulation.com.

Prescribing off licence

Clearly there are some drugs for which an indication outside the drug's licence is now accepted medical practice, but there is no incentive for the pharmaceutical company to apply for an alteration to its current licence. Non-adherence to the product licence as summarised in the Summary of Product Characteristics may therefore be justified if the licensed indications do not reflect current knowledge, the indications listed do not include well-proven uses of the drug, or the licensed indications are over-restrictive. Clearly there needs to be significant clinical advantage to using an unlicensed product over a licensed one. The legal responsibility for prescribing falls to the doctor who signs the prescription. Doctors are free to prescribe unlicensed drugs, or to prescribe drugs for unlicensed indications if they feel that it is in the patient's best interest. However, if a patient came to harm, the prescribing doctor might have to justify the use of the drug. Clearly the GP must recognise the limitations of their knowledge as recommended by the GMC, and provide 'all necessary medical care . . . as normally practised by a GP' under their terms and conditions of service and act in the best interests of the patient. The reasons for prescribing outside the licence should be documented in the record, and patients should be informed of the drug's unlicensed use or status and their consent obtained. If in doubt, it may be worth seeking advice from professional colleagues or from the local drug and therapeutics committee.

Patient group directions

Patient group directions (PGDs) are written instructions for the supply or administration of medicines to groups of patients who may not be individually identified before presentation for treatment. It is important to distinguish medicines given by nurses under PGDs from *nurse prescribing*. Until recently there was confusion about the legal position with regard to the administration of medicines by nurses, for example, to patients who had not first seen a doctor. The original Medicines Act 1968 was not written with this situation in mind. However, new legislation came into effect in August 2000, which clarified the position. To satisfy both legal and professional requirements, there should be agreed written directives for the administration of medicines such as infant vaccines, contraception and travel immunisations.

The *Health Service Circular HSC 2000/026*[28] states that:

> the majority of clinical care should be provided on an individual basis. The supply and administration of medicines under patient group directions should be reserved for those situations where this offers an advantage for patient care (without compromising patient safety), and where it is consistent with appropriate professional relationships and accountability.

There are detailed requirements which can be found in the above *Health Service Circular*, and further information is available from the NPC[29] (www.npc.co.uk/publications/pgd/pgd.pdf).

Useful information is also available from the Royal Pharmaceutical Society[30] (www.rpsgb.org/pdfs/factsheet10.pdf), the group protocols website (www.groupprotocols.org.uk/) which gives examples of PGDs in use in the NHS and includes a useful flow chart called 'To PGD or not to PGD', the MHRA website (www.npc.co.uk/repeat_prescribing/repeat_presc.htm) and a recent MeReC publication[31] (www.npc.co.uk/MeReC_Briefings/2003/briefing_no_23.pdf).

Storing medication

Medicines should be stored safely and securely out of children's reach. Vaccines need to be stored at the correct fridge temperature, which should be monitored and recorded daily. Doctors should be discouraged from accepting returned medication from patients and storing it in drawers in their consulting rooms, as children or others may get hold of these drugs. Advise the patient to return them to the pharmacy instead. Care should be taken to avoid excessive exposure to heat of drugs stored in the doctor's bag (as can easily occur in a car in the sun).

Acknowledgements

The author would like to thank his colleagues at the Medical Protection Society for their interpretation of the current controlled drugs regulations.

Further resources

Along with the references and websites mentioned in the text, the reader may find the following resources useful.

- *Drug Information Zone* – part of the NHS UK Medicines Information Agency (UKMI), which provides useful information on medicines (www.druginfozone.org).
- *Prescriptions Prescribing Authority* – can provide PACT data (www.ppa.org.uk).
- *Toxbase* – gives useful information on overdoses and poisons (www.spib.axl.co.uk/).
- *National Teratology Information Service* – provides information and advice about all aspects of toxicity and drugs in pregnancy (www.nyrdtc.nhs.uk).
- National Prescribing Centre (2004) *Saving Time, Helping Patients: a good practice guide to quality repeat prescribing.* National Prescribing Centre, Liverpool (www.npc.co.uk/repeat_prescribing/repeat_presc.htm).
- Department of Health (2003) *Building a Safer NHS for Patients: improving medication safety.* Department of Health, London.
- *Dispensing Doctors Association* (www.dispensingdoctor.org/).
- *Electronic Medicines Compendium* (includes pharmaceutical patient information leaflets and Summaries of Product Characteristics) (www.medicines.org.uk).

References

1 Department of Health (2001) *Building a Safer NHS for Patients.* Department of Health, London; www.doh.gov.uk/buildsafenhs
2 National Prescribing Centre and NHS Executive (1998) *GP Prescribing Support: a resource document and guide for the new NHS*; www.doh.gov.uk/nhsexec/gppres.htm
3 Department of Health (2000) *Pharmacy in the Future: implementing the NHS Plan*; www.doh.gov.uk/pharmacyfuture/index.htm
4 National Prescribing Centre (2002) *Modernising Medicines Management: a guide to achieving benefits for patients, professionals and the NHS*; www.npc.co.uk
5 British Medical Association and Royal Pharmaceutical Society of Great Britain (see current edition) *British National Formulary*; www.BNF.org
6 Rubin P (ed.) (2000) *Prescribing in Pregnancy.* BMJ Publishing, London.
7 Berry D, Knapp P and Raynor D (2002) Provision of information about drug side-effects to patients. *Lancet.* **359**: 853–4.
8 Department of Health (2004) *Management of Medicines: a resource to support the implementation of the wider aspects of medicines management for the National Service Frameworks for Diabetes, Renal Services and Long-Term conditions*; www.doh.gov.uk
9 Department of Health (2003) *Building a Safer NHS for Patients: improving medication safety.* Department of Health, London; www.doh.gov.uk/buildsafenhs/medicationsafety/index.htm
10 Royal Pharmaceutical Society of Great Britain (2003) *Professional Standards Directorate Factsheet 11. Dealing with dispensing errors*; www.rpsgb.org.uk/pdfs/factsheet1.pdf

11 Department of Health (2004) *Delivering the Out-of-hours Review: securing proper access to medicines in the out-of-hours period*; www.out-of-hours.info/downloads/short_medicines_guidance.pdf

12 Dispensing Doctors Association (2003) *Dispensing Guidelines*; www.dispensingdoctor.org/

13 Bates DW, Leape L *et al.* (1998) Effect of computerised physician order entry and a team intervention on prevention of serious medication errors. *JAMA.* **280**: 1311–16.

14 Royal College of General Practitioners and National Patient Safety Agency (2004) *In Safer Hands.* Issue 5. RCGP, NPSA, London.

15 Baker R *et al.* (2004) Investigation of systems to prevent diversion of opiate drugs in general practice in the UK. *Qual Safe Health Care.* **13**: 21–5.

16 National Prescribing Centre (2004) *A Guide to Good Practice in the Management of Controlled Drugs in Primary Care (England).* Preview Edition, November 2004; www.npc.co.uk/publications/Controlled%20Drugs%20November%202004.pdf

17 Department of Health (1999) *Drug Misuse and Dependence: guidelines on clinical management*; www.doh.gov.uk/drugdep.htm

18 Department of Health (2002) *Destruction of Controlled Drugs in GP Practices*; www.doh.gov.uk/pricare/cddestruction/index.htm

19 Royal Pharmaceutical Society of Great Britain (2003) *Professional Standards Directorate Factsheet: 1. Controlled drugs and community pharmacy*; www.rpsgb.org.uk/pdfs/factsheet1.pdf

20 Shipman Inquiry (2004) *Fourth Report – The Regulation of Controlled Drugs in the Community*; www.the-shipman-inquiry.org.uk/fourthreport.asp

21 Department of Health (2004) *Safer Management of Controlled Drugs: The Government's response to the Fourth Report of the Shipman Inquiry*; www.doh.gov.uk

22 Drug and Therapeutics Bulletin (2000) Drugs for the doctor's bag. *Drug Ther Bull.* **39**(9).

23 Rudland S and Jacobs A (1994) Visiting bags: a labile thermal environment. *BMJ.* **308**: 954–6.

24 Royal College of General Practitioners and National Patient Safety Agency (2003) *In Safer Hands.* Issue 2. RCGP and NPSA, London.

25 Green S, Goodwin H and Moss J (1996) *Problems in General Practice. Medication errors.* Medical Defence Union, Manchester.

26 British Society for Haematology (1998) Guidelines on oral anticoagulation (third edition). *Br J Haematol.* **101**: 374–87; www.bcshguidelines.com

27 Royal College of General Practitioners and National Patient Safety Agency (2004) *In Safer Hands.* Special focus: warfarin. RCGP and NPSA, London.

28 Department of Health (2000) *Health Service Circular HSC 2000/026.* Department of Health, London; www.doh.gov.uk

29 National Prescribing Centre (2004) *Patient Group Directions (PGDs): a practical guide and framework of competences for all professionals using PGDs*; www.npc.co.uk/publications/pgd/pgd.pdf

30 Royal Pharmaceutical Society of Great Britain (2003) *Professional Standards Directorate Factsheet 10. Patient group directions*; www.rpsgb.org.uk/pdfs/factsheet10.pdf

31 National Prescribing Centre (2004) *MeReC Briefing.* Issue number 23; www.npc.co.uk/MeReC_Briefings/2003/briefing_no_23.pdf

Chapter 26

An afterword: moving the patient safety agenda forward

Keith Haynes and Malcolm Thomas

Introduction

If you are reading this chapter and have come this far then it is likely that you are now one of the 'cognoscenti' of the risk management patient safety movement. Our hope is that your use of this book will have increased your interest in this important issue and perhaps even strengthened your commitment.

At this stage it is tempting to look back and summarise what has gone before, but there seems little point if you have reached this stage. We thought therefore that we might take the opportunity to reflect on the journey of the 'patient safety movement' to date and offer our personal perspective on some of the important next steps. We hope that this will serve as a suitable 'endpiece' to the journey so far.

'All changed, changed utterly'

There can be little doubt that the real fillip for patient safety and clinical risk management came with the introduction of clinical governance in the late 1990s. Clinical governance was the Government's immediate response to the GMC's hearing into the doctors involved in the paediatric cardiac surgery services at Bristol Royal Infirmary and to similar events at the time, including inquiries into cervical screening, histology reporting and gynaecological treatment. As a consequence, the Government found itself having to deal with a loss of public confidence in health professionals, and saw the need for a system that demonstrated their accountability. In quoting W B Yeats in his *British Medical Journal* editorial, 'All changed, changed utterly,' Richard Smith was correct in identifying that British medicine would be irrevocably changed by the events at Bristol.[1] Subsequent events and actions have confirmed that all roads lead from Bristol.

The publication in 2000 of the CMO's report entitled *An Organisation With a Memory* provided further stimulus to the debate about the need for improved patient safety.[2] It suggested that we know very little about adverse events because of the absence of effective reporting systems, and it made a number of recommendations to improve those systems. It set some quite specific targets

This chapter is a revised version of an article published in Volume 9 of the *Medico-Legal Journal of Ireland* in 2003, reproduced here with kind permission of Thomson Round Hall.

for reducing recognised risks in obstetric claims, deaths from suicide and deaths from the maladministration of cytotoxic drugs.

Subsequent plans included setting up the NPSA, which was charged with establishing a national mandatory reporting system and a research programme into patient safety.

Another recent CMO's report, *Making Amends: a consultation paper setting out proposals for reforming the approach to clinical negligence in the NHS,*[3] outlined proposals for reforming the way in which legal claims are made. The proposals emphasise preventing harm, reducing risks and improving safety so that the level of medical error is reduced. Interestingly, for the first time in such a report a connection is made between improving patient safety, a new 'duty of candour' (or open disclosure) and the potential to reduce the financial and human implications of litigation. In a climate where recent legal reforms have attempted to reduce the financial burden of rising litigation costs and damages but done little to address the root causes of litigation, any attempt to improve patient safety and reduce the human impact of litigation is to be welcomed.

More recently, in *Standards for Better Health,*[4] patient safety has been identified as a core standard requiring healthcare organisations to:

> continuously and systematically review and improve all aspects of their activities that directly affect patient safety; and . . . apply best practice in assessing and managing risks to patients, staff and others, particularly when patients move from the care of one organisation to another.

The evidence so far

Despite the very positive and well-intentioned initiatives of recent years to improve patient safety through effective clinical governance and risk management, some of the early evidence suggests that there is still some way to go.

CHI – now superseded by the Healthcare Commission – noted a number of emerging causes for concern.[5]

- Organisation-wide policies and strategies for clinical governance are not being formulated.
- In some instances, policies and strategies are not being implemented, or are being implemented only partially or ineffectively across areas of clinical governance activity.
- Organisations tend to be reactive rather than proactive. CHI observed that this occurs where organisations do not anticipate problems and threats to quality, responding only to those issues that cause particular public concern.
- Good practice and learning identified by CHI are not always shared across and between organisations.
- There are failures to communicate, from strategic to operational levels. In particular, boards and clinical leaders do not always share their vision, values and policies.
- There are barriers to communication between disciplines and staff groups within clinical areas. CHI identified this as a persistent theme which it felt undermined the effective delivery of healthcare.

Importantly, CHI identified that four of the seven components of their definition of clinical governance stand out as a cause for concern, including risk management.[5] CHI found that trusts are poor at managing risks to patients, and are particularly poor at putting in place effective adverse-event-reporting systems that staff are both trained to use and committed to using.

Most recently, the National Audit Office study *Achieving Improvements Through Clinical Governance: a progress report on implementation by NHS trusts*,[6] concluded that although the structures and organisational arrangements to make clinical governance happen were in place, progress in implementing clinical governance has been patchy, varying between trusts, within trusts and between the different components of clinical governance. The report does acknowledge achievements of clinical governance, which include clinical quality issues becoming more mainstream, more explicit accountability of both clinicians and managers, and more widespread transparent collaborative working. Nevertheless, most trusts still view clinical governance in terms of structures and process.

The report also recognises that risk management has developed substantially since 1999. The overall message is that there is still room for improvement.

We have also been led to believe that the US experience is much better and that there is much to learn from colleagues across the Atlantic. Although there was a flurry of activity after the publication of the seminal report *To Err is Human*[7] (which included Congressional hearings, an expression of support from President Clinton for mandatory reporting of serious incidents, and $50 million being allocated for research into the causes of medical error), a recent article in *The Washington Post*[8] demonstrated that there has been a lot of talk but very little action.

What needs to be done?

Patient safety and risk management are firmly on the agenda as never before in the UK. As such, the various initiatives will have an impact. The real issue is to identify a prescription that will allow the patient safety and risk management agendas to flourish and realise their full potential. To do this, a number of barriers will have to be overcome.

Healthcare: a high-risk enterprise

Albert Wu[9] suggests that there is no place for mistakes in modern medicine, and that society has entrusted clinicians with the burden of understanding and dealing with illness. Although it can be said that 'doctors are only human', technological advances and therapeutic innovations have created an expectation of perfection. Wu argues that patients, who have an understandable need to consider their doctors infallible, have colluded with them in denying the existence of errors.

Cyril Chantler has said that 'medicine used to be simple, ineffective and relatively safe. Now it is complex, effective and potentially dangerous.' This suggests that the price of the success of medicine in the last 20 years has been to create a 'safety paradox'. Healthcare staff are technically competent, committed to their patients and use sophisticated technology, but errors appear to be common and patients and staff are frequently harmed.

In our introduction to this book we acknowledged that healthcare is a risky business, but that nevertheless there was little appreciation of this during clinicians' formative years. You might be tempted to ask what place patient safety has in a culture of 'see one, do one, teach one'.

If this is the case, why then does the healthcare sector not behave like a high-risk enterprise? In fact, comparisons are commonly made between the healthcare sector and the aviation, nuclear power and petrochemical industries, but these comparisons can often seem facile, as those industries do not have to deal with the idiosyncrasies of the human condition. Nevertheless, there is the potential to learn a great deal from their preoccupation with safety. A starting point must be to recognise that modern healthcare is a high-risk enterprise, and to train healthcare professionals accordingly.

Education, education, education

Scant attention appears to be given to patient safety and risk management issues on current undergraduate medical and nursing courses. In a stakeholder study, Nicklin[10] noted that education commissioners made no reference to undergraduate training in risk management. Moreover, although they recognised the importance of the subject, they felt that the cost of training should be borne by the organisation or the individual. On average, just 4.75 hours were devoted to clinical risk training during the 3-year nursing course.

The NPSA and the NHS Confederation in their recent report, *Creating the Virtuous Circle: patient safety, accountability and an open and fair culture,*[11] call on educators to provide qualification courses for clinical staff at all levels which include patient safety and which promote an open approach to error. The report also recommends that undergraduate courses should introduce the basic ideas and goals of patient safety, and that patient safety models should be included in CPD. It goes on to suggest that educators must also teach practitioners about the personal factors that promote a wider, open approach and which are crucial to patient safety, such as leadership, teamwork and communication. Importantly, and boldly, it suggests that education should address and seek to shape those personal behaviours that can affect patient safety.

Embedding patient safety issues in our educational programmes has to be the key element in any prescription. Perhaps we need to see patient safety and risk management as being a matter of good clinical practice at root, and reaffirm a commitment to some of the basics, including good documentation, consent, safe prescribing and effective communication. However, our sense is that there is still a long way to go.

Balancing the quantity and quality agendas

Despite the efforts of the clinical governance movement to put quality firmly on the NHS agenda, much of that agenda is driven by a preoccupation with meeting performance targets linked to volume (e.g. waiting lists and times). The Government has reaffirmed its commitment to this agenda.[12] Achieving waiting-list targets and remaining in balance financially are still the main drivers for most Boards. However, it is perhaps worth a moment's reflection to note that the scandals which have damaged the reputation of trusts have been clinical in origin (at Bristol and Alder Hey, for example, and in the case of Rodney Ledward). We might also speculate as to what impact these ever higher levels of activity have on quality and patient safety. For any healthcare organisation, the quality agenda should be as important as its performance targets linked to volume – and perhaps even more so, given that higher rates of activity might conceivably create a higher-risk environment.

Sharing the patient safety agenda with the public

Depending on which continent you are from, the extent of medical error has been described as ranging from 3.7% to 16.6% per hospital admission.[13,14] It is estimated that in the USA there are 44 000–98 000 deaths a year due to medical error.[7]

Is this a debate that we could, and should, have with the public? The NPSA and NHS Confederation report[11] asserts that 'patients should also be encouraged to take greater responsibility and make sound decisions for their own care'. A useful illustration of this is the *Quality of Health Care Pack: 'Q Pack'*[15] prepared by the Agency for Healthcare Research and Quality (AHRQ). This pack aims to provide the public with practical advice on what they can do to prevent medical errors.

But is this a debate that the politicians want the public to have? It is time for politicians to demonstrate an understanding of the issues surrounding patient safety, as well as a greater commitment to the means of improving the situation. After all, they continually find themselves having to respond to media attention and public concern about scandals involving clinical care. Working on the root causes and not just the symptoms may pay dividends.

Supporting the second victim of medical error

The fear of blame and retribution is often cited as the reason for healthcare staff not reporting adverse incidents.[9,10] The healthcare organisations and media are all too ready to look for a scapegoat. It also remains a widely held view that doctors are treated differently to nurses for the same offence. The number of convictions for manslaughter has risen from two in the 1970s to 17 in the 1990s. In these circumstances, it is hard to convince healthcare professionals that the primary purpose of any adverse-event-reporting system is learning and not retribution. In a recent survey of GPs, 81% said that they did not trust their NHS trust or the Department of Health to run a blame-free system for reporting their mistakes.[16]

Many errors do not cause harm but are almost as important as those that do. Clearly, if we are to learn from mistakes, we need to know about as many errors as possible. Adverse incident reporting/significant event audit needs to be embedded as a natural component of good medical practice, with an emphasis on the system and the reality that we are all human and prone to error. The efforts of the NPSA to introduce root cause analysis are to be applauded as a step in the right direction, because this approach attempts to move us on from blaming the individual to reviewing the whole system. However, as the NPSA has observed, root cause analysis is unlikely to make as good copy as naming and shaming.[11]

In the mean time, the second victims of medical error may take some convincing. In our rush to create more and bigger bureaucracies, we have overlooked the need to put in place a supportive framework for vulnerable staff.

Celebrating success

The patient safety and risk management agenda is relatively new. To date, therefore, an evidence base for risk management has yet to evolve. However, let us reflect on the fact that the litigation crisis that we often hear about has hardly materialised. Indeed, the number of claims against GPs seems to have plateaued in the last 5 years, and the cost of claims against GPs actually decreased between 2000 and 2001.[3]

Risk management is a very practice-based discipline, and there are many excellent examples of risk management at work within healthcare organisations and in various educational programmes. This book was born out of much of this good practice. Such initiatives often go unnoticed, yet they are really what effective risk management is about. We should celebrate them and the major contribution that risk management has made already, while acknowledging that there is still some way to go.

References

1 Smith R (1998) All changed, changed utterly. British medicine will be transformed by the Bristol case. *BMJ*. **316**.

2 Department of Health (2000) *An Organisation With a Memory. Report of an expert group on learning from adverse events in the NHS*. The Stationery Office, London.

3 Department of Health (2003) *Making Amends. A consultation paper setting out proposals for reforming the approach to clinical negligence in the NHS. A report by the Chief Medical Officer*. Department of Health, London.

4 Department of Health (2004) *Standards for Better Health: health care standards for services under the NHS. A consultation*; www.dh.gov.uk

5 Commission for Health Improvement. *CHI's Combined Annual Report and Accounts 2001–2002. Growing a new organisation*; www.chi.gov.uk

6 National Audit Office (2003) *Achieving Improvements Through Clinical Governance: a progress report on implementation by NHS trusts*. The Stationery Office, London.

7 Institute of Medicine (2000) *To Err is Human*. National Academies Press, Washington, DC; www.nap.edu/readingroom

8 Boodman SG (2002) No end to errors. Three years after a landmark report found pervasive medical mistakes in American hospitals, little has been done to reduce death or injury. *The Washington Post*. **2 December**; www.washingtonpost.com/

9 Wu A (2000) Medical error: the second victim. The doctor who makes the mistake needs help too. *BMJ*. **320**.

10 Nicklin PJ (2001) *Perceptions and attitudes towards clinical risks: the findings of a stakeholder survey*. Unpublished paper. Medical Protection Society, London and University of York, York.

11 NHS Confederation and National Patient Safety Agency (2003) *Creating the Virtuous Circle: patient safety, accountability and an open and fair culture*. NHS Confederation, London; www.nhsconfed.org and www.npsa.nhs.uk

12 Department of Health (2004) *The NHS Improvement Plan. Putting people at the heart of public services*; www.dh.gov.uk/assetRoot/04/08/45/22/04084522.pdf

13 Brennan TA, Leape LL, Laird NM *et al.* (1991) Incidence of adverse events and negligence in hospitalized patients: results of the Harvard Medical Practice Study 1. *NEJM.* **324**(6): 370–6.

14 Wilson BH, Runciman WB *et al.* (1995) The quality in Australian Health Care Study. *Med J Aust.* **163**(9): 458–71.

15 Agency for Healthcare Research and Quality (2000) *Quality of Health Care Pack: 'Q Pack'*; www.ahrq.gov/consumer/pathqpack.htm

16 Survey by Doctors.net.uk reported in June 2004; www.doctors.net.uk/news/index.cfm

Index